*The Complete Guide to Relieving
Cancer Pain and Suffering*

The Complete Guide to Relieving Cancer Pain and Suffering

RICHARD B. PATT, M.D.

and

SUSAN S. LANG

OXFORD

UNIVERSITY PRESS

2004

OXFORD
UNIVERSITY PRESS

Oxford   New York
Auckland   Bangkok   Buenos Aires   Cape Town   Chennai
Dar es Salaam   Delhi   Hong Kong   Istanbul   Karachi   Kolkata
Kuala Lumpur   Madrid   Melbourne   Mexico City   Mumbai   Nairobi
São Paulo   Shanghai   Taipei   Tokyo   Toronto

Published by Oxford University Press, Inc.
198 Madison Avenue, New York, New York 10016
www.oup.com

Oxford is a registered trademark of Oxford University Press

Library of Congress Cataloging-in-Publication Data
The complete guide to relieving cancer pain and suffering / Richard B. Patt,
Susan S. Lang.—Rev. and expanded ed.
    p.   cm.
    Previously published in 1994 under the title: You don't have to suffer;
Lang listed as the first author on t.p.
Includes bibliographical references and index.
ISBN 0-19-513501-6
1. Cancer pain.
I. Lang, Susan S.
II. Lang, Susan S. You don't have to suffer.
III. Title.
RC262.L27 2004
616.99'406—dc22   2003017317

10 9 8 7 6 5 4 3 2 1

Printed in the United States of America
on acid-free paper

To yesterday's, today's, and tomorrow's cancer and pain patients, who deserve the best. And to my mother and father, who always did their level best: her passing humbled me and opened my heart to his love. And finally to my wife, Pauline, who means everything to me. *R.B.P.*

In loving memory of my mother, Beatrice Lang, and my in-laws, Jerry and Mickey Schneider. They taught me invaluable lessons of life, love, and death. *S.S.L.*

Contents

Preface

Tremendous strides have been made in the field of cancer pain and suffering since the first edition of our book one decade ago. Today almost every state has a cancer pain initiative—coordinated efforts of health care professionals to overcome barriers, promote education, disseminate accurate information regarding pain control, and advocate for the removal of regulatory and legislative barriers to allow physicians to more appropriately use pain control measures. In recent years numerous professional organizations also have forged collaborations and have issued updated pain guidelines and position papers that advocate the appropriate use of pain control treatments. The U.S. Congress has declared the years 2001 through 2010 the Decade of Pain Control and Research to help promote greater public and professional awareness of scientific, clinical, and personal issues concerning pain and pain management. And in April 2003 the National Pain Care Policy Act of 2003, H.R. 1863, was introduced into the House of Representatives to provide important federal recognition of pain as a priority health problem in the United States and to establish the National Center for Pain and Palliative Care Research.

Although tremendous scientific, medical, and educational advances have been made and public perceptions have changed, the undertreatment of pain associated with cancer is still a major public health problem, according to almost every professional society associated with cancer or pain. Inadequate knowledge, inappropriate attitudes on the part of health care workers and families, fears and misconceptions about narcotic drugs and the importance of pain relief for promoting health and well-being, a punitive and complex drug regulatory system, and problems with insurance reimbursement and drug delivery systems still abound.

As recently as 1998 researchers reported that more than a quarter of cancer patients in daily pain did not receive pain relievers.[1] When Kathleen M. Foley, one of the nation's most highly regarded and outspoken cancer pain experts from Memorial Sloan-Kettering Cancer Center and the Weill Cornell Medical College, testified before the Senate Committee on the Judiciary in 2000 on the state of pain relief in this country, she cited studies indicating that 37 percent of children dying of cancer were undertreated for pain; that although 40 percent of elderly cancer patients experience pain, less than one-quarter receive *any* pain relief; and that of ten thousand dying hospitalized patients, half suffered from significant unrelieved pain in the last days of life.[2]

We write this book for families and loved ones, hospice workers, and health care professionals, to help prevent this tragedy from recurring day in and day out. In this second edition we totally update and revise all the information on medications (including foreign medications) and medical interventions to relieve pain and other kinds of suffering associated with cancer, cancer treatment, and dying, as dozens of new medications and techniques are now available. We also have significantly expanded the sections on mind-body techniques, such as relaxation techniques, psychotherapy, meditation, yoga, biofeedback, and music therapy, among others, since research has substantiated the powerful role that such strategies can play not only in minimizing worry, pessimism, and depression but also in helping to arrest or perhaps even reverse the disease process and promote longevity.

This new edition also includes numerous forms that families can use for documents such as living wills and health care proxies, and we provide detailed appendices to refer readers to dozens of other resources.

This book is intended to serve as a reference for families and health care workers on how pain relievers work, what doctors need to know to do their job best, how other kinds of medications or treatment can contribute to comfort, and how to relieve side effects and other distressing symptoms, including depression and anxiety, all of which can contribute to the suffering associated with cancer. We also offer many comfort care tips.

We recommend that readers who are new to the needs of cancer patients be sure to read Chapter 1 to understand the importance of treating pain and why many doctors and other health care providers neglect to treat it appropriately. Chapter 2 is background information about cancer and pain, including types and causes of pain. Chapter 3 is critical to understanding how to describe different kinds of pain, learning how to make the most of a pain assessment, and understanding the strategies doctors use in treating cancer pain. Chapter 4 covers how to identify doctors who use modern approaches to treating pain and how to be assertive in ensuring that pain and suffering are being appropriately treated.

Chapters 5, 6, and 7 include detailed information about medications typically used to treat pain and should be used as reference. Chapter 8 discusses why medications that aren't widely known as pain relievers are often used in the treatment of cancer pain, and Chapter 9 is for reference, explaining the various high-tech options used for pain that is not controlled by conventional means.

Chapters 10 and 11 should be read carefully; they include many tips on how to relieve suffering other than pain, including the side effects from medications as well as treatments. Chapter 10 focuses on gastrointestinal problems (such as nausea and constipation), and Chapter 11 covers all the other symptoms that might arise. Chapter 12 covers nondrug approaches to relieving suffering, including relaxation exercises, coping skills, biofeedback, and so on. Chapter 13 focuses on special cases, most notably children, teens, and the elderly. Chapter 14 discusses the psychological aspects of both the patient and the caregiver. And, finally, Chapter 15 covers the process of dying: how to provide comfort to the dying patient, and coping tips for caregivers.

This book is not intended, however, to substitute for the care of a physician. We mean to educate and offer tips for comfort care, but not to prescribe a treatment plan for any particular patient. Only qualified health care providers are equipped to use the judgment required to treat a particular patient with a particular illness. This book is intended to serve as a tool to foster open communication between the health care team and the patient and family, and to foster self-education—not as a recommendation or prescription for any particular treatment.

We hope that our use of pronouns and references to family members and loved ones will not offend anyone. For simplicity's sake we use masculine pronouns, although obviously there are many female physicians and many female patients. Likewise, we often refer to family members as synonymous with caregivers. There are, of course, many nontraditional family units and loving primary caregivers who are not family members.

The dark ages of cancer pain are behind us. You might say we are now striving for a new era, an era of enlightenment when it comes to attending to the pain and suffering of cancer. We now have the means to relieve most pain in almost all patients. Now we just need the appropriate use of the arsenal of pain treatment options available to us so that *no one* suffers needlessly. Patients with cancer and their families and friends need to know that much of the pain and suffering of living with cancer can be success-fully treated.

Finally, there is the last frontier: the countless patients without cancer who suffer from undertreated chronic pain that will persist for years to come. Much of what we have learned about cancer pain can be and is being applied in large populations of cancer survivors and patients with other illnesses. Over the next decade we look forward to better distin-guishing what aspects of cancer pain control can be safely applied to these other groups.

Richard B. Patt, M.D., and Susan S. Lang

Acknowledgments

Humble thanks to my coauthor, Susan Lang, a true professional, for her patience, understanding, and hard work, and to our editor, Joan Bossert, for her continued support and confidence.   *R.B.P.*

Endless thanks to my father, Solon J. Lang, for his love and hard work, which gave me opportunity; to my husband, Tom Schneider, for his patience and abiding love and support; and to our daughter, Julia. And without the continued support of our editor, Joan Bossert, we never could have done it.   *S.S.L.*

A Note for Chronic Pain Sufferers
Who Don't Have Cancer

Although this book is about the pain and symptoms associated with cancer, much of the information presented is surprisingly relevant to people who don't have cancer but who suffer from unrelenting or progressive chronic pain. These materials include Chapters 3 and 4 on assessing pain and being an active health-care consumer, all of Part II that details medication use and much of Part III, including Chapter 12 on mind-body approaches to easing pain.

Just as cancer pain is still often severely undertreated, so too is chronic non-cancer pain that accompanies trauma, degenerative, infectious diseases, and other medical disorders as well as chronic pain that simply cannot be explained. Sufferers are commonly disbelieved and untreated, leaving them feeling ridiculed, humiliated, depressed, and even suicidal. Often amplified by the absence of the drama associated with cancer, the barriers to good pain management (Chapters 1 and 2) are largely the same for chronic pain. Below are some of the barriers that both patients with chronic pain and cancer pain experience in trying to obtain satisfactory pain treatment.

- Fears of addiction that are not based on scientific evidence but on anecdote or personal experience, outdated myths, and social conventions. Using opioids to treat pain does not transform people who were not inclined to become addicted into drug abusers. No drug is so potent that the values, behaviors, and sense of what is meaningful, which have been established over decades, suddenly erode. In fact, far less than 1 percent of patients become addicted to even the strongest medications when they are prescribed under close supervision for pain. Although the use of opioids has jumped more than 1,000 percent in the last decade, there has been no corresponding increase in the incidence of drug abuse.

- Medical education about pain control remains grossly inadequate.

- Although we are still unable to cure many serious medical disorders, the treatment of symptoms, including pain, is almost always an afterthought, if it is considered at all, preventing untold numbers from living fully with their disease and maintaining dignity and their best functional status.

- Inaccurate assumptions persist that the use of opioids for chronic pain might mask or hide important clinical findings. In fact, when pain is relieved, people remain articulate and can usually describe their problems much more accurately.

- A lack of understanding persists that patients in pain who take opioids are dependent on those medications for quality of life, just as diabetics are dependent on insulin. This does not constitute addiction.

- Fears of legal reprisals inhibit physicians from prescribing opioids as often as they should and in appropriate doses.

- Most doctors lack the skills, experience, and confidence needed to establish pain management strategies and address patients' fears.

- Both cancer and chronic pain can be complex and difficult to control; a pre-packaged set of recommendations will not produce consistent results. Good pain treatment often requires time-consuming adjustments and consultations.

- Patients who do not receive adequate relief from medications need to pursue other avenues, such as nerve blocks, implantable pumps, physical therapy, behavioral interventions, and vocational evaluation and training; these treatments usually involve the coordinated interaction of multiple specialists.

Just as with cancer, even when a cure is not achieved for the underlying disorder, that's no reason why aggressive treatment should not be sought to relieve pain and suffering and improve physical and mental functioning.

Chronic pain sufferers can glean a lot of other useful information from this book. Whether you have cancer pain or chronic pain due to an injury or an ongoing medical disorder, in this day and age you should be able to obtain adequate control of pain. If chronic pain is severe, chances are it interferes with sleep, nutrition, concentration, energy levels, mental health, sexual function, and social relationships. Chronic pain compromises quality of life. Just as with cancer pain, don't accept it. Below are some of the features common to both chronic and cancer pain that the informed patient should be aware of and which should be addressed by treatment.

- The need for a comprehensive pain assessment at the start of treatment (Chapter 3), familiarity with pain rating scales (Chapter 3) and the importance of being an active health care consumer (Chapter 4).

- The need to be knowledgeable and prepared to discuss pain rather than be stoic and silent. Recognize that pain is hazardous to health and is best addressed early on (Chapters 1–3).

- The need to find physicians who will not ignore pain but will prescribe opioids when appropriate.

- The willingness to take the extra time to explore the use of adjuvant analgesics, medications originally developed for purposes other than pain relief which may relieve certain types of pain (Chapter 8).

- The need to understand that achieving good pain control is a process that usually requires some time to establish, after which periodic adjustments are frequently needed. Some patients will benefit from an interdisciplinary approach (Chapter 3).

- Recognition of the trial and error strategy employed by most physicians treating pain (Chapter 3).

- Although efforts may be made to make only one or two changes at once, many patients benefit from simultaneous treatment with multiple medications, each of which is adjusted to achieve the right dose of the right drug in the right patient at the right time (all of Part II).

- Understanding how to balance a medication's relative effectiveness versus its side effects against the medication's expected actions over time (all of Part II).

- Awareness of the World Health Organization three-step analgesic ladder (Chapter 3).

- Understanding the desirability of achieving basal pain relief with long-acting medications administered on an "around-the-clock" schedule and the role of short-acting "as needed" medications for acute or breakthrough pain. Carefully selecting the route by which analgesics are administered, despite the perception that injected drugs are better (Chapters 2 and 3).

- Although using opioids for chronic pain is controversial, in many cases it is appropriate and patients on such medications should be carefully monitored to manage adverse side effects (constipation, sedation, rebound pain, and cognitive impairments) and to chart progress (Chapters 6 and 7).

- Understanding the differences among tolerance, dependence, addiction, and pseudoaddiction (Chapter 1).

- The beneficial effects of behavioral, nondrug approaches, including relaxation, cognitive therapy techniques, acupuncture, hypnosis, biofeedback, focused breathing, imagery, distraction, skin stimulation and massage, herbal remedies, and more (Chapter 12).

- For intractable pain, the possible need for a high-tech option, such as nerve blocks, epidural steroid injections, trigger-point injection, implantable epidural and intrathecal drug pumps, and spinal cord stimulation may be necessary and consultation with a pain specialist necessary (Chapter 9).

And, of course, the goal of good cancer pain management is the same as good management of non-cancer chronic pain: improved quality of life.

Part I

CANCER AND ITS PAIN

Pain is a more terrible lord of mankind than even death itself.

—Albert Schweitzer

1

How Cancer Pain Undermines Health and Treatment

To be struck with cancer, or to have a loved one afflicted with cancer, is one of the most frightening events imaginable. To endure the dehumanizing pain of cancer without relief is overwhelming. To helplessly witness that anguish in a loved one is heartbreaking. To discover later, however, that the suffering might have been prevented is perhaps the worst of all.

Uppermost in the minds of many cancer victims are fears and anxiety about pain. We are now finally entering an era in which these fears may finally be put to rest. Today we are equipped with a modern arsenal of drugs and techniques capable of eradicating cancer pain in most cases. Around the country, in doctors' offices and pain clinics, many patients are successfully being properly treated and relieved of most of the suffering from cancer and cancer treatment. Yet, tragically, many cancer patients are not appropriately treated for pain and side effects; too many people are unaware that modern approaches to treating pain are almost always successful.

Cancer Pain Is Needless, Yet Undertreated

Far too many physicians overlook and undertreat cancer pain, often because they are misinformed or fearful of reprimands for prescribing powerful painkillers. As a result, pain treatment methods that are relatively simple to use are still not adequately applied. Although this situation is improving daily, needed changes still come too late for many. Each minute of every day, people are dying of cancer and suffering needless pain in hospitals and clinics around the world. Many cancer patients try to keep a stiff upper lip; they bear an enormous physical and psychological burden, not realizing that everyone around them bears that burden too. Cancer patients don't suffer in isolation; their family, friends, and other caregivers who helplessly bear witness suffer along with them. Patients with cancer and their families and friends need to know that much of this pain is unnecessary and that they can take a proactive approach to make sure that they or their loved ones don't suffer needlessly.

Patients, families, and friends have a job to do: educating and asserting themselves. Armed with the facts presented here, they can learn to overcome their fears about the use of narcotic medications (also called opiates or opioids), ask for additional help when pain persists, and, ultimately, learn to adopt strategies that help doctors take full advantage of available resources to fight cancer pain. The bottom line: you never need to give up or assume that little can be done to ease the pain and suffering of cancer.

How Pain Is Harmful—Even Hazardous—to Health

There is no benefit from enduring cancer pain. Pain relief is of the utmost importance, not only for humanitarian reasons but also for medical reasons. Pain is harmful and debilitating. It interferes with eating, sleeping, mood, and maintaining a strong fighting spirit, which are all vital, especially in times of stress. It robs people of the energy needed to fight illness and hinders their ability to tolerate demanding cancer treatments—treatments that can affect their outcome. Pain also makes people irritable, anxious, fearful, angry, depressed, and sometimes even suicidal. In fact, pain is one of the major reasons why patients request physician-assisted suicide. Cancer patients in pain are twice as likely to be depressed, anxious, or have a panic disorder compared to those without pain. Pain also compromises general well-being, interfering with work, social relationships, recreational interests, mobility, and even the ability to take care of oneself, which in turn affects self-esteem, body image, and feelings of competence and control.

Perhaps most important, experts are finding that persistent pain can weaken or inhibit the immune system and may even influence tumor growth and the risk of death. Animal experiments have shown, for example, that the tumors in rats with pain that was not treated with morphine grew much faster than the tumors of rats that received morphine.

And a Johns Hopkins Hospital study showed that patients with pancreatic cancer whose pain was aggressively treated with a nerve block (which blocked pain signals) not only had less pain, used less medication, and were much more functional, but also lived considerably longer than the group receiving a placebo.[1]

Moreover, patients with pain are ranked lower on performance status (how well they function and get around), making them less likely to be candidates for experimental procedures or therapies.

Pain must no longer be regarded as just a side effect of cancer. Rather, it is a legitimate health problem that is part of the disease process and warrants ongoing treatment that is as aggressive as treatment of the tumor itself. You usually have only one chance to mount the most effective possible fight against cancer, and for the best chances of success, pain must be treated early and aggressively.

Most Families Will Be Affected

Despite the millions of dollars spent on research in the quest for a cure, each year 10 million people are diagnosed with cancer worldwide, including 1.3 million Americans, and 6 million will die from it.[2]

The second most common cause of death in the United States, cancer kills one in every four Americans, accounting for more than half a million cancer deaths each year; that's fifteen hundred a day, or more than one cancer death every minute.

American Cancer Society, *Cancer Facts and Figures,* 2003.

Men have a little less than a 1 in 2 lifetime risk and women have a little more than a 1 in 3 lifetime risk of developing cancer.[3] More than 85 million Americans living today will develop cancer.[4] The disease costs this country some $171.6 billion a year.[5]

When a person is first diagnosed with cancer, the first two questions that typically come to mind are "Am I going to die?" and "Will I be in pain?" But studies show that people think cancer is more painful than it really is. Granted, pain is one of the most common symptoms of cancer—about one-third of those in its early stages and up to 90 percent of those with advanced cancer will have pain that is severe enough to warrant treatment with strong pain medications. On any given day, about half of cancer patients experience pain; about one-third report moderate to severe pain.

Yet up to 40 percent of cancer patients receive inadequate relief.[6] Studies published in the *Journal of the American Medical Association* and elsewhere document that that one-fourth of U.S. cancer patients with daily pain receive no pain medication, and that up to half of dying hospitalized patients experience significant pain in their final days.[7] Elderly cancer patients are 40 percent more likely to be treated inadequately for pain; although almost 40 percent of the elderly in nursing homes report daily pain, only one-quarter receive pain medication.[8] Thirty-seven percent of children with cancer die suffering from undertreated pain.[9] Minorities and women are particularly vulnerable; studies show their cancer pain is much more likely to be ignored or sorely undertreated.[10]

Despite twenty-first-century technology and medical advances that offer a high quality of life despite cancer, up to 60 to 90 percent of those with cancer pain suffer unnecessarily—as many as 3.5 million people around the world every day.[11]

The World Health Organization, one of the strongest proponents of treating cancer pain aggressively, asserts: "Freedom from pain should become the right of every cancer victim, and access to pain therapy is a measure of respect for this right."[12]

"You have a right to request pain relief. In fact, telling the doctor or nurse about pain is what all patients *should* do. The sooner you speak up, the better. It's often easier to control pain in its early stages, before it becomes severe."

Source: National Institutes of Health, National Cancer Institute, "Get Relief from Cancer Pain," http://oesi.nci.nih.gov/RELIEF/RELIEF_MAIN.htm

---

In recent years, the American Academy of Pain Medicine, American Pain Society, American Cancer Society, National Comprehensive Cancer Network, American Society of Addiction Medicine, Drug Enforcement Administration, and many more authorities have issued consensus statements acknowledging that although preventing drug abuse is important, it is unrelated to and should have nothing to do with the aggressive treatment of cancer pain (and other chronic pain) with opioids. Ten years ago, the state of Wisconsin took the lead with its Wisconsin Cancer Pain Initiative; today every state participates in the American Alliance of Cancer Pain Initiatives, a national network of efforts to raise awareness of the proper use of pain control treatment (www.aacpi.org).

In 1989 the first Intractable Pain Act was passed in Texas to make sure that no Texan requiring narcotics for pain relief, for whatever reason, was denied them because of a physician's real or perceived fear of disciplinary measures for prescribing opioids. Many states have followed suit. Today, the U.S. Congress has declared the years 2001 through 2010 the Decade of Pain Control and Research to help promote greater public and professional awareness of scientific, clinical, and personal issues concerning pain and pain management. And in April 2003 a bill was introduced into the House of Representatives (H.R. 1863, the National Pain Care Policy Act of 2003) to provide important federal recognition of pain as a priority health problem in the United States and to establish the National Center for Pain and Palliative Care Research.

There is simply no reason for patients with cancer to feel they must endure pain as part of their disease.

Why So Many Still Suffer

About 85 percent of the time, cancer's agony can be treated with relatively simple measures, such as analgesics (painkillers such as morphine and other opioids) or other simple medication-based treatments that have been in use for years and require only a doctor's prescription. For the remaining 15 percent, the pain can be relieved in almost all cases with more complex treatments that have developed in the burgeoning new medical subspecialty of cancer pain management.

Despite the sophisticated, technically advanced health care available in the United States, many Americans wish for death simply because they hurt too much, with no promise of relief. These appalling conditions persist because myths, misinformation, and biases about narcotic use abound despite massive educational efforts by public health experts, including U.S. government and scientific agencies.

On one hand, patients think they shouldn't complain; on the other, doctors and nurses don't always take complaints seriously. Fears about narcotics, street abuse of drugs, and confusing regulations inhibit doctors from prescribing adequate doses of painkillers and patients from using them when they are needed. How puzzling it is that U.S. scientists must file intricate forms to ensure the comfort of laboratory animals while no such guarantees exist for humans with life-threatening illnesses.

How Fears of Narcotics and Addiction Undermine Pain Treatment

Advocating for more responsible control of cancer pain is not the same as minimizing the dangers of drug abuse. Experts stress that these two issues are unrelated, except that exaggerated concerns about drug abuse makes cancer patients innocent victims of the war on drugs. More appropriate than the "Just say no" slogan would be "Just say no to drugs . . . *unless prescribed by your physician for a legitimate medical disorder.*" Cancer pain often calls for the appropriate use of painkillers such as morphine. Until our culture distinguishes between legitimate and illicit uses of narcotics, many doctors will continue to be reluctant to prescribe these medications adequately and many patients will be reluctant to take them even when prescribed.

In fact, today's doctors do prescribe strong opioids more than ever, yet reports of abuse have actually fallen. In an article published in 2000 in the *Journal of the American Medical Association,* one of our most prestigious journals, researchers point out that between 1990 and 1996 medical prescriptions for treatment with the opioids hydromorphone, fentanyl, oxycodone, and morphine increased by 19 percent, 1,168 percent, 23 percent, and 59 percent, respectively, while reports of abuse of the first three of these drugs actually fell by 15 percent, 59 percent, and 29 percent, respectively, and for morphine rose by just 3 percent.[13] Certainly some drugs intended for medical treatment are still diverted and abused, but compared with other drugs of abuse, improper use of prescription medications is quite low.

Clinical experience also indicates that the risk of addiction is minute when narcotics are used in a medical setting to treat pain associated with cancer, burns, or surgery. "Addiction is essentially not a problem in cancer patients; it is extraordinarily rare that cancer patients will become addicted to [opioids] even if they're used extensively," says Robert C. Young, M.D., president of Fox Chase Cancer Center in Philadelphia, and president of the American Cancer Society. "One study showed that of over 11,000 patients treated for pain relief, only 4 patients [developed] . . . an addictive pattern . . . ; the second study showed that in 550 patients treated more than 40 days with [opioids] for pain management, there was not a single addiction among them; in practical terms, it's simply not a problem."[14]

Recent publicity about the misuse of the opioid OxyContin has added fuel to the fears about opioid use for cancer pain. Misuse of OxyContin and other drugs has skewed people's perceptions about these drugs when, in fact, the vast majority of people who are prescribed these medications by their doctors will not become addicted. Proper, routine oral use of OxyContin and other opioids does not produce a high or rush, which is why addicts who seek these feelings will crush and then sniff or inject the pills rather than swallow them, as patients seeking pain relief do. (Soon new formulations of OxyContin should reduce the risks of street abuse.)

The drug abuse problem will not be solved by reducing access to drugs that are helpful for the vast majority of cancer pain sufferers, since those who are addiction-prone will just seek other accessible drugs.

If the unfounded fears about the use of narcotics were dispelled, chances are that Jack Kevorkian's assisted-suicide movement and the euthanasia movement would fizzle out. The same drugs that destroy lives and families when they are abused can restore the lives and families of cancer patients when they are used properly, because they allow a return to a more active lifestyle that combats depression by promoting a greater capacity to fight disease and preserve quality of life.

Confusion Over Addiction, Physical Dependence, Tolerance, Withdrawal, and Pseudoaddiction

One of the major roots of the cancer pain problem is that far too many people, including many health care professionals, confuse *addiction* with *physical dependence* and other terms and hold outdated fears and unscientific ideas about the safety of opioids, which in some settings are actually safer than aspirin and acetaminophen (Tylenol). To dispel unfounded fears and promote the proper and appropriate use of cancer pain medications, it is critical that the terms *addiction, physical dependence, tolerance, pseudoaddiction,* and *withdrawal* be distinguished from each other.

Addiction is psychological dependence—a chronic neurobiological disease characterized by not being able to control drug use, craving and compulsively using drugs for nonmedical reasons, or continuing to use drugs despite harm. The need to obtain and use drugs completely controls the addict's life despite the presence or threat of physiological or psychological harm. As addict lose control over their drug use, they typically become increasingly less functional and more socially isolated. Addiction is extremely rare among cancer patients. Already fighting for their lives, cancer patients characteristically resent any additional threat to their fragile control and try to avoid drugs, often excessively, even when their use would help restore normal function.

Physical dependence refers to feeling sick and appearing ill when a drug that has been used consistently is abruptly stopped, when the dosage is dramatically reduced, or if a drug reversal agent or antagonist is administered. In contrast to addiction, which is rare in cancer patients, physical dependence is expected and usually inevitable, regardless of a person's character, values, or background, with the regular use of an opioid. Unlike addiction, which is psychological and behavioral, physical dependence is a biological response that is neither harmful nor dangerous, as long as it is recognized and managed properly. It is the natural result of the body growing accustomed to a medication (a process that also occurs with nonopioid drugs) and need not be feared. The development of physical

Sorting Out the Terms

Tolerance	Physical Dependence	Addiction
Almost always occurs with repeated use	*Almost always occurs with repeated use*	*Rarely occurs in patients with pain*
Body adapts to the effects of the drug over time (effect of the drug on breathing, nausea, and to a lesser extent pain becomes milder over time)	Body adapts to taking the drug and so may develop withdrawal (abstinence) symptoms (much like the flu) if medication is abruptly interrupted or dose largely reduced	A chronic neurobiological disease characterized by craving, inability to take the drug according to appropriate schedule, compulsive use of the drug, and/or continued use despite harm
Presents an extremely low risk of developing addiction (psychological dependence)	Presents an extremely low risk of developing addiction (psychological dependence)	Creates an obsession with getting and using a drug for nonmedical reasons; addicted people may report stolen/lost prescriptions, change doctors frequently, and/or also use nonprescribed psychoactive drugs
Drug is used only to relieve pain and usually does not cause a high	Drug is used only to relieve pain and usually does not cause a high	Drug is sought to get high, boost mood, escape from reality, reduce anxiety, and/or become sedated; drug may be used in different ways, such as injecting diluted drug or sniffing crushed tablets
Higher doses may be needed to maintain same painkilling effect	Withdrawal symptoms may occur when drug is stopped but cease when drug use is restarted, even in lower-than-usual doses; symptoms can be avoided if medication is tapered in gradually lowered doses	Desire for drug stems from psychological needs and choices (possibly from a genetic predisposition) and is not affected by risk to economic, social, and physical well-being
Drug use can help restore normal function	Drug use can help restore normal function	Instead of restoring normal function, drug use increases isolation and moves patient further from the mainstream of society

dependence shouldn't interfere with pain control, since any symptoms of withdrawal (also known as abstinence syndrome) that occur once the drug is stopped can be entirely avoided by reducing the dose gradually. The cultural stigma of drug use is so strong that many cancer patients are anxious to be drug-free once painkillers are no longer needed and so discontinue pain medications more rapidly than is advisable. Be sure to consult a physician before discontinuing such medications.

Tolerance refers to the body's adaptation to a drug's effects over time, including respiratory depression (slowed breathing), nausea, and pain relief. Larger doses of a medication may be needed over time to achieve the same effect. Tolerance is expected with the chronic use of some medications and is totally unrelated to addiction. Tolerance shouldn't interfere with good pain control.

One benefit of tolerance is that when higher doses are needed, the increase is usually safe. Since there is no limit to how much tolerance may develop, there's no reason to worry about using pain medications early in an illness. Opioids can cause respiratory depression in those who are "opioid-naive" or unaccustomed to the use of strong pain medications, but fortunately this is one of the first effects for which tolerance develops. As long as opioids are started in low doses, they can later be adjusted upward so safely that even accidental overdoses are usually well tolerated. Constipation is the only side effect for which tolerance fails to develop, and it can be easily treated with activity, diet, and the prescribed use of mild laxatives.

The problems caused by our undertreatment of pain are so rampant that a new term, *pseudoaddiction*, has been coined to describe the misinterpreted behavior of patients who, when undertreated, understandably continue to seek needed relief. Well-meaning physicians who underprescribe because of exaggerated fears of addiction create a self-fulfilling prophecy, forcing patients with unrelieved pain to seek comfort by whatever means are necessary. But in such cases patients are craving pain relief rather than drugs per se. The term *pseudoaddiction* is unfortunate, since it implies that the patient is at fault, when in fact it is tightfisted prescribing and the system's failure to identify and adequately treat pain that forces patients to doctor-shop and hoard drugs.

The fear of opioid addiction is so powerful that institutional barriers intended to prevent addiction serve only to interfere with legitimate pain relief. These draconian measures may have seemed justified in the days when the medical use of opioids was thought to carry a significant risk of addiction, but in light of current knowledge, we see that such measures only prolong suffering.

Irrational fears of addiction plague patients and their loved ones as well. Patients may be reluctant to comply with their doctor's instructions, especially if they detect any mixed messages sent by poorly informed health care professionals or family members about the dangers of pain medications. Parents are especially concerned that children and teens who have cancer will grow up to be addicts if they take pain medication. In fact, when parents of children dying with cancer were asked about their major concern regarding narcotics, many reported fear that their child would grow up to be an addict, even though the families were grappling with a life-threatening illness that was causing treatable pain.

Simple exposure to a powerful drug won't change the values and behaviors a person has developed over a lifetime. Besides, for addiction to take root, some reward or high must become so desirable that one craves it again and again, no matter what the cost. We now recognize that instead of the euphoria that addicts experience with drug use, patients with pain feel dysphoria, an unpleasant sensation of being a bit groggy, "off," or just not quite themselves. When someone is already experiencing a disease such as cancer, which robs life of its normalcy, the last thing he wants is more loss of control; as a result, cancer patients usually shun taking more drugs than are needed to control their pain.

Many patients, during and after their cancer treatment, will need daily medication for pain. The focus is on monitoring and managing cancer pain with chronic use of medications. Just as we don't accuse people with diabetes or hypertension of being addicted to the medications they take daily, neither should cancer patients and survivors be stigmatized or humiliated for seeking relief.

Cultural Barriers to Pain Management

Undertreatment of cancer pain also is perpetuated by the common belief that the ability to endure pain is a virtue and reflects a strong character. Our culture depicts heroes as able to withstand great pain without flinching or complaining. These images imply that the old stiff-upper-lip syndrome— remaining stoic, refusing to complain—is somehow good for you. Others who feel this way, including some doctors and even families, regrettably may feel obligated to "build the character" of the patient by withholding adequate pain relief.

The other side of the coin is patients who don't seek relief for their pain because they "don't want to be a bother" or they fear they will be perceived as being weak-willed or of weak character. When it comes to a fight for one's life, it is not always virtuous to be the "good patient," since we all know that it's the squeaky wheel that gets the grease. Because doctors' and nurses' time is limited, they will naturally spend more time with those who express their concerns and problems, which may mean less time for those who are hesitant to ask for pain relief. A patient can't be helped if the care providers don't know that a problem exists. Cancer treatment is not like grade school: there's no gold star for quietly suffering or waiting an extra hour before the next pain pill.

In truth, trying to keep a stiff upper lip ultimately appears to do more harm than good. Even the bravest soul can remain stoic in the face of relentless pain only so long. Continued denial eventually crumbles, leading to a loss of self-esteem. And the longer that adequate pain relief is delayed, the more likely it is that a syndrome of anticipation and memory of pain will develop: the trauma of unrelieved pain is so grueling that even when the pain is not so bad, the patient remains fearful that his nemesis is just around the corner. Work with children who need repeated painful injections has shown that if the first treatment can be achieved relatively painlessly, repeated treatments are much less traumatic. Conversely, if children learn that something hurts, they will go to almost any lengths to avoid repetition.

Our culture also tends to compartmentalize the mind and body, and views pain as separate from the disease. These Western medical notions may interfere with treating the pain as an integral part of treating the disease and, ultimately, of treating the whole person. Professionals who still regard pain management as a stepchild of medicine do not focus on pain problems unless forced to, failing to recognize how important symptom control is to cancer treatment and quality of life.

Training of Doctors and Nurses

Although many patients are undermedicated for cancer-related pain, it is by no means because doctors are incompetent or uncaring; rather, they are uninformed. Pain medication is improperly used or underused because medical education mostly focuses on disease and its treatment and not on symptom control. Student doctors are usually taught how to treat short-term or acute pain from surgery or trauma, but most do not learn how to properly use painkillers such as morphine, the cornerstone of cancer pain treatment, for chronic pain. Relatively few schools adequately teach the principles of opioid use and other cancer pain treatments.

Various surveys reveal that more medical residents fail the on surveys regarding cancer pain than pass, and that doctors still fail to follow basic principles of treating cancer pain such as around-the-clock scheduling, inappropriately using meperidine (Demerol), and failing to take advantage of skin patches, pumps, and other new ways of administering relief.

Too Many Believe Options Will Run Out

Starting an opioid does not mean the "beginning of the end" or that aggressive treatments will no longer be pursued. The truth is that patients may need painkillers to resume a normal life during treatment. Then there is what some call the money-in-the-bank syndrome, which refers to the mistaken concern that there is only so much pain relief available, and if it is used too soon, it won't be available later. Patients fear that if they start taking narcotics too early, the drugs won't be as effective later, when they are "really" needed. Yet pain can be controlled both early in the disease as well as later, if it progresses. Nevertheless, about half of patients do not follow their doctors' orders when it comes to taking pain medication because of unfounded fears about opioids.

Doses May Vary Widely

Another problem that contributes to inadequate treatment of cancer pain is that prescribing strong painkillers, while still a science, is often an inexact one, and frequently requires educated trial and error. Determining the correct drug and dose for a particular patient can be difficult and time-consuming; it often requires well-thought-out trial and error until most of the pain is relieved with few side effects. That's because pain, pain thresholds, and a person's response and tolerance to medications vary widely, even in patients with the same kind of cancer. Also, pain cannot really be measured objectively, so proper treatment requires good communication between patient and doctor. Patients must feel comfortable discussing their discomfort, and doctors must trust their patients' report of pain.

Doctors can't know in advance which medication in what dose will be best tolerated by a given patient, so careful observation and a willingness to try different options are needed. Making the challenge even more complex is the fact that what relieves the pain today may not be adequate tomorrow, either because the disease has progressed or because the person has developed a tolerance to the medication. Every patient is different: one person will stay on the same dose for years, while another may need adjustments weekly.

Narcotic Doses and Tolerance Have No Upper Limit

Unfortunately, many health care professionals fail to understand that opioid medications such as morphine have no "ceiling effect" or upper limit as tolerance develops or pain intensifies. Although customary or standard doses of narcotics are published in older medical texts, these are based on the needs of patients taking opioids for the first time for acute pain (like labor pain or pain after surgery), not for the ongoing treatment of cancer-related chronic pain. While a typical starting dose of oral morphine may be as little as 20 to 30 milligrams (mg) every four hours (or 8 to 10 mg intravenously), some patients need and remain more functional on the equivalent of up to 35,000 mg a day. So treating pain requires good judgment and regular adjustments, rather than a cookbook approach such as that for treating infection, which usually responds to standardized doses. Hitting the moving target of cancer pain is harder and requires regular assessments and good communication.

With all of our contemporary medical advances, there is still no blood test or X-ray to detect how "real" pain is or how much pain exists. Going by the patient's report is still the best approach. While this is almost always reliable, doctors are used to trusting objective laboratory or radiological tests, especially when the fast-paced tempo of today's medical practice doesn't allow for the familiarity and trust engendered by contact with yesteryear's family doctor. As discussed in Chapter 4, patients and their families can do a lot to help doctors be more effective and comfortable in treating their pain by keeping diaries and pain scores.

Undermedication Is the Norm

Since many doctors still undermedicate cancer pain, they compound the error by teaching young doctors to do the same. And other doctors feel pressured to adhere to the norm of low doses set by their colleagues.

Even when an adequate range of doses is prescribed, some studies of postoperative pain show that most patients still only receive as little as one-quarter of the prescribed amount. In hospitals, it is nurses who usually dispense medications, and many nurses have their own misconceptions about what are safe and proper doses. So despite good intentions, the tendency to underdispense often wins out.

Yet the times *are* changing: in 2001, a San Francisco doctor was successfully sued for $1.5 million for giving inadequate amounts of pain medication to a dying cancer patient.

Misinformation About Breathing Problems

One of the most persistent myths that interferes with the optimal use of opioids is that these drugs are bad for breathing. Opioids do indeed slow breathing (a phenomenon known as respiratory depression), but this effect is gradual, controllable, and usually beneficial, as severe pain tends to increase respiratory rate. Dangerous respiratory depression is almost always limited to patients who are not yet accustomed to regular treatment with opioids, and then only when excessive doses are prescribed or are combined with other depressant drugs. Respiratory depression is not a serious risk when using low starting doses that are gradually adjusted upward. Tolerance develops in just a few days, so the threat becomes less and less of a problem. At somewhat increased risk for breathing problems are those with sleep apnea (intermittent cessation of breathing during sleep), the obese, and those using other depressant drugs, such as aggressively administered sedatives. Yet even in these circumstances, opioids can be used safely when steady doses are administered to counteract pain.

A relatively new finding that has revolutionized how doctors view the relationship between opioid use and breathing is the recognition that when opioids are properly used, they can actually improve the quality of breathing, especially in the very ill. The proper use of morphine is now a recognized treatment for shortness of breath and can improve breathing problems, especially in those with rapid or painful breathing. When patients are undertreated for pain, especially in the chest area, their ability to breathe deeply and cough is inhibited by their pain. The careful use of opioids in this setting allows patients to breathe more efficiently and clear their airways of excessive mucus. Also, rapid breathing is extremely inefficient because it does not allow sufficient time for oxygen from the lungs to get to the bloodstream. Shortness of breath can also trigger air hunger and panic. The use of opioids may slow breathing sufficiently to improve the efficiency of oxygen transport, thus easing panic and improving the efficiency of respiration. Thus morphine and other opioids are increasingly used in patients with breathing difficulties, even when pain is completely absent. Unfortunately, exaggerated concerns about respiratory depression still sometimes keep ill-informed doctors from prescribing enough medication to soothe the pain.

Underutilized Options

The frontiers of medical science are rapidly expanding, and keeping up with them is a challenge. Doctors who have mastered the use of simple painkillers (effective for most patients) may be unaware of different ways to administer morphine, of alternative drugs, and especially of effective drug combinations. For example, adjuvant analgesics are drugs that aren't normally regarded as painkillers but can relieve specific types of pain or enhance the painkilling effect of opioids. Also, electrical stimulation, nerve stimulation, surgical procedures to cut nerve pathways, and nerve blocks (see Chapter 9), as well as nondrug approaches such as relaxation training, biofeedback, hypnosis, acupuncture, and massage, used alone or in combination with painkillers, may help relieve pain, but are usually prescribed only by pain specialists.

The Need to Discuss Pain

A busy doctor may not ask a patient about pain, assuming that if the problem exists, the patient will bring it up without coaching. *Patients should not wait for a doctor to ask about the pain.* Sometimes the doctor may ask, "How are you?" to open a conversation, and the customary polite response of "Fine" may be recorded in the chart as "No pain today."

Patients are often reluctant to complain. They may feel that time with the physician is limited and their highest priority is to talk about curative treatment. They don't want to distract the doctor from this mission or bother or annoy him with their complaints. Some deny the pain in their effort to deny the disease and its possible progress. If pain has intensified, patients may not want to admit it; instead, they want to tell the doctor they feel better. Or perhaps they don't want to complain because they believe that their "good" behavior will be rewarded and that "bad" behavior will be punished. Yet reporting information about pain is vital—not only for diagnosing problems but to help improve a patient's physical and psychological status. Pain interferes with proper rest, nutrition, and a good attitude, which are never more important than during a cancer illness.

Many physicians and groups are so concerned that patients are not being asked about their pain that they have endorsed the American Pain Society's campaign to regard pain as "the fifth vital sign." Thus, when doctors or nurses measure blood pressure, pulse, temperature, and respiratory rate, they should also ask about the presence of pain, its severity, and the patient's satisfaction with its treatment.

But don't wait for your doctor to ask. Complaining about pain is not a weakness and shouldn't be an embarrassment. Patients and families who are reluctant to discuss the cancer pain problem are doing themselves and their doctors an enormous disservice.

Communication Between Patient and Medical Team

Often a doctor will prescribe a painkiller, usually a mild one at first, and the patient will passively accept that treatment, whether it works or not.

Myths and Truths about Cancer Pain

Myth	Truth
Cancer causes severe pain, and I just have to accept it.	Many cancer patients never experience pain, and those who do can almost always get relief.
Morphine and other narcotics will cause addiction	Cancer patients almost never become addicted to pain medications.
If I use morphine or another narcotic now, it won't work as well later. I should wait as long as possible.	Morphine and other narcotics neither lose their effectiveness nor have a maximum dose. If pain gets worse, the dose can be gradually increased indefinitely until relief ensues.
Morphine and other narcotics are too strong and will make me groggy, confused, and delirious and will cause other side effects.	Confusion and hallucinations are very rare when doses are selected carefully; drowsiness is common but not inevitable, and if it occurs, it usually resolves in a few days. Other side effects, such as nausea and constipation, can be avoided or easily treated.
My doctor will view my complaining about pain negatively.	Though sometimes true, this is not an excuse to suffer in silence, since it is now clear that pain is bad for health. Doctors need to be informed in order to help you.
Talking about pain will distract the doctor from my cancer treatment.	Relieving pain is part of your cancer treatment. Good pain control means better rest, which helps your body fight the disease.
Continuing or recurring pain means the cancer is worsening.	Pain is entirely unrelated to the progress or status of the underlying cancer in one-third of cases; it may be due to injury to nerves and other structures, a result of cancer treatments (chemotherapy, surgery, and radiation), or from an unrelated or indirect cause such as excessive bed rest, muscle strain, migraines, or stress.

(continues)

Myths and Truths about Cancer Pain (*continued*)	
Myth	*Truth*
I don't want any shots, so I'll endure the pain.	More than 90 percent of medications for treating cancer pain can be taken by mouth or other noninvasive means, like a skin patch. Injections are sometimes an option but are almost never essential.
I will lose control if I take morphine or similar drugs.	Although drowsiness is common at first, very few cancer patients feel high or lose control when they take pain medication properly. When maintaining control is an especially important concern, it should be recalled that uncontrolled pain is one of the key factors that reinforce feelings of powerlessness.

Patients need to communicate frequently and effectively with their doctor if relief is not obtained or if side effects supervene. Together doctor and patient need to persevere until adequate relief is achieved. And remember, oncologists are not the only ones who can help—oncology nurses, physician assistants, anesthesiologists, pharmacists, psychologists, and social workers have invaluable advice about symptom control and are often part of the primary doctor's team.

Some medications, most notably the opioids, begin to work immediately, while others (mostly nonopioid medications) may take several days or even weeks before their effects are established and can be fully evaluated. Have clear expectations about how long it will be before a prescribed treatment is expected to become fully effective (called "latency to effect") so that you can report if the treatment does not seem to be working. In the case of opioids, an experienced physician will know after just the first few doses whether the proper drug and dose have been selected, and can make immediate changes to continue the process of achieving pain control. Likewise, report any side effects—most often they are minor, are to be expected, and will resolve with a little patience and reassurance, but sometimes a drug may need to be stopped or its dose changed. No one wants to be a bother, but remember that it is your doctor's job to attend to these issues, and he can't help if he is not well informed. Don't wait until the next scheduled visit to report problems.

Patients Often Don't Tell Doctors When They Don't Follow Recommendations

Some patients hesitate to take their medications around the clock, on a fixed schedule, as pain medications are often prescribed. Instead, they believe, incorrectly, that they should tough it out as long as possible. By that time, however, even the strongest painkillers are much, much less effective. Instead of a steady relief, an erratic drug schedule can trigger a roller coaster of pain. Patients may wait until the pain is intolerable, and then, because they have waited so long, medications may or may not relieve it, or may cause unpleasant side effects because medication use is erratic instead of stable. Even if the pain subsides, the patient anticipates that the next wave is around the corner, so anxiety builds and the memory of pain remains fresh. *It is far more effective to maintain a moderate level of a painkiller in the bloodstream so that it can act preventively.* In this way, the patient achieves a steadier quality of relief. The only way to accomplish this goal is to take medications as prescribed and on schedule.

How Pharmacists May Unintentionally Contribute to Undertreatment

Pharmacists also contribute to the undertreatment of cancer pain when they retain old-fashioned ideas about opioids. Studies show that many pharmacists don't know that it's lawful to prescribe for cancer pain on a long-term basis and an acceptable medical practice. Many are still unaware of what constitutes legitimate dispensing practices for controlled substances in patients with cancer, or they don't understand the distinctions among addiction, physical dependence, and tolerance.

Many pharmacists make patients feel guilty about taking opioids and may increase the chances that the patient won't comply fully with their doctor's instructions. Also, the opioids are highly regulated substances, and dispensing them means additional paperwork. Busy pharmacists have been known to overinterpret regulations and may refuse to fill prescriptions because of a simple spelling error or some other technicality. If this occurs, try to be patient, since they too are burdened by overly restrictive regulations.

However, *do not accept* being treated with a lack of dignity. Unfortunately, because of pharmacists' fears of being duped by drug addicts, patients with legitimate needs may be inappropriately humiliated when they are just trying to follow doctors' orders. This is especially common when patients are younger or do not appear very ill. If difficulties arise, simply request calmly and respectfully that the pharmacist telephone your physician for clarification.

Also, many pharmacists, especially in urban areas, don't stock morphine and other opioids because they fear theft. In more isolated areas, pharmacies may not stock up on opioids because of burdensome paperwork and relatively few requests. This reduced availability makes it difficult for many nonhospitalized patients, especially those who lack energy, to get needed medications. Although it's a good idea to call pharmacies in advance to find out if needed medications are available in adequate quantities, many pharmacists are reluctant to respond to such queries truthfully, and especially to patients they don't know, due to fears of robbery. Although pharmacists will occasionally indicate that needed medications cannot be ordered or would take too long to get, requests that such medications be ordered should be honored (wholesalers can almost always routinely provide any medication within twenty-four to forty-eight hours). Remain polite but firm and persistent. Try using the same pharmacy regularly, calmly identifying yourself and your problem, and discussing your concerns with a manager. You may need to use a hospital-based pharmacy or one recommended by your doctor. Fortunately, as a result of the virtual revolution that is ongoing to legitimize pain treatment, more and more pharmacies now routinely stock a great variety of pain medications and are more understanding of the patient's predicament, especially once the patient is known to them.

Increasingly, pharmacists are appreciating the positive role they can play in treating patients' pain. Recognizing the cancer patient's plight, some pharmacies have sprung up that specialize in providing these previously stigmatized drugs and can even manufacture or compound custom doses of a medication that your doctor may prefer.

You Have a Right To:
- Enjoy appropriate pain relief without unacceptable side effects
- Have your reports of pain believed
- Have your doctor try to relieve numbness, tingling, or burning sensations
- Ask your doctor repeatedly about changing prescriptions, times, or doses
- Request treatment with stronger medication
- Get immediate help
- Understand the medication plan
- Get expert advice
- Accept nothing less than the best pain control possible
- Enjoy life despite cancer

Laws Intimidate Many Doctors from Prescribing Adequate Pain Medication

As discussed, cancer pain patients are innocent victims of the war on drugs, a campaign to discourage the illegal and recreational use of certain drugs. Regulations to tightly control morphine and other opioids are intended to curb abuse and not to interfere with the practice of medicine, yet many doctors find the stringent regulations confusing, inhibiting, burdensome, and threatening. To prescribe opioids, many states require doctors to fill out time-consuming triplicate prescription forms that they must register for and order at their own expense. One copy goes to state regulators, who look for "abnormal" patterns of prescribing, which can have a chilling effect on doctors' prescribing behavior. Such prescriptions cannot be refilled automatically or by telephone and must be carefully accounted for; they are also very constrictive. If the patient's name is spelled incorrectly or if a doctor needs to change the quantity of the drug rapidly or wants to prescribe more than a week's worth of a drug on an urgent basis, there may be delays, frustrations, and fears of being investigated.

The cumbersome triplicate prescription program may be abandoned in the future, but what's in store may not be much better. Although New York State, for example, is phasing out the triplicate prescription pads and shifting to a computerized system, morphine and similar medications must still be prescribed on state-issued forms and will be monitored. Although such review systems do not directly prevent physicians from prescribing controlled substances, many doctors avoid prescribing them altogether or are reluctant to increase doses if their patients get sicker or more tolerant of the medication because many of the laws regulating controlled substances are ambiguous. Although high dosing is necessary for some cancer patients, it is still not the norm. Many doctors fear that if they prescribe opioids at all, they may attract the unwanted attention of regulatory agencies. Even if a doctor is cleared of wrongdoing, such an investigation could be damaging professionally and could incur high legal costs.

Even When Cure Is Unlikely, Comfort Is Critical

Millions are spent each year on cancer treatments, yet only a fraction of that goes to pain relief research and palliative treatments for cancer patients who will probably not get better. Focusing on curing cancer is essential, but such a single-minded focus overshadows important efforts to promote lifestyle changes and early detection. In recent years, more attention has been focused on comprehensive cancer care, which includes early

Why Cancer Pain Is Often Undertreated

Regulations and Laws

- Try to control drug abuse with stringent controls that inadvertently inhibit the medical use of opioids.
- Require cumbersome, time-consuming triplicate prescription forms that are intimidating, while ambiguous laws inadequately distinguish between illicit and legitimate medical use of opioids
- Inhibit physicians from prescribing large doses of opioids for fear of an investigation, community perception of wrongdoing, or sanction
- Vary widely from state to state, resulting in confusion between the legitimate and illicit use of opioids

Medical Staff

- May have inappropriately low expectations for successful pain relief.
- May have inadequate training for treating chronic pain
- May have unfounded, exaggerated concerns about addiction in cancer patients
- May be misinformed about breathing problems and other side effects of opioids
- May confuse addiction, physical dependence, tolerance, and pseudoaddiction
- May have misconceptions about tolerance and the need for larger doses over time
- May believe pain should be severe before it is treated
- May view complaints about pain as indicative of weak character that must be strengthened
- May give pain management a low priority.
- May undermedicate on a regular basis and thus perpetuate the practice in trainees

Patients and Families

- May think that complaining about pain is a sign of weakness and that stoicism is a virtue
- May erroneously believe that worsening pain means the disease is progressing
- May fear that the doctor will be distracted from curative treatment or will resent taking time to address problems regarding pain
- May fear addiction if opioids are used
- May view a patient who asks for opioids as drug-seeking
- May fear the side effects of opioids
- May not comply with instructions because they are overwhelmed, fearful, and ill-informed
- May try to be a "good patient" and not complain or imply that the doctor is at fault

Health Care System

- Is geared toward curative therapy and gives low priority to ensuring comfort
- Often requires patients to change doctors or institutions because of insurers' mandates, resulting in poor coordination of care
- Inhibits pharmacists from stocking morphine and other opioids because of additional paperwork, the risk of investigations, and the potential for theft

detection, curative treatment, life-extending palliative treatments, symptom control, and even bereavement services for the families of cancer victims. This perspective acknowledges that patients' quality of life could be radically improved if cancer pain relief and palliative care (which deals with patients' psychological, social, and spiritual well-being as well as their physical comfort) were given more attention throughout the course of an illness. The overall five-year survival rate for a diagnosis of cancer still hovers near 50 percent (as it has for fifty years), and patients should not be abandoned just because they are not currently receiving potentially curative radiotherapy or chemotherapy. More doctors need to focus on treatment of the person, rather than just the disease; in that way, a person's comfort, dignity, and wholeness are kept in mind.

The Pain Management Revolution

The epidemic of undertreated pain has affected so many patients and has left so many families with a legacy of suffering that a virtual revolution is gaining ground exponentially: it's a movement of health care activists committed to improving cancer pain treatments. And this revolution is finally being endorsed by the administration of our health care delivery system. As of 2002, Medicare covers pain treatment costs, a move that may pave the way for private insurers and make it much easier to identify and find local doctors who specialize in pain treatment.

On the professional health care front, the Joint Commission on Accreditation of Healthcare Organizations, the premier association that evaluates hospitals, has adopted the improvement of hospital-based pain treatment as its latest initiative, effectively establishing a standard to which hospitals must adhere. The new standards assert patients' rights to the system's best efforts to render them free of pain and affirms that effective pain management is an essential component of health care. In addition, the state cancer pain initiative movement now includes all fifty states and has formed the American Alliance of Cancer Pain Initiatives to develop policies to improve the cancer pain problem. In the past few years, nearly every professional society and scientific organization concerned with the plight of the cancer patient has taken a strong and unequivocal stand on eradicating cancer pain, and most have issued guidelines intended to promote positive change.

Also, expertise in treating cancer pain is becoming much more widespread, largely as the result of teaching programs such as the AMA's Education for Physicians on End-of-Life Care (EPEC) curriculum. Cancer pain guidelines for doctors and patients (in English and Spanish) released by the federal government's Agency for Health Care Policy and Research (now

You Don't Have to Suffer!

- Cancer pain is dehumanizing.
- Pain relief restores dignity and control.
- Better pain control improves sleep, appetite, and mood.
- Treating the pain may help you fight the cancer and may improve survival.
- Treating the pain, even with strong medications, does not signify "giving up."
- Cancer pain is a medical problem with medical solutions.
- Cancer pain is often undertreated but can be relieved.
- Cancer pain is a family problem, too.
- The patient is the ultimate authority on the pain.
- "Toughing it out" is unnecessary and just doesn't pay.
- Treating the pain makes it easier to cope with the problems that won't go away.
- Many different medications can help.
- Strong medications needn't be saved until later stages of the illness; they don't stop working.
- Addiction is not well understood, even by doctors. It is rare in cancer patients.
- While medication side effects are common, they can be treated.
- When medications fail, high-tech treatments often work.
- Treatment is best aimed at the whole person: body, mind, and spirit.
- Effective pain treatment can usually be administered by your primary care doctor or oncologist.
- If a doctor is unwilling or unable to treat your pain, a referral to a pain specialist is warranted.
- Even if pain cannot be eliminated, it can almost always be controlled.

You have a right to expect freedom from cancer pain.

the Agency for Healthcare Research and Quality) with the American Pain Society have further helped legitimize needed changes, and attendance at professional meetings and conferences on pain control is soaring. Increasingly, hospitals are pulling together multidisciplinary teams to diagnose and treat pain, including cancer pain. California and the Veterans Administration require pain to be assessed as the "fifth vital sign," and this may become more widespread. In some areas, license renewal is contingent upon completion of education in pain management; in California, legislation encourages doctors treating dying patients to prescribe opioids "without fear of prosecution." And finally, the palliative care and hospice movements, with their basic premise of maximizing quality of life for terminally ill patients, are becoming more widely accepted (see Chapter 15).

While these activities have begun to foster a new environment that promises to one day make the tragedy of unrelieved cancer pain an unsightly historical footnote, much remains to be done to help legions of today's patients and their physicians overcome a legacy of misunderstanding.

The Right to Request and Obtain Adequate Relief

Changing human behavior is difficult—just look at how hard it is to stop smoking, lose weight, and exercise regularly. Thus it is difficult for doctors, despite education, to change their prescribing habits, especially when they feel threatened by regulatory agencies. Change is slow, and consumers cannot take for granted that they will receive state-of-the-art pain relief. If pain remains unrelieved or the patient cannot rest and sleep comfortably, family caregivers must persevere and ask for help from the doctor or medical team until comfort is achieved.

To ensure that a loved one does not suffer, consumers must learn what is available and appropriate for their unique situation, and how to be an advocate to work successfully to see that the pain is relieved. To ensure optimal relief, consumers need to know what to expect in the course of cancer pain treatment.

We must abandon old-fashioned notions about toughing out pain and begin to understand that pain undermines our body's best defenses against disease, not to mention the psychological and emotional suffering and toll on the quality of life that pain extracts. No one should suffer in vain and no patient should wish to die because of our failure to use the weapons we have to relieve pain.

Don't accept that you have to suffer.

Speak up. Tell your doctor or nurse when something's not working.

Plan for pain control. Understand your options and the potential side effects of each alternative.

Make sure your doctor shares your concerns. If a doctor says, "You're just going to have to live with it," look for a new doctor.

Be informed.

2

Understanding Cancer and Pain

> *In short, the right drug at the right dose given at the right time relieves 80 to 90 percent of pain.*
>
> —World Health Organization

A diagnosis of cancer is usually unexpected and is always a frightening and overwhelming experience. Few families possess the knowledge needed to undertake the many very difficult decisions that will be required; with referral to new doctors, busy medical offices, and changing insurance requirements, it is easy to feel bewildered, confused, and helpless. In addition to providing basic information about cancer and its treatment, this chapter will discuss the various kinds of pain that are associated with cancer.

What Is Cancer?

In cancer, a tumor—a mass of abnormal tissue—begins to grow in some part of the body. The tumor consists of many cells distinct from normal cells, and these tumor cells serve no useful purpose. The growths, known as neoplasms (meaning "new growths"), may be benign or malignant. Benign growths are usually harmless and are not cancerous. Malignant neoplasms, on the other hand, continue to grow, will eventually spread (metastasize), and are potentially deadly.

What makes malignant cells so dangerous is their tendency to grow uncontrollably and to metastasize, competing with normal cells for vital nutrients and interfering with the body's normal functions. As a malignancy grows, it may invade or destroy tissues nearby or spread elsewhere, such as to the lungs, liver, or bone, by means of the bloodstream or lymphatic system.

Understanding the Diagnosis

Cancer is not one disease, but in fact a group of more than one hundred diseases that are classified according to where and how the growth occurs, as well as specific microscopic and other features. Luckily, with the variety of radiological, laboratory, and other medical tools now available, doctors can often diagnose cancer early in the disease process if a patient consults the doctor as soon as he notices persistent changes in his health status. Thus, familiarity with cancer's most prominent early warning signs is extremely important.

Warning Signs of Cancer

- A change in bladder or bowel habits that persists for more than two weeks
- A lump or mass in the abdomen, chest, breast, underarm, neck, groin, pelvis, or elsewhere
- Unusual bleeding (nosebleeds, bleeding gums, rectal or vaginal bleeding), discharge, or drainage (from the rectum, genitals, nipple, or a lump in or under the skin, or in the urine, sputum, cough, or vomitus)
- The appearance of a new skin lesion (sore) or a change in the size or appearance of an established mole or wart
- A sore that bleeds or simply doesn't heal
- Hoarseness, shortness of breath, or a nagging cough that persists beyond a few weeks
- Chronic heartburn, indigestion, or swallowing problems
- Abdominal bloating, distension, or tenderness
- Unexplained lethargy, weakness, paleness, dizziness
- Frequent, repeated, or persistent infections
- Loss of appetite or weight
- Swollen lymph nodes, especially in the groin, neck, or underarm

---

Cancer can be characterized according to a number of criteria:

- *Type and site of cancer.* Where a cancer starts (such as lung, liver, or breast), also called the cancer's primary site, as well as the type of cell within the growth (histology) are among the most important features that define a cancer and its usual behavior.
- *Cell growth and metastases.* Depending on their cell type, location, blood flow, response to treatment, and other factors, tumors are more or less likely to grow relatively slowly or more rapidly (aggressively).

- *Ability to metastasize.* Depending on their type, some tumors are more or less likely to extend locally or spread to distant organs via the lymphatic system or bloodstream.
- *Stage at diagnosis.* Doctors classify cancers as early, middle, or late phases of the disease. The stage of cancer is defined by how much cell growth is seen at the original site of the disease and how much tissue is involved beyond this site. Whether lymph nodes or distant organs are involved is crucial to treatment recommendations and the probability of a successful outcome.
- *Treatment options.* Depending on many factors, certain cancers may be more or less likely to respond favorably to treatment with surgery, chemotherapy, radiation, or all three. Recommendations to pursue various treatment options depend on additional factors, including an individual's age, general health, and preferences.

Oncologists (cancer specialists) use a shorthand to pull these characteristics together and define a tumor's stage and site: T0 to T4 to rate the size of a primary tumor, N0 to N3 to distinguish whether nearby lymph nodes are affected, and M0 to indicates an absence of distant metastases and M1 if distant deposits exist. Depending on these characteristics, a tumor is assigned a stage ranging from stage 0 to stage IV. For example, a tumor with local growth that is limited to the primary site and which has not invaded lymph nodes or other organs might be evaluated as stage I (for early disease), T1 (for a very small tumor), N0 (no involvement of nearby lymph nodes), M0 (no distant metastases).

The doctor can explain the exact kind of cancer that has been diagnosed and the nature of its usual behavior. But remember that doctors talk of averages—some people are lucky and do better than average, and some fare worse. While doctors try to put this information in plain language, sometimes it may seem too technical, or the patient may be too upset or distracted to be fully attentive. Feel free to ask questions of oncology nurses, physician assistants, pharmacists, and other health care professionals to confirm your understanding of the situation and to investigate the possibility of a second opinion. In addition, many organizations provide free educational material (see Appendix 1).

Depending on the nature of your cancer, you may ultimately be attended by several kinds of doctors. A medical oncologist is an expert on chemotherapy and usually supervises the treatment team, but you may also need a radiation oncologist (who specializes in radiation therapy) and a surgical oncologist (a surgeon who deals especially with cancer). Depending on the nature of the cancer and the involved body region, subspecialist care may

be warranted, such as that of a gynecological oncologist (for female problems), a urological oncologist (for male problems), or a head and neck oncologist. It is also important that your regular family doctor remain informed
of your progress and choices. If you have pain that does not easily respond
to simple measures, a pain specialist (usually an anesthesiologist) or palliative care specialist may be consulted.

Cancer Treatments

Once a diagnosis is confirmed, treatment recommendations are tailored
to the particular type of cancer. The cancer site and stage, cell type, growth
characteristics, and individual health differences are all considered in rec-
ommending the most appropriate treatment. The goal of any treatment is
to kill or remove as many cancerous cells as possible, while minimizing
the risk of damage to normal cells.

Surgery may be indicated to attempt removal of the entire tumor (curative surgery) or, when this is impossible, part of the tumor (debulking
surgery). Reducing the size of a tumor may make it more responsive to
other treatments, a strategy referred to as adjuvant therapy. Adjuvant chemotherapy and radiotherapy are sometimes considered before surgery to
enhance the likelihood of removing the cancer in its entirety. Even if a
tumor is thought to have been completely removed, chemotherapy, radiation therapy, or both are often prescribed after surgery in an effort to ensure that microscopic deposits of circulating cancer cells have been
destroyed. Surgery may also be considered to biopsy (to diagnose whether
a growth is cancerous), to determine the kind of cancer present, to prevent
further growth of a hormonally dependent cancer (by removing a particular organ that secretes the hormone that is triggering the cancer growth),
and in some cases to reduce pain.

Radiation therapy, administered in about half of all cases of cancer,
uses targeted X-rays, gamma rays, or electron beams to bombard specific
sites of cancer. By breaking parts of the cell, radiation interferes with the
ability of cancer cells to continue dividing and spreading. Side effects can
occur and, depending on the area being treated, may include mouth sore-
ness, skin changes, nausea, bone marrow problems, and (rarely) the risk
of developing new tumors later; less common complications are described
later in this chapter (see "Cancer Pain Syndromes Associated with Cancer
Therapy" on page 45). Radiation is also often used to reduce pain by shrinking a tumor even when a cure is no longer possible (palliative radiotherapy), especially when cancer has spread to the bone, and to manage
other symptoms such as bleeding and swelling.

Chemotherapy uses oral or injected drugs to destroy cancerous cells or slow their growth while harming as few normal cells as possible. Often used in combination with surgery or radiation to ensure that as many cancer cells as possible are destroyed, and although less effective than radiation for symptom control, chemotherapy is also sometimes used to relieve pain when tumors press on nerves, parts of the lymphatic system, or veins. Side effects may include nausea, vomiting, mouth sores, and baldness (alopecia). Less common complications are described later in this chapter.

Other Important Terms Associated with Cancer

Here are some of the most important terms that come up when cancer is diagnosed:

- *Metastasize.* As indicated above, cancer cells that spread through the body are said to be metastasizing. When a cancer has originated in one area but then spreads to another site, the secondary sites are called metastases. Metastases can be local or distant: a local metastasis (or local extension) means the cancer has spread near the primary tumor, usually just by gradual infiltration into more normal neighboring tissue. On the other hand, a metastasis may be to a distant organ, spread usually through the blood or lymphatic system, most commonly to bone, liver, lung, or brain. The lymphatic system, much like the body's system of veins, is distributed throughout the body and returns materials from the body's tissues back to the circulation. While it normally helps filter disease, the lymphatic system may also be implicated in the spread of cancer from one region to another. In fact, swollen lymph glands can be an early warning sign of a developing tumor. Metastasis is a very serious complication of cancer and usually makes treatment of the disease much more difficult and urgent.
- *Oncologist.* We've already mentioned that a doctor who specializes in cancer is an oncologist; the science of cancer is called oncology. Subspecialties within the field of oncology include medical oncology, radiation oncology, gynecological oncology, surgical oncology, and so on.
- *Biopsy.* A biopsy is often a minor surgical procedure in which a doctor will remove a small bit of tissue from a growth for a pathologist to analyze whether the growth is benign (noncancerous) or malignant (cancerous) and to identify other cellular features.

Increasingly, biopsies may be nonsurgical. By placing a small needle in the troublesome area under X-ray guidance, a bit of tissue can be removed and analyzed. Called either a needle biopsy or fine needle aspiration (FNA), this is sometimes an office procedure and is usually performed by an interventional radiologist or pathologist.

For other terms, see the Glossary at the end of this book.

What Is Pain?

Like hiccoughs, pain is one of those occurrences that we just don't give much thought to unless it's present and persistent. When first asked, most patients will just say their pain "hurts." One of this book's jobs is to help you think about pain more critically, so that you can provide doctors with the information they need to provide more effective treatment.

Pain is an unpleasant sensation or emotional experience that is triggered by tissue damage or the threat of tissue damage. But how intensely a particular person will perceive pain depends on his psychological state as well as other predispositions and traits, as outlined in the following pages.

Basically, pain has two components: (1) A *sensory component* that involves the transmission of the pain signal (electrical impulses and chemical events) from the hurt or threatened tissues to the spinal cord and brain (which together make up the central nervous system). Scientists use the technical term *nociception* to describe this complicated transmission process, which involves the release and modulation (balancing) of a variety of chemicals, hormones, and neurotransmitters (the body's chemical messengers), many of which are still undergoing intense study today. The signals generated from the damaged area are further processed in the spinal cord and ultimately converge on specialized sites in the brain where they are interpreted as pain. (2) A *reactive component* (sometimes called an affective or emotional component) that involves how the person responds to the pain, which is dependent on the person's pain threshold and his pain tolerance. A person's pain threshold is the intensity of the stimulus a person considers painful. Pain tolerance, on the other hand, is how intense or how long the unpleasant sensation can persist before the person experiences the sensation as pain.

A person's perception of pain also depends largely on how the uncomfortable sensation is filtered, altered, or distorted by that person's thoughts, feelings, and memories of past experiences. For example, depressed or anxious patients tend to have lower thresholds of pain (see box below and Chapter 14). Other factors may play a role as well, such as age (some research suggests that older people and those with a history of heavy alcohol or drug use, for example, may need more painkiller to dull pain) and race (Asians may need less morphine than whites, on average).

Also, the context in which pain occurs is relevant. Prior experiences with cancer or pain or the meaning of the pain can influence pain perception. If a woman with breast cancer remembers witnessing a relative with breast cancer die in agony, she may be terrified that she'll be just as sensitive to pain. On the other hand, the meaning of pain to a highly paid football player who is badly injured in a game is very different. He may feel less pain because he is thinking of his bonus or knows his pain is not a threat to his life. Likewise, the meaning of pain to a mother in childbirth is very different from the meaning of pain to a cancer patient. Even among cancer patients, pain in the first blush of disease is usually more manageable and often is even ignored in the imperative to fight the tumor, while pain that accompanies advanced cancer, when chemotherapy may no longer be a viable option, may seem more relentless and toxic given the absence of distraction and the concerns that the pain generates.

Although pain is probably the second most common ailment (after flulike symptoms) for which a doctor is consulted, it has historically been neglected. Because pain always results from another primary disorder, our cure-oriented system has only recently come to view pain as a bona fide medical problem. Historically, no one has been accountable for pain treatment, and patients were shuffled back and forth from the primary care provider to numerous specialists, making patients feel increasingly hopeless, depressed, and abandoned. Fortunately, this sad state of affairs is rapidly changing. Doctors can now take advanced fellowship training and obtain board certification in pain management, and increasingly, patients' reports of pain, especially when related to cancer, are being taken more seriously.

Since pain can't be objectively measured by, say, blood tests or X-rays, and is rarely accurately perceived by observers, doctors have no way of knowing how much of the pain is from physical insult or psychological distress. But doctors increasingly agree that this distinction should not even be addressed, since no matter which predominates, the suffering needs to be addressed. As scientists become increasingly aware of how enmeshed mind and body phenomena are, they are viewing pain as an authentic experience and a legitimate medical disorder, regardless of its physical or psychological components. If a patient complains of pain, those complaints should be taken seriously, even when the source is uncertain.

Influencing Pain Threshold	
Factors that can lower pain threshold (when pain is more distressing and harder to endure)	*Factors that can raise pain threshold (when pain is less distressing and easier to endure)*
Discomfort	Relieving the symptoms
Sleeplessness	Sleep
Fatigue	Rest
Anxiety	Using antianxiety medications
Fear	Understanding
Anger	Sympathy
Sadness	Diversions
Depression	Reduction in anxiety; antidepressants
Boredom	Elevation of mood
Social abandonment	Companionship
Tenseness	Relaxation/breathing exercises, imagery, and skin stimulation
Isolation	Empathy
Lack of movement	Exercise
Pain	Using analgesics (painkillers)

How Pain Occurs and Is Detected

In almost all cases, pain starts with some injury or damage to a body part. The table below shows the terms used to describe the source of the pain and how the pain is typically manifested. *Nociceptive pain* arises from injury to the body's peripheral tissues (as opposed to the nervous system) and is distinct from the other main category of pain, *neuropathic pain* (that originating in nerve injury). The two types of nociceptive pain are *somatic pain* and *visceral pain*.

Neuropathic pain occurs when elements of the nervous system are damaged (peripheral nerves, spinal cord, and brain) and may persist even when there is no obvious injury in peripheral somatic or visceral tissues. Neuropathic pain is usually a bizarre, unfamiliar experience and is often described with words that we don't typically associate with pain, such as *tingling* or *jolts*.

How Pain Is Triggered

Our body's tissue is made up mostly of cells, and when cells are injured—for example, by physical trauma, chemical burns, or reduced blood flow—their damaged walls release a variety of chemicals, including an especially

Types of Pain		
Kinds of Pain	*Sources of Pain*	*Descriptors of How It Feels*
Nociceptive pain	Injuries to body's peripheral tissues—that is, anywhere in the body but in the nervous system (including spinal cord and brain); responds to analgesics	Dull or sharp aching pain
Somatic pain	Connective tissue such as skin, muscles, bones, and ligaments	Aching, sharp, dull, or gnawing
Visceral pain	When internal organs (intestines, lungs, heart, liver, spleen, and blood vessels) are distended (stretched or swollen), twisted, or deprived of blood (ischemia)	Pulling, stretching, tightness, heaviness, or dragging and pressure
Neuropathic pain	Pain from within the nervous system; doesn't respond well to opioids and anti-inflammatory drugs but does respond to selected anti-depressants and anticonvulsants	Tingling, burning, numbness, electrical shocks or jolts, even itching

important parent compound, arachidonic acid. This substance, a fundamental building block of the body, is broken down into a complex series of chemicals called prostaglandins. These chemicals, among others, trigger pain receptors (also called nociceptors), which react by initiating electrochemical signals that are transmitted to the spinal cord and brain. Prostaglandins released after an injury also make nociceptors even more sensitive, leading to inflammation (irritation) and even more pain, which is why, for example, a finger that's been accidentally cut or banged with a hammer becomes red, swollen, and extrasensitive to touch after it has been hurt. The signals initiated by the nociceptors are like a code, carrying information related to how severe the injury is, what kind of damage has occurred, and where the trouble is located.

The idea of cellular receptors is relatively new. Scientists believe these are specialized proteins on cell walls that, depending on their structure and character, react only to very specific stimuli, chemicals, or drugs. When an injury occurs, specialized pain receptors are stimulated, initiating a long chain of events, culminating in pain. Other related receptors, which possess different structures, are stimulated by pain medications and related substances, initiating signals that ultimately result in the relief of pain. The receptor and the chemical or event that activates it ("turns it on") have been compared to a lock and key. The receptor is like a lock that in its resting state passively prevents the activity that it controls or mediates. Only when the receptor encounters the special substance that activates it (the "key that fits the lock") does it respond, in this case by initiating a signal that, after being influenced or modulated by numerous other chemicals and events, is ultimately interpreted as pain or pain relief.

How Pain Is Detected

Once the pain signal has been initiated, a very complex series of events is set into motion, which is only now beginning to be fully understood. Imagine a complex matrix of electrical switchboards that modulate and integrate electrical signals traveling back and forth from the periphery to the entire expanse of nerves outside the spinal cord and those linked to it. Once impulses initiated by peripheral injury are received at the spinal cord, they release a variety of other chemicals, which further modify the signal, which goes on to stimulate impulses that travel to the thalamus (another way station) in the brain. The brain acts like a computer, deciphering the encoded message, and ultimately interpreting the signal as pain. As a result, signals are sent back to the periphery, initiating activities such as withdrawal, exclamations like "ouch," and other manifestations of suffering. At each step of this convoluted path, the signal triggers complex chemical, electrical, and structural responses that further modify the original signal and create their own repercussions, which ripple through the body's nervous system and the peripheral tissue over which it reigns.

How Pain Relief Strategies Can Interrupt Pain Signals

One very effective way to relieve pain during the initiation of its signals is to prevent the formation of the prostaglandins (the pain-stimulating break-

The Vicious Cycle of Pain

If pain becomes chronic, it can plunge a person into a vicious cycle of painful problems.

Nervous System Changes

When nerves that conduct pain rebuild after an injury, repair is often incomplete or disordered, and nerve fibers sometimes connect to and may abnormally excite other kinds of nerves. As a result, pressure on one spot can trigger pain elsewhere, or pain can be associated with muscular twitching, swelling, changes in skin color, and local temperature changes.

Spasm and Muscle Tension

Pain often leads to local muscle spasm, a normal reflex that signals the need to avoid movement until healing occurs (a process called splinting). If excessive, however, spasm can be problematic—by increasing tension, spasm can incite pain in neighboring parts, leading to a self-perpetuating cycle of pain and spasm that, if uninterrupted, can contribute to chronic pain.

Psychological Stress

The stress from pain boosts the release of "fight-or-flight" hormones such as norepinephrine, which over time can contribute to fatigue, exhaustion, and depression.

Depression

Exhaustion and stress from unrelieved pain leave us feeling hopeless and helpless, which can intensify depression. Depression increases our sensitivity to physical pain, discourages us from engaging in distracting, enjoyable activities, and is associated with suppression of circulating levels of serotonin, a chemical that boosts mood.

Disturbed Sleep

The above problems interfere with initiating and maintaining restful sleep, which leads to more exhaustion and is thought to deplete endorphins, the body's own opioidlike substances, which otherwise help to boost mood and blunt pain.

Awkward Postures and Deconditioning

To avoid pain, we may rest excessively and assume unhealthy positions that can strain other muscles, which can lead to spreading pain and even total body pain. As disused muscles get weaker, discomfort increases and we become even more reluctant to use the muscles when a return to normal activity is required to restore function and reduce pain.

down products of arachidonic acid), and that's just what aspirin and other anti-inflammatory drugs, such as ibuprofen (Advil) and naproxen (Naprosyn), do. They have little effect on the brain and work mostly in the periphery to prevent the nociceptors (pain receptors) from becoming overly sensitive.

The spinal cord and brain contain other paths that can be interrupted or modified to control pain. Morphine and the other opioid drugs, as well as the body's own opioidlike substances (endogenous opioids such as endorphins and enkephalins), help to suppress pain messages primarily within the spinal cord and brain, thereby blunting or diminishing the perception of pain and the body's responses.

Thus, aspirin (and other anti-inflammatory drugs) and narcotic drugs (opioids) suppress pain by two distinct mechanisms that can be complementary. As we'll see in later chapters, this is why they are often used together to treat cancer pain.

Comprehensive pain strategies not only need to intercept the transmission of pain signals with medications and other techniques but also need to include relaxation exercises and attention to attitude, mood, sleep habits, isolation, and physical activity.

Types of Pain

In general, the pain of cancer patients (and other patients) may be divided into acute and chronic pain.

Acute pain can be regarded as a vivid message that an injury has occurred or that an abnormality is developing, thus signaling the body to react so as to avoid further injury—for example, the reflex to remove a burned hand from the hot handle of a pot, reactive muscle spasm that immobilizes a sprained ankle, or the need to seek to medical treatment or testing for a persistent stomachache. Once the cause of pain has been established, the pain can be said to have outlived its purpose, so it no longer is sending beneficial warning signs. In the case of cancer, its cause should be treated, and it is safe to alleviate the pain with symptomatic treatment.

When pain occurs in a person with cancer, it is often incorrectly assumed to be due to the tumor pressing on some pain-sensitive structure. This is often not the case—one-quarter to one-third of the pain experienced by cancer patients is not a direct result of the tumor but is a side effect of cancer treatment, such as scarring or nerve injury after surgery, pain from getting on and off a radiation table, or nerve or joint injury from chemotherapy.

Chronic pain may be harder to bear because the patient often feels like there's no end in sight. Even when very severe, acute pain (for example, after surgery) can be tolerated if we know it's bound to get a little better each day. That is why acute pain in the early stages of cancer is usually well tolerated; during aggressive cancer treatment, patients are often distracted from the pain, so it can more easily be ignored. Pain that is chronic and unrelenting with no end in sight, on the other hand, is much harder to tolerate, even when it is not as severe. With time, coping mechanisms wear out and frustration and depression mount. Although it may

Acute versus Chronic Pain

Acute Pain	Chronic Pain	Chronic and Acute Pain
Sharp and intense; comes on suddenly but passes in several days to up to several months.	Can be dull and achy to agonizing; persists and often worsens over months.	Both can occur together. When cancer patients have pain, the most common scenario is chronic pain (low-level if treated effectively) with intermittent superimposed bouts of acute pain. The acute pain episodes may be due to a new source of discomfort, increased movement or activity, a recently developed psychological condition, or an undertreated chronic pain condition, resulting from arthritis, for example.
Stems from a particular spot (well localized).	Starts off as acute pain but over time becomes difficult to pinpoint, describe, and cope with.	
Autonomic (or automatic) responses include dilated pupils, flushed or pale skin, heavy perspiration, rising blood pressure, and a rapid pulse and hyperventilation. Patient grimaces, rubs, or protects area of pain.	Autonomic responses become less conspicuous over time as blood pressure and pulse return toward normal, and the patient doesn't look like he hurts as much.	
Responds predictably and well to appropriate therapies.	Cause is usually more difficult to diagnose and therefore treat.	
Serves a useful, protective biological purpose by signaling the body to react and to avoid further injury.	Has outlived its warning value; like a broken doorbell that continues to ring, it serves no real value.	

not be as sharp as acute pain, chronic pain can be severe and may exact a serious toll on a patient's personality, lifestyle, and activities, affecting his mental, emotional, psychological, and sexual well-being, as well as impairing appetite and sleep. Without appropriate treatment, sufferers may show signs of depression, may experience feelings of hopelessness, and may withdraw from social activities altogether.

Terms That Describe Pain

Doctors often use specific terms to describe pain. Becoming familiar with these descriptors may help patients and families communicate more effectively with physicians and their team.

Constant pain or *basal pain* refers to pain that doesn't let up and should be treated with medication that is taken regularly, around the clock (ATC) or on a time-contingent basis, rather than just when it hurts the most. (The difference between "around the clock" and "as needed" pain administration is discussed in Chapter 3.) This strategy helps to prevent pain rather than treating it after its intensity is already well established, a much more difficult task.

Types of Pain		
Type of Pain	*Definition*	*How It's Treated*
Constant or basal pain	Steady, constant pain	Medication prescribed to be taken in scheduled doses or when needed
Breakthrough pain	Despite pain medication, pain sometimes breaks through	Rescue doses are prescribed to be taken when needed, perhaps before activity that tends to trigger the pain
End-of-dose failure pain	When pain occurs regularly before next scheduled dose is due, that is, rescue doses are needed frequently	Dose of regularly scheduled medication is increased
Intermittent pain	Unpredictable pain that occurs irregularly	Intermittent injections, pain-killing "lollipops," or anesthetic procedure

Breakthrough pain is pain that intermittently "breaks through" an otherwise effective preventive medication schedule. When it is related to a specific activity, such as eating, going to the bathroom, laughing, or walking, it is called *incident pain*. Breakthrough pain is best managed with extra doses of rapid-onset short-acting medicine for when the pain breaks through the baseline medicated comfort; these extra doses are called escape or rescue doses or may be referred to as a bolus. These extra doses are taken on an as-needed or symptom-contingent basis (often written as PRN, an abbreviation for the Latin term *pro re nata*). When incident pain is relatively predictable, that same extra prescribed dose is best used just before engaging in the pain-provoking activity.

End-of-dose failure refers to breakthrough pain that usually occurs just before the next scheduled dose of around-the-clock medication is due. This usually signals that the dose of ATC medicine is too low and needs to be raised or given more frequently. When rescue doses are needed frequently, it suggests that the prescribed dose of basal or ATC medication is insufficient and should be increased, after which the need for frequent escape doses should diminish.

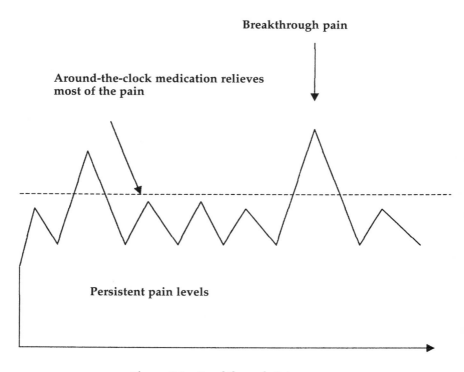

Figure 2.1   Breakthrough Pain

Intermittent pain is unpredictable and occurs irregularly, on and off. Taking medication around the clock may be ineffective for intermittent pain because relief may be inadequate during painful episodes and sedation may be troubling during pain-free periods. Intermittent pain, therefore, is one of the few instances in which an as-needed (PRN) prescription for medicine is usually best. Unfortunately, pain that is truly intermittent and comes and goes abruptly may have disappeared by the time most oral pain medications start to work. As a result, severe, intermittent pain may be best treated with a novel approach, such as using injectable pain medications; Actiq, a new, lollipop-like form of the opioid medication fentanyl, or an anesthetic procedure that will diminish pain by dulling the nerves involved in its transmission.

Who Has Cancer Pain

Not all cancer hurts. In fact, many cancer patients will experience relatively little pain. In the early stages of the disease, only one out of ten patients has pain that is strong enough to affect mood and activities. In intermediate-stage cancer, about half of patients will suffer moderate to severe pain, and when cancer is advanced or terminal, 75 to 90 percent of patients have chronic pain that is severe to excruciating. *But remember, when treated correctly, the vast majority of cancer pain victims—from 90 to 99 percent—can expect satisfactory pain relief.* Most important, these encouragingly high success rates are based on patients' own reports, not just on the observations of doctors or nurses.

Why Cancer Pain Is Different

Chronic pain that is not related to cancer—such as pain from arthritis, back injuries, or gastrointestinal disorders—is very different from the pain of progressive cancer. One reason is that cancer pain is more liberally treated with a greater variety of therapies and usually responds well, while treatment options for most chronic noncancer pain are more restricted and satisfactory relief is usually more elusive. For example, morphine and other narcotic drugs are used routinely in cancer and are extremely effective; addiction is considered a remote risk. In contrast, the use of morphine for chronic pain is highly controversial and remains infrequent or even the last resort, both because it appears to be much less reliably effective and because concerns about addiction are pervasive. Attitudes have changed rapidly in recent years, and today's patients with chronic noncancer pain are much more likely to be treated with opioids than in the past, but such treatment remains stigmatized and guarded, often leaving patients feeling humiliated, like failures or criminals. In the case of chronic pain unrelated to cancer, patients often need to be encouraged to live with some or all of their pain because there is no cure. If there is any good news with cancer, it is that the pain can be controlled.

Pain versus Suffering

Before we discuss specific cancer pain syndromes (characteristic presentations that arise as a consequence of different cancer types), it's important to first understand the differences between pain and suffering, two broad concepts that are closely related. Pain is more intimately related to the actual injured tissue and the signal that is generated. Suffering, on the other hand, includes pain and can be a consequence of it, but it is more closely related to our interpretation of the pain signal and our responses to it.

Psychological, cultural, and socioeconomic factors all play important roles in how we react to significant life events, including how much we suffer when we experience pain. *The relative contributions of these psychosocial components, however, do not make the pain that underlies them any less authentic, real, or valid.* The powerful influence of our mind, though, may help explain why the pain from tumor growth or tumor recurrence may be much harder to tolerate than pain that stems from scarring in cancer that has been cured, since these types of pain have such different meanings and significance. Suffering, therefore, includes feelings that are linked to the problems of being ill with cancer and the stress that arises from them. Terminal cancer patients often suffer more, for example, if they believe their pain can't be controlled, but once it has been demonstrated that, in fact, their pain can be relieved, their suffering diminishes. Often a referral to hospice or a pain specialist is sufficient to render pain easier to manage, since the simple assurance that someone will be specifically accountable for managing pain reduces anxiety. Childbirth is another example that shows the difference between pain and suffering: although its pain is undeniable, childbirth is associated with little suffering because the experience is usually viewed as part of a joyous event.

In expressing suffering, patients may exhibit attention-seeking behaviors, such as remaining disabled despite improvement or constantly looking for a different doctor. Other examples of how psychological factors influence suffering include:

- Depression that stems from feelings of helplessness, isolation, physical disability, fatigue, the actual or threatened loss of wellness, income, and identity, and fear of death
- Anxiety about treatment, outcome, expenses, and the welfare of family members
- Anger at being ill; at friends and family for not being supportive enough; at doctors for being unavailable or unable to cure the patient; and at health care facilities for delays, blunders, or insensitive treatment

Thus, although a person's response to pain—his so-called pain behavior (grimacing, crying, limping, asking for help)—may appear to be a direct result of the damage caused by cancer, this behavior is always strongly influenced by psychological factors, a fact that patients sometimes resist acknowledging. But perhaps this is an artificial distinction. Most experts would now argue that you can't have pain without the influence of psychological factors. In fact, more and more scientists are convinced that we cannot separate mind from body and that effective treatment, especially for cancer patients, must consider the mind and body as a whole.

The relationships between pain and feelings or mood are complex. If a depression is effectively treated through counseling or antidepressants, the severity of pain problems and their associated distress often significantly subside. If depression persists, even aggressive pain therapy with morphine or surgery often fails to significantly relieve pain, because a strong psychological component of pain remains.

How Feelings Can Affect Pain

One doctor tells the story of a woman with persistent pain that didn't seem to respond to treatments that ordinarily work well. After days of trying various medical therapies without success, a staff member finally spoke with the patient in greater depth and discovered that the patient was terribly anxious about what would become of her beloved poodle if she died. The social services staff pursued this issue, and after reassurance that a caring foster home was available for her dog, the patient's pain responded much more favorably to treatment and, along with her anxiety, rapidly subsided.

On the other hand, persistent pain can trigger depression—cancer patients in pain have been found to have higher rates of depression than otherwise similar cancer patients who had no pain. It is not surprising that when pain is well managed, depression often resolves or becomes easier to treat.

What's vital to remember here is that regardless of the extent to which psychological, emotional, and spiritual factors trigger or influence pain, the pain and suffering are just as authentic, legitimate, and real to the person who is experiencing them. In working with a patient who has pain and suffering, therefore, caregivers need to understand that, if they are to be successful, efforts to relieve pain must take into account the full range of reasons for the patient's suffering. (See Chapter 14, "Dealing with Feelings.")

Why Cancer Hurts

Tumors themselves do not hurt. Pain is caused either by the effects of the cancer treatments (such as chemotherapy, surgical scarring, and radiation), the effects of the tumor's growth (intruding on neighboring tissues or invading other tissues distant from the tumor's primary site), other conditions that occur along with the cancer (such as herpes zoster, commonly known as shingles, a condition that chemotherapy patients are more susceptible to, or back pain from prolonged bed rest), or side effects from therapies and medications (such as getting on and off the radiation table, constipation, or nausea). In addition, of course, many patients with cancer may have long-standing chronic pain due to an unrelated condition such as arthritis or an old back injury. Since chronic pain is so often undertreated, many cancer patients are surprised and pleased to learn that these old pains they have been told to live with can in fact also be relieved.

Like virtually all medical therapies, almost all treatments for cancer are associated with some risk of toxicity or side effects and complications. In an effort to destroy all of the cancer cells, some healthy cells may be damaged as well, but since many therapies have an excellent chance of helping the patient, these are risks that most patients are willing to take. After successful treatment, patients may live long and healthy lives, and although some may experience lasting complications (such as pain) from their cancer treatments, it is also reassuring that not all the pain associated with cancer is from tumor growth, but rather may be related to treatments.

Cancer Pain Syndromes Associated with Cancer Therapy

As we've said, one of the challenges of designing the best cancer treatment involves destroying as many tumor cells as possible while preserving the integrity of normal cells. Still, some injury, either temporary or permanent, usually occurs to normal cells and may produce pain, which can be transient or, in some cases, lasting. This is why it is wrong to always assume that more pain in the cancer patient means the tumor has gotten worse. Pain from cancer therapy is, in fact, much more common than has been realized, and as we've already mentioned, accounts for about one-quarter to one-third of the pain reported by cancer patients. Fortunately, however, like the other pains associated with cancer, treatment-related pain can be successfully treated, even when it is chronic.

Although we list many of the possible problems that may arise in the cancer patient, it must be remembered that there is an enormous diversity in the experiences of cancer patients, and although we discuss many different syndromes below, the likelihood of any patient experiencing more than a few is very low. We list many here so that a patient who is having a particular problem can find it described and may be reassured to recognize that it is not a freak occurrence but the possible effect of a particular treatment.

Specifically, these pain syndromes stem from the following three categories: pain from surgery, pain from chemotherapy, and pain from radiation therapy.

Pain from Surgery

In addition to the self-limited pain that follows most operations, amputation and surgery on the chest (thoracotomy), breast (mastectomy), neck (radical neck dissection), and rectum, in particular, may cause lasting pain. Usually, pain is from nerve injury and may be described as "numbing," "burning," or "shooting"; it is often accompanied by hypersensitivity of the skin near the operated region. It has recently been recognized that pain after amputation is much more common than was previously thought. In the past, patients used to think they were going crazy when they felt sensations in the part of the body that had been removed (called phantom limb pain). It has also recently been recognized that similar pain may follow breast, colostomy, and head and neck surgery (phantom breast pain, phantom anus pain, and even phantom tongue pain).

Pain from Chemotherapy

Certain types of chemotherapy are more likely than others to cause pain. Here is another reason to make sure pain is fully discussed with the doctor. This kind of pain can often be relieved or eliminated by adjusting the chemotherapy. Polyneuropathy (damage to many small nerves), especially common after treatment with the drugs vincristine and vinblastine, may be first felt as jaw pain, but most commonly causes tingling sensations in the feet and hands, as well as stomach problems (autonomic neuropathy). Taxol, a popular, relatively new chemotherapy drug, is also commonly associated with polyneuropathy, as well as myalgias (muscle aches) and arthralgias (joint pain). Granulocyte colony-stimulating factor (G-CSF), or Neupogen, is a treatment that has been recently developed to counter low white blood cell counts that can be caused by chemotherapy. Given as a weekly subcutaneous injection, it is very effective, but it may cause severe bone pain for several days, especially in the ribs, low back, and sternum or breastbone. Steroids are commonly used in cancer treatment and, when taken for a long time, can weaken the bones (a condition called osteoporosis or excessive bone resorption) and even destroy the bone, especially the hip joints (called aseptic necrosis). If steroids are withdrawn too quickly, joint pain (pseudorheumatism) can result as well. Painful, sensitive mouth sores (known as stomatitis and mucositis) can be caused by many types of chemotherapy, especially when combined with radiotherapy or bone-marrow transplantation. This kind of pain is usually very severe but lasts only days to weeks in most cases. The recognition and treatment of mucositis is crucial so that treatment does not interfere with nutrition.

PAIN FROM RADIOTHERAPY

Radiation therapy can cause a variety of symptoms, usually related to the area that is being treated. In addition to fatigue, bleeding problems, skin injury, nausea, and diarrhea, there may be pain in the skin, bone, or near nerves. Pain can result from actual injury to these structures or may be due to indirect causes, such as scarring and fibrosis (excessive and thickened connective tissue) or injury to blood vessels that supply these structures. The spinal cord is very sensitive to radiation, and occasionally injury here may produce bizarre pain in the lower half of the body, sometimes accompanied by numbness and even paralysis or bladder problems (incontinence). Occasionally, years later, radiation therapy can even produce new tumors on nerves that are included in the treatment field.

Cancer Pain Syndromes Caused by Tumor Growth

One of the most common sources of pain in cancer patients is a result of the effects of tumor growth, which accounts for almost 80 percent of the pain in hospitalized cancer patients and about 60 percent in outpatients. Again, although many different syndromes are described here, the likelihood of a particular patient experiencing more than a couple are very unlikely.

Specifically, pain from the cancer itself is caused by the cancer:

- Invading nerves, blood vessels, bones, or parts of the lymphatic system

- Pressing on nerves, causing compression
- Obstructing hollow organs such as the gastrointestinal tract, trachea, or ureter
- Blocking blood vessels, which can cause poor circulation and swollen, engorged veins
- Killing, infecting, or inflaming tissues
- Pushing on tissues, causing them to become swollen or distended

The type of pain depends on exactly where the tumor damage occurs. The part of the body that is injured and the probable mechanism of pain will help determine what type of medications will help. Here is a general overview of the various pain syndromes associated with cancer.

Bone Pain

Tumor invading bone is the most common cause of cancer pain, although interestingly, spread of cancer to the bone is not always associated with pain (silent metastases). Bone metastases are especially common with cancer of the prostate, breast, thyroid, lung, or kidney but can occur with almost any tumor. A test called a bone scan is often used to identify tumors that have spread to the bone, but plain X-rays, CAT scans, and magnetic resonance imaging (MRI) may also be used. Although many types of tumors in bone are not painful, when they do cause pain, the pain often flares up at night and is worse with movement or when the body bears weight. Typically, bone pain feels like a dull, deep ache or like a gnawing pain; it may cause muscle spasms or spells of stabbing pain. All of the body's bones, in a sense, can be considered part of the same organ or organ system, so once a single bone has shown evidence of tumor spread, patients shouldn't be surprised to find that the cancer has spread to other bones, even though only some of the bone lesions may hurt.

Occasionally, headaches occur with tumors in the bones of the outer skull, and when bones near the base of the skull are affected facial pain and nerve abnormalities may arise. Back pain is common when lung, breast, prostate, bladder or kidney cancers metastasize to the spine. Persistent, deep, boring pain in the hip or thigh sometimes signifies that tumor invasion of this region has caused or may soon cause a fracture (pathologic fracture or impending fracture), and may be a reason to consider surgery to avoid being bedridden. Pain involving the bones of the spine may signify that a compression (crush) fracture has occurred. Pain from vertebral compression fractures usually gets better with time, and treatment with surgery is usually not considered unless there is also injury to the spinal cord.

Bone pain is often treated with anti-inflammatory agents (NSAIDs) and opioids (narcotics) and usually responds especially well to radiation therapy or a radiation-like treatment with a bone-seeking isotope injection, such as strontium-89 (Metastron) or samarium (Quadramet), when feasible.

Pain Due to Nerve Damage

Pain from nerve damage, which affects 20 to 40 percent of patients, may be associated with hypersensitivity and is often described as burning, tingling, numbing, pressing, squeezing, or itching. It may even trigger pain in numb areas. Patients often describe nerve pain as a bizarre experience, different from the sensations they usually associate with pain. Nerve pain can be extremely unpleasant, even intolerable.

Usually nerve pain is constant and steady. Sometimes, in addition to the continuous pain, sudden intermittent pains occur, often described as shooting, like a lance stabbing (lancinating), electrical, or jolting in nature. In trying to understand pain better, doctors have compared these types of pain to a seizure or convulsion and have found more than a few similarities. Pain does not cause seizures, but both nerve pain and seizures are electrical phenomena; like a seizure, pain from a nerve injury may be sudden and unpredictable in onset and duration. This similarity is why doctors use anticonvulsants such as gabapentin (Neurontin), carbamazepine (Tegretol), valproic acid (Depakote), and phenytoin (Dilantin) to treat shooting pain.

Many patients with nerve pain also experience associated problems, such as bladder or bowel weakness, an impaired sense (poor taste, smell, hearing, or feeling, or vision problems), or motor, balance, or reflex problems. Some patients also suffer from what is known as alodynia, that is, an unpleasant abnormal sensation, such as that experienced with shingles, in which a patient exhibits unusual pain sensitivity from something as ordinary as light touch, which doesn't normally cause pain; this may result from contact with clothing, bedsheets, or even the wind.

Unfortunately, nerve pain often responds relatively poorly to narcotic drugs such as morphine when they are used alone. Sometimes, however, it can be relieved by combining drugs, such as by adding certain types of antidepressants (tricyclic antidepressants), anticonvulsants, muscle relaxants (like baclofen), orally administered local anesthetics (sodium channel blockers such as mexiletine), and drugs known as alpha-adrenergic antagonists. Still, in all these cases, relief is unpredictable, and new combinations or adjustments of medications may be needed every few weeks, during which time the drug dosages may be raised steadily to find the right dose. Sometimes rubbing the painful area with topical medicines that contain aspirin, chloroform, or capsaicin can help nerve pain as well. (See Chapter 8 for more details.)

More invasive techniques such as nerve blocks may provide short-term relief, and sometimes a series of these injections (usually performed by a specially trained anesthesiologist) may provide prolonged periods of relief. In special cases, long-term electrical stimulation of the spinal cord or brain can be used to provide long-term relief as well.

Muscle Pain

Until recently, muscle pain had been underrecognized in cancer patients, largely because even modern tests do a poor job of identifying damage to muscles. When muscles are injured, the pain may be described as dull, aching, and sore, often accompanied by stiffness and local tenderness. Although it may feel like a cramp, muscular cancer pain is usually more severe and persistent than a typical cramp.

In general, muscle pain (like the pain of the flu) does not respond extremely well to morphine and similar drugs, or even to traditional muscle relaxants (Soma, Robaxin, Parafon Forte, or Flexeril), which may just be sedating. Stronger muscle relaxants, developed for the treatment of multiple sclerosis and spinal cord injury—baclofen (Lioresal), tizanidine (Zanaflex)—may be helpful when started in low doses. Typically, doctors treat muscle pain with the NSAIDs (for example, aspirin and ibuprofen), in addition to quinine, diazepam (Valium), baclofen (Lioresal), phenytoin (Dilantin), dantrolene (Dantrium), and carbamazepine (Tegretol).

Physical therapies such as mild exercise, gradual stretching, heat or ice, ultrasound, TENS (transcutaneous electrical nerve stimulation), relaxation exercises, and massage may also help to relieve such pain. (See Chapter 12 for details.) Many patients obtain relief when a local anesthetic or steroids are injected into persistent areas of pain, a relatively minor procedure called a trigger point injection. (See Chapters 9 and 8, respectively.)

Abdominal Pain

When the superficial nerves just beneath the abdominal wall are involved, pain tends to be well localized but may radiate out in bandlike patterns and be associated with hypersensitivity and altered sensation. Abdominal pain may also stem from tumors in the liver, pancreas, stomach, intestines, or pelvis.

Tumors in the liver tend to result in constant, dull, dragging pain, especially over the right upper abdomen, and often a feeling of fullness. It may also express itself in the midback, or in the right shoulder if the diaphragm is irritated. Such a tumor may also cause reduced appetite, nausea, and vomiting.

Pancreatic tumors tend to cause relentless, boring, aching pain in the midabdomen that spreads to the midback and often is relieved by curling up, by lying down in the fetal position, or by sitting, either in an easy chair or slumped over a table, and may be aggravated by lying flat with the legs outstretched.

Tumors in the stomach give rise to pain similar to that of pancreatic tumors or a burning pain like that of ulcers.

Intestinal tumors may block the bowel, causing colicky (crampy, spasmodic) pain, bloating, nausea, and vomiting.

In the pelvis, tumors may be caused by bowel, ovarian, or uterine cancer, or by tumors in the abdomen that are outside specific organs. Such pain tends to feel vague and hard to pinpoint, yet causes fullness, pressure, dragging, or discomfort on both sides of the body. In some patients, pelvic pain may be intermittent and shooting or feel like a red-hot poker in the rectum. When a tumor affects the bladder, the pain may be spasmodic or burning, and can cause a sense of fullness of the bladder.

When blood vessels or areas of the lymphatic system become blocked by a tumor, pain may also arise. When an artery is blocked, for example, the patient may feel numb or weak in the area; as an area becomes deprived of blood and oxygen because of the blockage, a deep, aching pain may be felt. Moving the area may be particularly uncomfortable. When veins or lymph vessels are obstructed, an area may become engorged, causing swelling and tightness; sometimes the area affected may look bluish or red. Some of these conditions, especially when rapidly progressive, are medical emergencies, requiring an urgent consultation with a doctor. A particularly common site for painful blockage of a vein (called thrombosis) is the calf. A deep venous thrombosis (DVT) in this area usually causes swelling of the foot and tenderness involving the fleshy part of the back of the calf.

Headache

Usually headache in the cancer patient is a preexisting problem or relates to stress and has no specific relation to the underlying cancer. Nevertheless, headache is a prominent feature in about 60 percent of patients with brain tumors. When due to a brain tumor, headaches often feel steady, deep, dull, and aching but are rarely rhythmic or throbbing. They are usually intermittent and may be worse in the morning or with coughing or straining. Usually the severity of the headaches that occur with brain tumors is only moderate and is rarely severe enough to awaken patients from sleep. Often such headaches are helped by aspirin or steroids, cold packs, or rest. The sudden onset of headache that is associated with nausea, vigorous or projectile vomiting, confusion or sleepiness, or an irregular breathing pattern or pulse may signal a neurological emergency—increased intracranial pressure from the rapid swelling of brain tissue within the skull's rigid encasement—and requires rapid assessment and treatment.

Other Head and Neck Pain

Splinting is a medical term that refers to the body's tendency to immobilize an injured part to minimize pain and promote healing, a protective reflex that is usually adopted unconsciously. Pain in the neck and head area is sometimes problematic because it is often triggered by swallowing, eating, coughing, talking, and other movements of the head that are relatively involuntary, thus making splinting impractical and sometimes impossible. Head and neck pain, however, may respond well to a variety of therapies, including radiation, NSAIDs, opioids, anticonvulsants, and antidepressants. Nerve blocks, neurosurgery, and the administration of opioids near the brain (intraventricular opioids) may also be effective but are considered only infrequently.

Other Sources of Pain Associated with Cancer

Other Conditions

Pain may also result from other conditions that occur at the same time as the cancer (comorbid conditions) and which may or may not be directly related, such as arthritis, gastrointestinal disorders, and long-standing back pain; these account for pain in about 3 percent of hospitalized cancer patients and 10 percent of those cared for at home. Some physicians also consider problems related to the side effects of cancer therapies as another category of pain, such as discomfort due to muscle spasms, muscle wasting from inactivity, constipation, mouth sores from dehydration, and other causes, such as bedsores (also called decubitus ulcers). These problems are discussed more fully in Chapters 10 and 11.

"Benign" Pain

As we've indicated, patients are sometimes fearful of admitting ongoing pain for fear that it means that their condition has worsened. This natural tendency toward denial underscores the importance of recognizing that not all pain associated with cancer means a tumor has grown or recurred or that the cancer has progressed. We have already discussed how treatment of the tumor can cause pain by injuring normal neighboring tissue; scarring can also cause pain. Doctors sometimes call such discomfort benign pain, even though it can produce ill effects if untreated. However, even if pain is not directly related to cancer, it is best not to label it as benign, since no matter what the cause, persistent pain is always undesirable and inconsistent with well-being. Muscle spasm is a good example. Spasm (or splinting) is a protective reflex that causes us to hold an injured body part still, and thus this reflex serves a purpose, at least for a time. Sometimes muscle spasm persists longer than is necessary and can become the main source of pain: an injury produces spasm, but the spasm may tug on nearby areas, producing additional pain and spasm, triggering a vicious cycle of pain and spasm that persists beyond the original injury and may continue until it is interrupted by treatment. This type of pain is not associated with the tumor having progressed, but for proper treatment to be initiated, the doctor must be made aware of the existence of the persistent pain. In this case, under doctor's counsel, it may be safe to push through the body's alarm system and to stretch and exercise despite the pain. Even though physical therapy or rehabilitation may make the pain temporarily worse until the stiffness has improved, the resulting pain is not a signal that new harm is brewing.

Finally, increased pain may simply be a result of the development of tolerance to painkillers, which is common with prolonged use and can be remedied by adjustments coordinated by your doctor.

Good Pain Treatment Is Good Cancer Treatment

Regardless of the source of the pain, it should be treated, not only to make the patient more comfortable but, as discussed in Chapter 1, because it is harmful to health, impairs quality of life, and interferes with the ability to fight cancer.

Remember: suffering is needless and will only make things worse. Pain treatment should be a high priority, not relegated to the back burner. It is as essential to treat pain as it is to treat the cancer itself, because unrelenting pain can influence the course of a cancer illness. The cancer and pain should be viewed as inseparable.

3

Assessing Pain and Planning
Treatment Strategies

Living with unnecessary pain decreases your overall quality of life. It may make you less active or depressed. You may have difficulty sleeping, working, or spending time with family and friends. You may erroneously equate your pain with advancing cancer and begin to feel hopeless. Because you need all of your energy to get through your cancer treatments and get healthy again, living with cancer pain is simply foolish.

This chapter provides an overview of how doctors assess cancer pain, what patients should expect from a comprehensive pain assessment, and the general approaches doctors use to tackle cancer pain.

Strategies to Relieve Pain

While there are many ways of addressing pain problems, each technique pertains to one of three basic strategies doctors use to relieve cancer pain.

Strategy 1: Attacking the Source of the Pain

Whenever possible, the first and best way to relieve cancer pain is to eliminate or modify the source of the pain by removing or shrinking the cancer that is causing the pain, with surgery, radiation, or chemotherapy (including hormones). However, these approaches are sometimes impractical and even unsafe. First, each of these kinds of treatments has some risk.

Second, many patients are not candidates for surgery, especially if the cancer has spread or if a patient's overall condition is poor. Finally, not all tumors respond well to radiation and chemotherapy. Even when they do, treatments sometimes have to be limited because they can cause reduced blood counts and may make patients feel run-down. Also, most of these treatments produce pain relief only slowly, and some may actually worsen pain or, as a side effect, cause new pain.

Nevertheless, these strategies are often very effective in relieving pain, even when a complete cancer cure is unlikely. Since these antitumor strategies to control pain involve shrinking the tumor, except for surgery they rarely work instantly; it takes time to safely shrink a tumor, and so pain relief may be slow. Some doctors still make the mistake of relying on an either-or principle, instead of properly combining strategies. That is, the goal of anticancer treatments can be curative (in pursuit of a cure) or palliative (used to relieve symptoms without a hope of a cure). Either way, painkillers should be used and tapered as the effects of the cancer treatment start to take hold. Sometimes (e.g., after starting tamoxifen, a breast cancer treatment, or after administering Neupogen, a treatment to boost white blood cell counts) analgesics are needed to relieve initial flare-ups of pain, at least temporarily.

Even if pain isn't relieved, it doesn't mean a poor response to the antitumor treatment: pain commonly persists even after very effective antitumor treatment (including surgery), especially when the tumor has produced scarring or fibrosis, or when its bulk has chronically stretched, bruised, or infiltrated nerves and other pain-sensitive structures. Sometimes powerful anticancer treatments produce their own new pain, an unfortunate complication.

Strategy 2: Distorting the Pain Message with Analgesics

The most common way to relieve pain is to alter the perception of pain at the level of the spinal cord and brain, where the pain messages are ultimately received and interpreted, with painkillers or analgesics, such as morphine. Even though patients may fear that doctors will view their pain as "in their head," in truth, all pain *is* in the head. No matter how or where it hurts, pain is ultimately recorded in the brain, which acts like a computer interpreting the meaning of all the sensations we experience. Morphine and related drugs alter the perception of pain in a selective and reversible way, with no permanent damage or changes. Pain is blunted, and with proper use individuals can continue to function normally, and often much better, once an individualized medication treatment program has been established.

Strategy 3: Interrupting the Pain Signals

The third way to treat cancer pain, which is used much less frequently, is to use a nerve block of some sort that interrupts the pain signal somewhere between its source (usually the tumor) and the central nervous system (which includes the spinal cord and brain) where the signals are received. This approach is like cutting an electrical wire to interrupt a circuit, and resembles a dentist's injection of novocaine.

To treat cancer pain, neurosurgical and anesthetic procedures can numb, cut, burn, or freeze nerves or nerve centers. Such blocks can be administered by injecting chemicals nearby, such as local anesthetics for short-term relief, steroids for intermediate relief, and (when appropriate) nerve-damaging alcohol or phenol for longer-term and even occasionally permanent relief. Since these treatments have greater risks and aren't as reliably reversible, they are appropriate for only a small proportion of patients. (See Chapter 9 for details.)

Before any of these approaches are used, however, physicians must first assess the pain situation by gathering information about the underlying cancer, the pain, and the person experiencing it. Some doctors will ask about characteristics of the pain, others will use formal questionnaires, and many will request the presence of a family member or friend to share their observations and assist with planning.

Since every person's pain is different, each treatment plan will be different as well. What worked for a friend, who may even have had a similar cancer, may not be appropriate for a specific patient. Just as many people can't buy suits off the rack, drug therapy must be tailored for an optimal fit.

How to Prepare for a Pain Assessment

To ensure the best treatment, you need to accurately convey all relevant information about the disease, prior treatments, other medical conditions, lifestyle and coping methods, medication use, and other vital information.

Bring Details

An assessment usually begins with a basic history and may include questions about marital and work status, ability to complete activities of daily living, exercise levels, network of support, cultural and ethnic background, psychological and social strengths and weaknesses, spiritual beliefs, health problems other than cancer, allergies, medication use, prior surgery, and the abilities and health of your spouse or significant other (including the ability to care for the cancer patient, to drive, etc.). Remember, the more the doctor knows, the better he can help.

Bring a Companion

When possible, the patient should bring someone else to the pain assessment, ideally the person responsible for the patient's overall care. That person can serve as the patient's advocate and actively participate in decisions. Many doctors encourage whole families to come, since ill patients are often distracted by their pain, deny the seriousness of their illness, or may find it difficult to concentrate or adequately communicate their concerns. A companion can ensure that all questions have been answered, take notes, and be prepared to review them with the patient later.

Patient and Family Checklist for Doctor's Appointment

Bring to the appointment:

- A companion who is prepared with questions, paper, and pen
- A list of important events in the medical history, especially involving the cancer
- A summary of cancer treatments and recommendations so far
- A list of medications (or the bottles in a bag) and allergies to medications
- Completed pain questionnaire and/or diary
- List of problematic symptoms
- Notes on the patient's outlook and emotional well-being
- A tape recorder (with permission)

Provide Details about the Pain

Most people find it difficult to discuss their pain and may be taken aback when pressed for details. Some just say, "It just hurts; I can't describe it." Pain specialists list more than seventy-five words to characterize pain (see below). Pain from a toothache is very different from the pain of a burn or a fresh surgical incision. Your physician needs to especially know whether the pain is burning, tingling, numbing, or electrical in character because some of these features may reflect nerve damage, which is treated differently from other types of pain.

Although many pain clinics use formal pain questionnaires, many doctors don't. Basically, measures of pain attempt to assess three dimensions: (1) pain intensity, location, and character, (2) pain relief, and (3) psychological distress or mood. Review the following table, which gives you a vocabulary for your pain.

How It Feels	Where Pain Is Probably From	Technical Term for Type of Pain
Aching, sharp, dull, knifelike, throbbing, pulsing, gnawing	Soft tissue: muscle, bone, ligament, fat, and skin pain	Somatic Nociceptive
Pressure, pulling, tugging, dragging, heaviness, twisting, fullness	Internal organs or blood vessels	Visceral Nociceptive
Tingling, burning, searing, flickering, numb, pins and needles, itching, crawling, sensitive	Nerves	Neuropathic
Miserable, annoying, unbearable, exhausting, tiring, agonizing, torturous	Pain that is strongly influenced by emotions, anxiety, or depression	Psychosomatic (which does *not* mean it isn't real)

Words for Describing Pain

Flickering	Tugging	Splitting	Miserable
Quivering	Pulling	Constant	Intense
Pulsing	Wrenching	Unremitting	Unbearable
Beating	Hot	Tiring	Spreading
Pounding	Burning	Exhausting	Radiating
Jumping	Scalding	Sickening	Penetrating
Flashing	Searing	Suffocating	Piercing
Shooting	Shooting	Fearful	Tight
Pricking	Lacerating	Frightful	Numb
Boring	Electrical Jolting	Terrifying	Drawing
Drilling	Tingling	Punishing	Squeezing
Stabbing	Itching	Grueling	Tearing
Lancinating	Smarting	Cruel	Cool
(piercing)	Stinging	Vicious	Cold
Sharp	Dull	Killing	Freezing
Cutting	Sore	Wretched	Nagging
Lacerating	Hurting	Blinding	Nauseating
Pinching	Aching	Annoying	Agonizing
Pressing	Heavy	Troublesome	Dreadful
Gnawing	Tender	Rasping	Torturing
Cramping	Taut		
Crushing			

How Intense Is Your Pain?

Pain Intensity Scale
0 No pain   1 Mild   2 Discomforting   3 Distressing   4 Horrible   5 Excruciating

Source: Reprinted from the McGill Pain Questionnaire. © 1970 by Ronald Melzack, Ph.D., and used with permission of Dr. Melzack.

Here are several of the most well-known pain questionnaires. Choose the one you feel most comfortable with, and bring it along to your doctor's appointment.

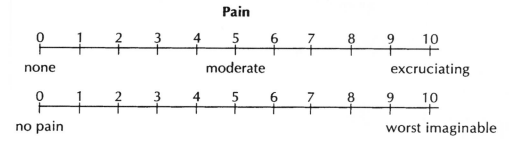

Figure 3.1   Visual Analog Scale

For children under seven and some adults, the face scales below are very useful since they don't rely on language.

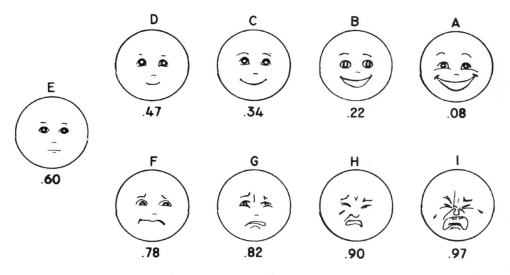

Figure 3.2   McGrath's Face Scale

Children are presented with one of three different randomly ordered face sheets. They select the face that best represents how they feel in relation to their pain, from the "happiest feeling possible" (little pain) to the "saddest feeling possible" (great pain). The numbers represent the magnitude of pain affect (between 0 and 1) shown in each face based on previous research on children.

Source: From P. A. McGrath, *Pain in Children: Nature, Assessment, and Treatment* (New York: Guilford, 1990), p. 76.

The Brief Pain Inventory (which takes only about fifteen minutes) is quick and one of the most useful tools, as it also includes questions on functional status and quality of life.

STUDY ID# _____   HOSPITAL# _____

DO NOT WRITE ABOVE THIS LINE

Brief Pain Inventory (Short Form)

Date: ___/___/___   Time:_____

Name: _____ _____ _____
                    Last   First   Middle Initial

1) Throughout our lives, most of us have had pain from time to time (such as minor headaches, sprains, and toothaches). Have you had pain other than these everyday kinds of pain today?

1.   Yes   2.   No

2) On the diagram, shade in the areas where you feel pain. Put an X on the area that hurts the most.

Right   Left | Left   Right

3) Please rate your pain by circling the one number that best describes your pain at its worst in the last 24 hours.

0	1	2	3	4	5	6	7	8	9	10
No Pain										Pain as bad as you can imagine

4) Please rate your pain by circling the one number that best describes your pain at its least in the last 24 hours.

0	1	2	3	4	5	6	7	8	9	10
No Pain										Pain as bad as you can imagine

5) Please rate your pain by circling the one number that best describes your pain on the average.

0	1	2	3	4	5	6	7	8	9	10
No Pain										Pain as bad as you can imagine

6) Please rate your pain by circling the one number that tells how much pain you have right now.

0	1	2	3	4	5	6	7	8	9	10
No Pain										Pain as bad as you can imagine

7) What treatments or medications are you receiving for your pain?

_____

8) In the last 24 hours, how much relief have pain treatments or medications provided? Please circle the one percentage that most shows how much relief you have received.

0%	10%	20%	30%	40%	50%	60%	70%	80%	90%	100%
No Relief										Complete Relief

9) Circle the one number that describes how, during the past 24 hours, pain has interfered with your:

A. General Activity

0	1	2	3	4	5	6	7	8	9	10
Does not interfere										Completely interferes

B. Mood

0	1	2	3	4	5	6	7	8	9	10
Does not interfere										Completely interferes

C. Walking ability

0	1	2	3	4	5	6	7	8	9	10
Does not interfere										Completely interferes

D. Normal work (includes both work outside the home and housework)

0	1	2	3	4	5	6	7	8	9	10
Does not interfere										Completely interferes

E. Relations with other people

0	1	2	3	4	5	6	7	8	9	10
Does not interfere										Completely interferes

F. Sleep

0	1	2	3	4	5	6	7	8	9	10
Does not interfere										Completely interferes

G. Enjoyment of life

0	1	2	3	4	5	6	7	8	9	10
Does not interfere										Completely interferes

Pain Research Group
Department of Neurology
University of Wisconsin-Madison

Figure 3.3   Brief Pain Inventory

Several other scales are used with children: the "Oucher," which shows a scale from 0 to 100 and six photographs of a four-year-old's face depicting different levels of pain; pain drawings or pain maps, where children color where they hurt (using four different colors that represent varying intensities of pain); a poker chip assessment, in which children are given four red poker chips, which represent "a piece of hurt," and are asked how many chips their pain has; a pain "thermometer"; and a list of pain words for children and teens.

While there's no "best" pain tool, any of these (or other) scales give patients and doctors a consistent way to communicate about pain on an ongoing basis. A Mexican investigator, Dr. Ricardo Plancarte, has even popularized an effective fruit scale that asks "whether your pain is more like the size of a grape or a watermelon," for use with farmers who don't read well.

Pain Word List for Children and Teenagers

Sensory Words	Sensory Words	Emotional Words
Aching	Hot	Awful
Hurting	Cramping	Deadly
Like an ache	Crushing	Dying
Like a hurt	Like a pinch	Killing
Sore	Pinching	Crying
Beating	Pressure	Frightening
Hitting	Itching	Screaming
Pounding	Like a scratch	Terrifying
Punching	Like a sting	Dizzy
Throbbing	Scratching	Sickening
Biting	Stinging	Suffocating
Cutting	Shocking	Evaluative Words
Like a pin	Shooting	Annoying
Like a sharp knife	Splitting	Bad
Pinlike	Numb	Horrible
Sharp	Stiff	Miserable
Stabbing	Swollen	Terrible
Blistering	Tight	Uncomfortable
Burning		Never goes away
		Uncontrollable

Source: Reprinted from D. Wilkie, W. Holzemer, M. Tesler, et al., "Measuring pain quality: validity and reliability of children's and adolescent's pain language," *Pain* 41 (1990): 151. Reprinted with permission of Elsevier Science and authors.

What to Tell a Doctor about Pain

Here are some questions that can help you identify what to tell the doctor about the pain:

- Where is the pain? Is it in a single spot or more than one place? Which is the worst pain?
- Does the pain ever radiate—shoot or travel—from one location to another? Are there any secondary pains?
- Did the pain predate the cancer? Is it chronic pain, like arthritis or migraine pain? If a new pain, is it like pain that you've had before?
- Is the pain constant (uninterrupted and always present)? Intermittent (comes and goes)? Or constant (perhaps at a low level) but punctuated with periods of severe pain, especially with movement or activity (which is the most common mode of all)?
- How severe is each pain on average? How severe is it when it subsides (least pain experienced)? How severe is it at its worst? Try using a 0-to-10 scale; 0 means no pain, and 10 is the worst pain imaginable.
- What kind of pain is it? What words best describe it (*burning, aching, stabbing, piercing,* etc.)?
- When does each pain start (during the night, when getting out of bed, etc.)? How long does it last? Are there any patterns to it?
- What tends to aggravate the pain—for example, what movement or position?
- What helps relieve it? Do heat, cold, massage, distraction, position, activities, or medications have any effect?
- How does the pain affect activities, energy level, appetite, sexual habits, movement, posture, mood, and sleep?
- Are there any other changes associated with the pain? Is there numbness or weakness?
- Is there leakage of urine or soiling of undergarments?
- Is the skin near the area ever affected—for example, are there changes in the temperature, color, or texture of the skin, and has sweating or the growth of hair or nails changed?
- Have any painkillers ever been used in the past? Were any of them particularly effective or ineffective? How long were they effective? Were there side effects? Are any being used now? What other medications are being taken?
- What would the patient do differently if the pain didn't exist? What new activities would the patient engage in?

Keeping a Pain Diary

A pain log not only helps doctors diagnose a pain problem but also helps measure progress. After only a few days' entries, a pattern may emerge, such as the pain occurring at a particular time of day or after a particular activity. By using a numeric scale (0 to 10, with 0 being no pain and 10 the most severe pain imaginable) to measure and record the pain day by day, or by using one of the other assessment tools regularly, you can help the doctor know whether to increase, decrease, or change medications. Also, your confidence and self-esteem may increase as you see how the pain diminishes.

Caregivers also find it useful to log medication use, doctors' visits, toilet habits (for example, last bowel movement), and other problems.

Keeping a journal to record thoughts and feelings also can be helpful, especially for patients and family members who find it hard to express themselves aloud. Life-threatening illnesses are passages in people's lives, both for the patient and for the caregiver; an openness to the experience and the expression of feelings can help launch gratifying communication with others.

Daily Pain Diary							
Date	Pain level 0–10 (mild, moderate, severe)	Activity that triggered pain	Medication taken and dose	Other pain relief methods used	Pain level 0–10 (mild, moderate, severe) after medication	Side effects experienced	Other comments (other symptoms, moods,problems)
Midnight							
1 a.m.							
3 a.m.							
5 a.m.							
7 a.m.							
9 a.m.							
11 a.m.							
Noon							
1 p.m.							
3 p.m.							
5 p.m.							
7 p.m.							
9 p.m.							
11 p.m.							

Convey All Symptoms

Cancer has been called a multisymptomatic disease, which means that it can affect different patients in many different ways, often at once. Here is a list of some of the symptoms people with cancer describe; each is important for the doctor to know about.

Symptoms That Cancer Patients May Experience

Systemwide Symptoms
Loss of appetite (anorexia)
Weight loss (cachexia)
Tiredness/weakness
  (fatigue, lassitude)
Loss of strength Weakness
  (asthenia)
Difficulty initiating and
  maintaining sleep
  (insomnia)

Neurological Problems
Drowsiness
Confusion, disorientation
Hallucinations
Headache
Muscle weakness
Altered sensations (numb-
  ness, tingling, etc.)

Respiratory Problems
Difficulty breathing (dyspnea)
Shallow, rapid breathing
  (tachypnea)
Irregular breathing with breath-
  holding (periodic apnea)
Cough
Hiccoughs (singultus)

Gastrointestinal Problems
Difficulty in swallowing
  (dysphagia)
Nausea
Vomiting
Dehydration
Constipation
Diarrhea
Leakage of stool (inconti-
  nence)
Sensation of the frequent,
  usually unsuccessful
  need to pass stool,
  accompanied by pain,
  cramping, and straining
  (rectal tenesmus)

Psychological Problems
Irritability
Anxiety
Panic
Depression
Dementia

Urinary Problems
Inability to control urination (inconti-
  nence)
Painful urination (dysuria)
Bladder spasms (tenesmus)
Difficulty urinating (hesitancy,
  frequency, urgency, etc.)

Other Bedsores; dry, sore mouth

Symptoms to Report to Your Doctor, Especially If Onset Is Sudden or Rapid

Knowing the condition of the patient includes taking into account the whole person—the well-being of the body, mind, and spirit. This kind of approach helps the doctor determine just what is going on so he can begin to sort out what problems are caused by the cancer, the cancer treatment, or medications. Painkillers sometimes produce side effects, which can prevent doctors from prescribing high enough doses. If kept informed of symptoms, however, the doctor can usually help reverse or prevent them, so higher doses of a painkiller may be prescribed when necessary.

People often just endure the side effects of medications, thinking incorrectly that they must. For example, constipation almost always occurs with painkillers, and nausea is common with chemotherapy. By simply adding a laxative when an opioid is prescribed and an antinausea medication during chemotherapy, the patient can easily achieve the relief he craves and needs. Even fatigue, weight loss, and sedation can be made more manageable with currently available products and methods.

Inform the Doctor and Other Staff Immediately
If Any of These Symptoms Suddenly Occurs for the First Time

Hallucinations
Severe confusion or disorientation
Severe trembling, uncontrolled muscle movements, convulsions, seizures
Numbness, tingling, or weakness in feet, legs, or trunk, with or without incontinence
Sudden breathlessness or painful breathing or coughing
Inability to urinate (retention) or to control urination (incontinence)
Inability to control stool (fecal incontinence) or no bowel movement for several days
Unrelieved nausea, vomiting, or diarrhea
Any combination of hives, itching, skin rash, wheezing, or facial swelling

---

Be Prepared for Psychological Questions

As discussed in Chapter 2, suffering is more than physical discomfort and usually involves psychological issues such as moodiness, anxiety over family and financial burdens, and fears about illness, pain, disfigurement, loss of mental and physical control, and death. To treat pain comprehensively, doctors need to address psychological concerns, even though these matters may seem unimportant, too personal, or beyond help (denial). Patients shouldn't be surprised or offended if asked about personal and cognitive styles (how the patient explains the world to himself), coping mechanisms, depression and anxiety, whether these feelings preceded the illness (preexisting) or were brought on by the illness (secondary or reactive), a history of excessive concerns about health and illness (hypochondria), a preoccupation with one's looks and attractiveness (body image), and so forth. Doctors also need to be informed of any history of drug or alcohol use because patients with such histories may tolerate or respond to analgesics and other drugs differently than others.

The Goals of Pain Treatment

The overall goal of any pain management plan is to enhance quality of life, improve the patient's ability to maintain or resume normal activities, and allow the patient to focus on the things in life that give it meaning. The priorities usually are:

1. *To provide a good night's sleep.* Plenty of pain-free sleep at night is important because when sleep is abnormal we become less tolerant to pain. Also, if you don't sleep well at night, you will nap often during the day, which makes it harder to sleep the next night. Medication may be needed to resume a normal circadian (rhythmic) sleep-wake cycle, but it must be complemented with efforts to reduce daytime naps. Discuss these issues with your doctor, since fighting cancer, especially in the elderly, is hard work, and some daytime rest may still be advisable.

2. *To relieve pain while resting.* The next step is to ease pain during wakeful rest, which usually requires long-acting medications prescribed around the clock (discussed later in this chapter).

3. *To relieve pain triggered by movement.* The next, and sometimes most difficult, goal to achieve is to relieve pain that is triggered by specific activities, such as getting out of bed, turning over, bathing, and so on. Referred to as breakthrough pain, incident pain, or pain on movement, this type of pain is usually best managed with prescribed doses of a relatively rapid-onset, short-acting medication with or before the pain-provoking activity (called a rescue dose or escape dose—see below).

These priorities are usually addressed in this order, with getting a good night's sleep being paramount. Once that is accomplished, the doctor will then attempt to relieve the pain that persists during rest and finally that which accompanies movement.

Drug Therapy: The Cornerstone of Pain Treatment

Pain medications are used commonly for acute or chronic pain for patients of all ages, including infants and the elderly, and will relieve pain in about 90 percent of cases. The World Health Organization (WHO) began a revolution in cancer pain therapies with its recommended "ladder" of medications for the appropriate sequence of therapies. It suggests that doctors treat mild cancer pain with mild painkillers and progress to more potent ones as needed, adding supplemental medications that can enhance pain relief or relieve medication-related side effects as necessary.

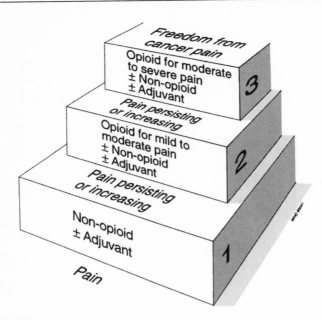

Figure 3.4   The WHO's basic pain strategy, called the "analgesic ladder," is now used worldwide to treat cancer pain.

Source: Reprinted with permission of the World Health Organization.

The Basic Pain Strategy: The Painkiller Ladder

The WHO's basic pain strategy, now used worldwide to treat cancer pain, suggests the following steps:

Step 1: Nonsteroidal Anti-inflammatory Drugs (NSAIDs)

These drugs, useful for mild to moderate pain, include aspirin, acetaminophen (Tylenol, etc.), and ibuprofen (Advil, Motrin, Rufen, Nuprin, Medipren, among others). In fact, there are almost twenty different NSAIDs.

Until recently, the various NSAIDs did not differ greatly from each other, and while most still don't, a doctor may suggest trying different types (medication rotation), because one may work better or be better tolerated in one person than another. Unfortunately, there's no way to know in advance which will be better for a particular person until they are tried, a process of educated trial and error with careful observation.

New specialized NSAIDs, dubbed by the media as the "superaspirins," include agents such as rofecoxib (Vioxx) and celocoxib (Celebrex); they are technically called COX-2 inhibitors (see Chapter 5) because they work preferentially on one of two enzymes involved in the mechanisms associated with pain. While they are not necessarily more effective for pain, they are somewhat less likely to cause complications such as ulcers and bleeding, which is particularly important to the elderly or those with a history of alcohol abuse or liver and kidney problems. However, insurers often insist that doctors fill out time-consuming forms justifying their use because of their dramatic additional expense.

Surprisingly, when taken in the right dose (not too high or too low) at the right time (around the clock, as directed), the NSAIDs are often quite effective for even severe pain—especially pain that stems from bone tumors, bone metastases, and local inflammation (tissue irritation).

Often, an adjuvant medication (a complementary or helper medication), such as certain antidepressants, anticonvulsants, and muscle relaxants, may enhance the effects of the more traditional painkillers. Medications to prevent nausea or constipation may also be prescribed.

When taken on schedule continuously, relief is quick, often within twenty-four hours. If there is no noticeable benefit within forty-eight hours, or if side effects such as stomach problems, blood-thinning effects (bruising, bleeding), or drowsiness occur, the doctor should be informed so that an escalation of the pain treatment strategy to the next logical step can be planned.

Even when they aren't strong enough to eliminate the pain, as long as pain is reduced and there are no serious side effects, NSAIDs should probably still be taken, but usually in combination with a stronger (opioid) medication. Since the two relieve pain by different mechanisms, taken together they can produce an additive or synergistic benefit, so that less opioid medication is ultimately needed.

Step 2: Opioids Conventionally Used to Treat Moderate Pain: Mild or Weak Opioids

Codeine (usually prescribed as Tylenol #3) is the prototype and most familiar of these drugs, with propoxyphene (the active component of Darvon and Darvocet) the most common alternative. Despite the historical popularity of these agents, today other so-called weak opioids are usually preferred, including hydrocodone (Vicodin, Lortab, Norco, etc.), dihydrocodeine (Synalgos DC), tramadol (Ultram), and oxycodone (Percodan, Percocet, Roxicodone, OxyFast, OxyIR). Most of the weak opioids come combined obligatorily with aspirin or acetaminophen. This limits how much can be taken (usually two tablets every three to six hours)—not because of the narcotic, but because too much aspirin or acetaminophen can cause serious health problems.

Actually, the distinction between weak and strong opioids has little scientific basis, since higher doses of the so-called weak agents produce effects similar to those of lower doses of strong agents. The distinction is more cultural in nature, resulting from our drug-phobic society and its excessive concern about prescribing morphine and other potent opioids. These agents are really only considered "weak" because safe doses are limited by the need to avoid a buildup of acetaminophen and aspirin. While these agents have a definite role for mild and moderate pain, a doctor's preference for prescribing weaker drugs (and patients' reluctance to advance to stronger ones) can sometimes cloud decisions about which alternative would be the most effective and safe. It is usually wiser to rely more on products with a higher proportion of hydrocodone (instead of a higher proportion of acetaminophen) because it is safer and allows for more flexibility in increasing doses, yet this practice is still unfortunately often ignored.

One of the most common errors made by well-meaning physicians who still harbor exaggerated concerns about the risks of addiction is to maintain patients on these weaker opioid medications, often in spiraling doses, when a stronger one would better relieve the pain and—because excessive acetaminophen and aspirin are avoided—may actually be less risky.

Again, at this step, adding an adjuvant medication (most commonly antidepressants, anticonvulsants, and sometimes steroids) can improve pain relief without increasing the opioid dose and, as a result, limits the risks of potential opioid side effects such as nausea, sleepiness, itchiness, and constipation. When pain remains inadequately quelled at maximum recommended doses and, despite dose increases, pain persists for more than twenty-four to forty-eight hours, the next step on the ladder should be considered. See Chapter 6.

Step 3: Opioids for Severe Pain: Strong Opioids

Despite many new alternative opioids, morphine is still usually the drug of first choice and is most commonly recommended for severe pain, not only because of years of experience using it, but also because it is available in a wide variety of dose formulations and can be administered in a variety of ways, including intravenous, subcutaneous, intramuscular, and spinal injections; rectal suppositories; immediate-release and controlled-release pills and capsules; and so on. Nevertheless, as with all opioids, some patients have problems with morphine (there is no best drug for everyone), such as persistent nausea, drowsiness, or dysphoria (feeling strange or unpleasant). While the fear of taking morphine is not a sufficient reason to reject its use out of hand, if true problems occur, doctors will suggest one of several strategies. Since side effects, especially nausea and grogginess, are common but usually short-lived whenever *any* opioid is first started, the preferred approach to mild side effects is usually to stick with regular administration. This gives the body a chance to become accustomed and immune to these effects, although an antinausea medication may be recommended for a few days, to allow tolerance to develop. A common physician error, however, is to continue the regular use of antinausea medications beyond a few days even though nausea usually resolves spontaneously.

Also, the drowsiness that occurs is often catch-up sleep, because the pain is finally relieved after having disrupted sleep for a long period. If troublesome side effects persist, other similar opioid drugs can be substituted. A small proportion of patients (especially the elderly and those with kidney problems) are predisposed to the buildup of morphine metabolites; while not dangerous, this may explain grogginess or nausea that doesn't easily wear off. When side effects are not excessive but pain relief is inadequate at a given dose, more morphine (or a similar opioid) is prescribed, a safe and effective practice, since there is no maximum dose for the strong opioids. See Chapter 7.

Again, the adjuvant analgesics as well as an NSAID can continue to be useful at this step because they can enhance pain relief without increasing opioid doses. Similarly, some adjuvant drugs can help reduce anxiety or side effects. See Chapter 8.

Step 4: Surgical and Other Anesthetic Measures

Despite good pain control when the ladder approach is applied thoughtfully, some 10 to 20 percent of patients will benefit from additional, more aggressive pain control techniques at some stage of their treatment.

Although the WHO ladder addresses only medication-based approaches, more aggressive treatments are now available and included in guidelines formulated by the American Society of Anesthesiologists and the U.S. government's Agency for Health Care Policy and Research as additional steps.

Usually administered by trained pain specialists, anesthesiologists, or neurosurgeons, these more aggressive procedures include specialized injections, finely tuned removal of nerves, and more complex surgical therapies that are discussed in detail in Chapter 9.

During Steps 1 to 4: Supplemental Measures Used
Throughout Pain Treatment

Many techniques, from relaxation and cognitive skills to new forms of transcutaneous electrical nerve stimulation (TENS), as well as psychological, behavioral, and cognitive therapies (hypnosis, relaxation, guided imagery, traditional counseling and psychotherapy, physical therapy including the use of massage, and newer forms of bodywork such as acupuncture) can often be safely integrated with more traditional treatments. These are described further in Chapter 12 and should be discussed with the physician.

Individualizing Pain Strategies

Regardless of the prognosis for curing the cancer, the prognosis for controlling the pain is excellent. But effective pain treatment is not a hard-and-fast science that is determined in one visit to the doctor. The first prescription and dose is a test, and—depending on a patient's degree of illness, tolerance levels, and other factors—the dose may need to be increased until it relieves the pain. Sometimes just a day or two is adequate to determine whether the dose needs adjustment, but sometimes this can take a week. The first try rarely provides satisfactory pain relief with few side effects, but each change in dose or medication in the right direction is a sign of success. Even when treatment is satisfactory, adjustments are frequently needed as illness recedes or progresses, or as the patient builds a tolerance to some medications. Cancer is a dynamic disease, and its pain is like a moving target, making treatment, like so many things in life, a work in progress. The road to good pain control usually has a few detours or bumps, maybe even a few dead ends. Don't become discouraged.

When a New Drug Is Started

- Expect some trial and error.
- Ask when you will start feeling the drug's effect.
- Ask if the dose can be varied (raised, lowered, taken more or less frequently) without contacting the medical team. If so, how much can it be changed, and how often?
- Ask what kind of side effects might be expected. If unwanted symptoms occur, can the doses be tapered without calling the medical team? If so, by how much?
- Ask if cold medications or over-the-counter analgesics, such as those used for headache, may be taken. Many contain aspirin, which should be avoided by patients on chemotherapy, and many others contain high doses of acetaminophen, which may not be appropriate. Allergy medications may induce drowsiness and could compound the sedative effects of narcotics.
- Tell the doctor if any herbal therapies are being used, since the effects and interactions of some supplements can be unpredictable.
- Call if the pain is not relieved adequately in a reasonable time.
- Call if any side effects can't be tolerated or persist.

Remember: Treatment can always be adjusted or modified.

If a drug therapy does not seem to work or causes persistent or serious side effects, no one is to blame, and the failure of one drug is no indication that another won't work or even that the same medication won't work well at another time, combined with others, or taken in another way. For example, often a medication will unexpectedly produce a side effect, but the same drug can be safely restarted at another time in a lower (less effective) dose and, surprisingly, can then be gradually raised to the previously problematic dose with excellent results and few, if any, side effects.

Allergies versus Side Effects

Side effects of a medication, such as nausea, vomiting, or itchiness, are quite common but often confused with an allergic reaction. Side effects can make a patient miserable, but they are usually not dangerous or life-threatening and can minimized by changing the dose, means of administration, or other factors. An allergy, however, is a whole-body hypersensitivity response that invokes specific immune responses and can range from annoying to a medical emergency. An anaphylactic reaction can cause wheezing and difficulty breathing, hives, swelling, low blood pressure, and even shock. Though such a reaction is potentially life-threatening, epinephrine and other life-support measures are usually effective. Medication-related side effects, however, are self-limiting and do not respond to epinephrine. True allergies to opioid medications are extraordinarily rare.

"Shotgun" versus "Sniper" Approach

Pain therapies have to be adjusted on a regular basis, and, depending on the nature of the pain and how distressed the patient is, the doctor may make one change in treatment or a number of changes at once. The latter usually results in quicker improvement but makes it more difficult to assess what worked and what didn't. Occasionally, a short hospitalization is warranted to get pain and other symptoms under better control. When multiple changes are recommended, make sure each step and its rationale are clearly outlined.

Use a Problem-Solving Approach

As soon as pain relief wanes or side effects cannot be controlled effectively, the team should be contacted to raise the dose (if pain is the problem, this is usually the preferred and first route), add an adjuvant medication (to treat side effects or to reduce the dose of painkiller, which should reduce side effects), or switch medications. Thus, using a pain diary to monitor changes as they occur is critically important.

Informing the Medical Team

Inform the medical team about any and all changes in your condition—physical, psychological, emotional—and be sure they are treated (e.g., nausea, constipation, dry mouth, etc.). Insomnia should be treated most vigorously!

Discuss Alcohol

Even if it's minor, ask the doctor (in private, if you are the caregiver and if it's necessary) about the health effects of the patient's use of alcohol and other drugs. Although an occasional drink is usually okay and perhaps even therapeutically relaxing once medication is stabilized, alcohol in combination with a narcotic can be dangerous. Intoxication under any circumstances, however, is not only unsafe but may give the doctor cause not to treat the pain as aggressively with narcotic medications. Be sure to discuss these issues with the doctor, no matter how embarrassing

Tell the Patient Everything

Sometimes family members and other caregivers don't know whether to tell the patient everything about his condition and treatment. Realize, however, that it is the patient's right to know everything. Communicate all decisions to the patient, whether or not you think the patient understands or cares.

Try Medications by Mouth First

At first, drugs should be administered by mouth or with a skin patch to preserve the patient's mobility, independence, sense of control, and self-esteem. Only when mouth sores develop or swallowing becomes difficult should other means be explored.

Be Prepared for Higher Doses of Opioids

It is standard and normal to increase opioid doses as time passes. "Recommended" or "maximum" doses listed in textbooks were not intended for cancer pain; these doses are often useful starting points, but more medication will usually be required over time. With no single right dose for many analgesics, the appropriate dose will vary from patient to patient and over time. Once a drug, or combination of drugs, is prescribed, if it is not relieving the pain, its dose should first be increased under a doctor's supervision until a ceiling dose is reached (which will not occur with the opioids) or until side effects are unmanageable or unacceptable. The ceiling dose is a level above which increases in the medication no longer provide added pain relief but only increase side effects or toxicity. Since opioids

How Pain Medications Are Administered

Route	Medical Abbreviation
By mouth	PO
Liquid, pill, capsule, caplet	
Lollipop (lozenge, oralette)	
Rectal suppositories	PR
Skin patch (transdermal)	TTS
Injections	
Intravenous	IV
Patient-controlled analgesia	PCA
Intramuscular	IM
Subcutaneous (under the skin)	sub q, subcu, SC, SQ
Under the tongue (lozenges)	SL
Through the nose (nasal sprays)	IN
Epidural, spinal	
High-tech options (nerve blocks, implanted pump, etc.)	
These methods are detailed in Chapter 9.	

usually have no ceiling, the dose can always be raised to reestablish effectiveness. If a new medication is needed, the patient should then be switched to a stronger or more suitable medication.

Expect Treatment with Multiple Drugs

Expect several drugs for pain to be prescribed; ask if they are not. (See Chapter 8.) A laxative should be prescribed as soon as opioid therapy begins. Ask if it is not offered.

Antinausea medications (antiemetics) are needed in up to 40 percent of cancer patients, at least for a time. Anticipate their need and have nausea treated as soon as possible, should it develop. Also, as discussed, adjuvant drugs may be prescribed.

Frustration and Problems

Although not all doctors have the background, interest, or temperament to treat pain carefully, a knowledgeable doctor from any specialty can help up to 90 percent of patients achieve good control of pain. But even with a well-informed doctor, the process can be time-consuming and frustrating for everyone involved. The key to success is to accept up front that doctors rarely will get it all right the first time, usually through no fault of their own. Continue to work with the health care team until you are satisfied.

Consider whether it makes sense to ask the doctor about consulting a pain specialist or a local or regional pain clinic. (See Appendix 1 for where to find pain specialists.)

As-Needed versus Around-the-Clock Prescriptions

Many studies show that far too often doctors prescribe doses of painkill-ers that are both too low and administered too infrequently. To compound the problem, nurses may then reduce the already deficient doses that have been prescribed. These doctors and nurses are not heartless (far from it) but are usually responding to antiquated concerns about addiction and insufficient teaching in medical and nursing schools.

As-Needed Prescriptions: A Questionable Approach to Cancer Treatment

Although still an effective way to control some kinds of pain, prescribing pain medication for cancer patients on an as-needed basis (abbreviated PRN) is no longer regarded as appropriate in most cases. By the time a cancer patient needs the medication, pain has spiked inappropriately high. Patients who try to tough it out, thinking that they should be stoic or that delaying their medication will help them somehow (such as by prevent-ing addiction), could actually make matters worse.

When a patient is hospitalized, an as-needed order can unnecessarily trigger a confrontation between the patient and nurses who incorrectly ex-pect a dose to last four to six hours. Yet patients often experience the return of pain earlier than expected and may be in agony, pleading for the next dose or suffering in unnecessary silence. Because of exaggerated fears of addiction, a well-intentioned but ill-informed nurse may postpone the next dose of pain-killer as long as possible. By the time the pain is finally treated, it may be so severe that a much larger dose is needed to relieve it, which also boosts the chances of triggering a side effect, such as nausea or mental confusion.

Also, the as-needed method requires patients to wait for the pain to return before they can request additional medication. Since doses are of-ten too low or too widely separated, patients may become preoccupied with their pain, becoming "clock watchers," anxious and fearful that the pain will return before the next dose is allowed.

It is ironic that this clock watching, brought about by undertreatment and as-needed dosing, is often interpreted as addictive behavior. The ap-pearance of the very problem we are trying to avoid (addiction) seems to be triggered by undertreating, not overtreating, the pain. Actually, when undertreated cancer patients seek additional medication, it is not addic-tion but a manifestation of pseudoaddiction, a problem that is caused by the treatment (or undertreatment) itself. These unfortunate individuals are actually seeking relief from pain, not more medication, and will usu-ally stop taking pain medications altogether when their pain resolves.

Prolonged as-needed treatment is like a bad roller coaster ride—the patient's level of comfort is always changing, as periods of relief occur, but often with side effects, and the pain always returns. Even after more effective therapy is started, patients may maintain an anticipation and memory of pain that remain very hard to shake.

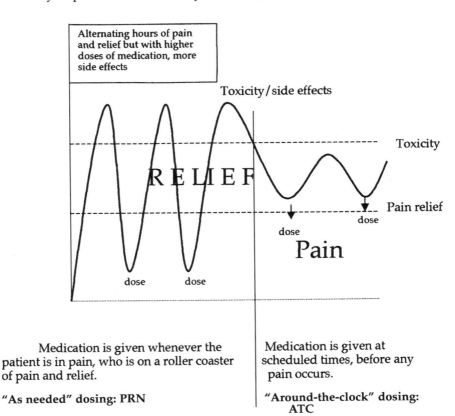

Medication is given whenever the patient is in pain, who is on a roller coaster of pain and relief.

"As needed" dosing: PRN

Medication is given at scheduled times, before any pain occurs.

"Around-the-clock" dosing: ATC

Figure 3.5   "As needed" and "Around-the-clock" Dosing

Around-the-Clock Prescriptions: The Approach of Choice for Cancer Patients

Most often, pain from cancer is relatively constant. It is therefore logical that around-the-clock pain is best treated with around-the-clock dosing of a long-acting medication, often supplemented with a short-acting drug if the pain breaks through. Studies show that administering pain medication at regular intervals and in sufficient doses to prevent severe pain usually results in a lower overall dose being needed, with better relief and fewer undesirable side effects.

Cancer pain specialists now recommend that adequate doses of all the analgesics—including NSAIDs and opioids—and medications for constipation, nausea, and vomiting be taken before pain and other symptoms worsen. Once pain and related symptoms are well established, medication to prevent them should be prescribed proactively around the clock.

How Drugs Are Chosen

Although cancer pain specialists typically follow the WHO analgesic ladder, at least as a guideline, which drug they prescribe on each rung of the ladder depends on the individual patient, doctor, and even community and institutional standards. This is especially true since many insurers have introduced preferred formularies—lists of drugs that, all things being equal, member doctors are encouraged to use rather than other products that are less effective or cost more. Doctors take many factors into account when selecting medications, including the patient's age, type of cancer, other medical problems, and analgesic history (what worked in the past to relieve pain, what didn't), as well as their own familiarity and experience with particular medications. No one drug on each rung of the ladder is better than another for every patient every time. What one patient tolerates well may cause side effects in another. If side effects interfere with treatment, another, equally potent medication is often prescribed. What has been ineffective or problematic in the past may be ideal at another time. And under different circumstances, medications may best be administered by another route, at a different starting dose, or combined with other medications.

Understanding Palliative Therapy

When cancer causes pain, the first thing a doctor will try to do is to eliminate or shrink a tumor as much as possible, using radiation, surgery, or chemotherapy, alone or in combination. Although the patient's comfort is important, it is considered secondary to curing the cancer, especially at the start of treatment, when chances for a cure are best. But even when a cure isn't possible, chemotherapy, radiotherapy, or surgery may be recommended to alleviate pain and other symptoms. Many cancers may be incurable, but few are untreatable.

Undertaking palliative treatment by no means implies that the patient is giving up or succumbing to the illness. Instead, it reflects a shift of the goal from cure to enhancing comfort and quality of life. There is increasing evidence that good palliative care (attention to symptoms) also often indirectly extends survival because of its beneficial effects on quality of life, functional status, and mood.

Pain is the primary focus of palliative treatments, but other symptoms such as persistent nausea, coughing, breathlessness, or painful swallowing also can be reduced by treatment. (See Chapters 10 and 11 for discussions of treatment strategies for various side effects and other symptoms.)

When considering palliative treatments, ask:

- How likely is the patient to become more active as a result of treatment?
- Have previous treatments with radiation, chemotherapy, or surgery made further treatment riskier or less likely to be effective?
- How do the probable short-term discomforts and any need for rehabilitation balance against potential long-term benefits?
- How demanding is the treatment? Is hospitalization required?
- How long will it take before results are established? (Sometimes radiation is given daily for up to a month, and another month may pass before results are fully realized.)
- What are other options?
- What is the estimated life expectancy, with and without the treatment? (This is, admittedly, a difficult question for everyone to contemplate.)

Palliative Radiation

Radiation can very effectively be used to reduce pain, especially pain that is well localized. Radiotherapy, administered by a radiation oncologist, is particularly effective for:

- Bone pain, especially when it stems from breast, lung, bladder, kidney, or prostate cancer
- Pain from a primary or secondary tumor that involves the brain or spinal cord
- The control of bleeding due to tumors
- Reducing the pain, discomfort, and odor from tumors that ulcerate the skin, such as certain breast cancers, head and neck cancers, anal cancers, and skin cancers
- Relieving difficulty in breathing (dyspnea), coughing, or chest pain due to tumors blocking the bronchial tubes, esophagus, or trachea
- Reducing the pain caused by large liver tumors

- Relieving pain from tumors pressing on nerves or growing into nerves or on the spinal cord, causing back pain, leg weakness, shooting pains, sphincter problems, or numbness
- Relieving headaches due to inoperable brain tumors that cause excessive pressure in the skull
- Shrinking tumors that are blocking hollow organs or tubes, such as the bronchial tubes, esophagus, bile ducts, ureters, lymph channels, blood vessels or gynecologic, gastrointestinal, or upper digestive tracts, or when problems arise from tumors growing in small, constricted spaces

Within the limits of safety, palliative radiation treatments are designed to be convenient and efficient for patients so that they need not spend a great deal of time and energy going to and from therapy.

Palliative Chemotherapy

Although systemic treatments with chemotherapy and hormone therapy for malignancies are commonly used in attempts to eradicate the cancer, they are often overlooked in treating cancer pain. One reason may be that doctors tend to divide cancers into "curable" and "incurable" categories and then treat the disease accordingly. Nevertheless, an incurable (though not necessarily untreatable) situation can sometimes be managed with chemotherapy. Although cases vary widely, by the time the pain of advanced disease requires an aggressive pain strategy, many oncologists shy away from chemotherapy because it can't produce a cure and can make an already sick patient even sicker. Even without a cure, palliative chemotherapy or hormonal therapy can alleviate pain, albeit slowly, from a growing tumor and sometimes can slow down disease progression. Because of its risk, cost, and usually slow effect, controlling pain with chemotherapy should be considered only in very specific situations.

Among the cancers that respond most promptly to palliative chemotherapy are:

- Small-cell lung cancer, which accounts for about one-quarter of lung cancers
- Multiple myeloma, which affects the bone marrow and surrounding tissue
- Colon cancer, the third most common cancer among adults

Hormone therapy, a type of chemotherapy, is usually well tolerated in patients with hormone-responsive tumors and can often produce excellent pain relief with few side effects. Often two or three different hormones need to be tried, especially in prostate or breast cancer, before getting the desired response. Cancers that respond particularly well to palliative hormonal therapies are:

- Breast cancers that have spread widely (metastasized) to the bone or vital organs (lungs, liver), particularly estrogen- or progesterone-receptor-positive cancers.
- Prostate cancer, the third leading cancer among men, that has spread to the bone and causes pain; surgically removing the testicles (orchiectomy) can also change hormone levels and diminish pain
- Endometrial cancer
- Cancer of the testes

These are generalizations, however, and many factors influence the choice of therapies.

CONCURRENT THERAPY

Even when trials of palliative treatment with radiation or chemotherapy are undertaken, most patients will still need treatment with medications for pain, at least until the effects of the other treatments become established.

WHEN TO START

Difficult questions arise when considering a course of chemotherapy or hormonal treatments for pain. All medical treatments have potential risks and benefits. How likely are toxic effects, how strong might they be, and how well will the patient tolerate them if they do occur? If there's only a small chance of significant improvement, devastating side effects (nausea, vomiting, fatigue) could seriously deteriorate quality of life, and sometimes even bring a risk of death. Sometimes, for example, chemotherapy can be more dangerous than the cancer itself, and risky treatment should be avoided if the only reason for pursuing it is so that the patient and family feel as though something is being done. Choosing not to pursue anticancer therapy is not the same as doing nothing; acknowledging an unwelcome reality and emphasizing symptom control can be a very courageous act that can yield important dividends. It is difficult to justify a small chance of just marginal to mild benefits against the near certainty of some toxic effects, especially when more easily reversible and adjustable treatments with pain medications may get the job done with less risk. Another consideration is that the patient's prior success in coping with chemotherapy, since the ability to cope often decreases with each successive treatment, especially when results have been disappointing in the past.

If a cancer is incurable but not actively causing problems, it may be best to reserve a systemic approach until it's needed to reduce pain and discomfort later on. This is also true when pain does become a problem and stems from a tumor that is known to respond well to chemotherapy but is localized and can be treated by radiation or even surgery. Although this may sound contradictory to earlier statements made about not putting off pain treatment, in this case we're talking about putting off chemotherapy for when it might be most effective.

A logical, stepwise approach cannot be described here because each treatment decision requires careful tailoring to each individual case; when considering palliative treatments for pain, doctors must take into account many factors.

WHEN TO STOP

Pain relief takes time to be established. Once chemotherapy is under way, however, a common pitfall is to see it through even when it is clearly not helping.

Although it is often not said out loud, chemotherapy is frequently chosen primarily for psychological reasons, so the patient and family feel that something is being done and they are not giving up. Since palliative chemotherapy may result in only a small boost in the quality or length of life, patients and families must continually assess its risks versus benefits and express concerns about whether to continue, postpone, or stop treatment. While maintaining a positive attitude remains extremely important, ethical considerations demand that truthfulness prevail. Patients often repress their awareness of harsh realities if they fear that expressing it would upset their care providers; yet, surprisingly, they may be relieved to clear the air. Even when bad news will cause distress, it is usually better addressed earlier rather than later. Understandably, devoted family members are often overprotective, but they may underestimate their loved ones' capacity to overcome hardships in even the worst circumstances. With time and a compassionate approach that still leaves some room for hope, human beings' capacity to deal with adversity is extraordinary. It is generally best to acknowledge the truth, to grieve in whatever way feels right, and together to seek the strength to persevere. Realistically hoping for the best while avoiding untruths that can come between otherwise strong partnerships is a delicate balance. Although difficult, when a complete cure is unlikely, patients should be encouraged to value the time they have and concentrate on small goals—such as uninterrupted sleep, sufficient comfort, and energy to play with grandchildren or to attend church.

Palliative Surgery

Occasionally, surgery may be the best way to relieve a particular pain or symptom, but it should be considered only if there is a reasonably good chance that it will significantly improve the patient's quality of life or allow lower doses of medication that trigger unpleasant side effects. Palliative surgery may be used to eliminate the source of symptoms (such as the removal of a breast that contains a painful lump, or removal of the ovaries or pituitary gland to prevent hormone-dependent breast or prostate cancer from getting worse) or to improve the outcome of radiation or chemotherapy by reducing the volume of malignant tissue (debulking surgery). Surgery may produce easier access for chemotherapy or radiation treatment by allowing the placement of an intravenous port through which medication may be administered without injections. Or surgery can be used to interrupt or modulate the transmission of pain impulses (such as a nerve block—see Chapter 9 for more details).

Palliative surgery is commonly considered when:

- The intestines are blocked, which interferes with eating and produces unrelenting abdominal distention, nausea, vomiting, and pain (an intestinal bypass or colostomy may relieve these symptoms when obstructions are irreversible and laxatives, analgesics, and antinausea medications have proved ineffective).

- The biliary system is blocked, preventing the flow of bile from the liver and causing abdominal pain and jaundice (yellow skin and eyes); a surgical bypass or a stent may be considered in such cases.

- The urinary system is blocked; a urinary diversion called a nephrostomy, ureterostomy, or cystostomy or a urinary stent may be recommended in these cases.

- Fluid builds up in the abdomen (ascites) or around the heart (pericardial effusion), or lung (pleural effusion); in such cases a shunt can drain the fluid.

- The veins of the circulatory system are inadequate for intravenous access; an intravenous catheter or port can be inserted into the neck or chest, or sometimes a less invasive alternative called a PIC line can be used.

- Blood flow through an artery is blocked or inadequate, or it is necessary to deliberately block blood flow to a tumor (embolization), and this results in ischemia (poor circulation), ulcers, or gangrene; an arterial graft or bypass, or even amputation, depending on the situation, may be used.

- A tumor is large, causes pain, and doesn't respond to other treatments.

- Tumor infiltration weakens bone structure, causing or predisposing the patient to a fracture; surgery using pins, cement, or a prosthesis can stabilize the bone and sometimes allow a very ill patient to walk again. Such fractures usually occur in the lower extremities, so spinal or epidural anesthesia can be used instead of general anesthesia.

- Tumors compress the spinal cord; a decompressive laminectomy may be recommended to prevent permanent paralysis.

Just because surgery can be performed, however, doesn't mean it must be. In fact, hospice patients generally do well through the end of their lives relying only on medical management, even if the conditions described above arise.

4

On Being an Active Health Care Consumer

How effectively pain is controlled depends on many factors, especially the strategy employed by the doctor and the patient's relationship with the doctor. Even an effective strategy will fall short if communication with the doctor is poor, because the patient's changing needs can't be met. This chapter will help families:

- Determine what to look for in a doctor
- Assess the doctor's attitude toward pain and pain management
- Encourage a doctor to take pain problems more seriously
- Become good consumers of health care
- Learn strategies to communicate pain problems
- Cope with doctors who are reluctant to medicate pain adequately
- Help doctors to be most effective in helping the patient

Why Is It Difficult to Discuss Pain with Doctors?

Although they may be excellent physicians, most oncologists are very busy and often preoccupied with life-and-death decisions. They also may minimize the importance and impact of a patient's pain or inaccurately judge its severity. Regrettably, in many cases how a nurse, doctor, or oncology fellow assesses a patient's pain has little relationship to the patient's self-scoring of pain intensity.

Doctors sometimes prescribe pain medication with an inappropriately low expectation for satisfactory relief and then pass those low expectations on to their patients; some overlook residual discomfort once they've prescribed a medication. Study after study has shown that far too many doctors—including the majority of oncologists—end up giving their patients far too little pain medication or are unfamiliar with proper dosing or alternatives when basic pain relief treatments don't work.

Because the body adjusts to it, chronic pain can slip by a doctor's notice if the patient doesn't speak up. Doctors easily spot acute pain because it triggers autonomic responses: the heart races (tachycardia), blood pressure goes up (hypertension), the patient sweats (diaphoresis) and may become pale, and the pupils may dilate. Chronic pain is harder to identify because the body adapts to pain over time and the autonomic responses are no longer triggered. Inexperienced doctors may say the patient doesn't look as if he is in pain.

A good doctor to turn to for pain treatment is one who:

- Does not doubt or second-guess your experience of pain
- Does not assume he is the best judge of how much you hurt
- Does not presume that he is the best judge of how much pain you should endure before he prescribes adequate medication

---

Studies show that doctors, nurses, and even spouses often underestimate the amount of pain a patient has. Without any reliable "pain detector" test available, experts insist that the patient should be the best authority, unless there is a definite reason to be concerned (recent history of alcohol or drug abuse, new confusion, etc.). If the patient is not asked, he needs to volunteer information on how much pain there is and how the medications affect him (ideally documented by a pain diary). Regardless of whether the doctor can determine the source of pain , analgesics should be started to enhance comfort and begin to empower the patient as soon as possible.

Communication with Doctors

When family members take an active role in helping the doctor and other health care professionals manage the pain of a loved one with cancer, they

Dos and Don'ts of Pain Relief	
Do	**Don't**
Assert yourself! Tell the doctor that it hurts.	Skip scheduled doses.
Expect some trial and error: call the doctor if the medication isn't effective enough or side effects are too unpleasant.	Be stoic; enduring pain does *nothing* to help your condition, yourself, or your family.
Keep calling the doctor whenever pain and side effects are not adequately addressed. Doctors expect frequent contact with pain patients.	Accept *anything* but adequate relief.
Take the medication as prescribed.	
Keep a log or pain diary.	
Ask for another doctor if your pain problems persist or are neglected.	

can be assured of the best possible quality of life for the patient, even during the worst of times. By working closely with doctors, families can avoid many of the all-too-common and unnecessary agonies of cancer, including the sinking feeling of looking back with regret that more was not done.

Families can help by being vigilant about identifying and treating pain problems aggressively. Communication with the medical team must be open and responsive to the patient's changing needs: since pain and other symptoms are often a moving target, providing relief is best regarded as a work in progress.

Communication Among Family and Friends

When a loved one is stricken with cancer and is seriously ill, a network of support is often created and a vigil is maintained. Too often supporters, who may have other obligations to balance including their own health, become exhausted. Some of this fatigue is often needless. Friends and family members may be afraid to ask for help from others, unaware that these others feel helpless, too, and given the chance would enjoy the opportunity to rally around. Overwhelmed by their own fear and needs, family members may unconsciously compete for attention, adopting the role of the martyr or vying to be seen as the "good" son, daughter, or spouse.

Even in the best of circumstances—when love is the main motivator—family members can literally make themselves sick with stress at a time when openness and a level head are most needed. How stress is handled around the patient can affect the doctors and nurses, who are stressed themselves. Families must strike a balance between advocating for their ill loved one and being mindful of the numerous concerns that may preoccupy their doctors and nurses, including other patients' illnesses; their own (often neglected) families and sensibilities; pressures to keep up with new developments, to avoid errors and lawsuits, and to cope with arcane hospital policies; interactions with other staff; mounting paperwork; long hours, and so on.

Complying with the Doctor's Recommendations

Although doctors expect patients to follow treatment recommendations and to tell the doctor what they didn't do and why, only half of patients follow their doctors' recommendations. In their sincere attempts to help patients, doctors become frustrated when patients don't comply and don't tell them. Patients need not follow blindly whatever the doctor says, but the responsible thing to do is to tell the doctor if the patient or family disagrees or finds it too difficult to comply. While it is tempting to avoid confrontation by telling the doctor what you think he wants to hear, this will ultimately interfere with treatment and establishing a trusting relationship. Doctors may find it frustrating to find out at the next appointment that a recommendation was not followed and that up to a month may have been lost. Patients and families need to speak up immediately if they do not agree with or do not understand a recommendation because then the doctor will have the opportunity to help the patient understand his choices better, or may make alternative recommendations that suit the patient better. Once home, if the doctor's recommendations can't be followed for whatever reason, inform the office so that an alternative or contingency plan can be developed.

Not complying with the doctor's instructions also can be dangerous, such as not taking a laxative regularly as prescribed, which could lead to an upsetting, even life-threatening, emergency. Although the transition from being an independent well person to being an ill patient with a shopping bag full of medications can be overwhelming, it is not an adequate excuse for not following the doctor's instructions (or informing the office if the patient can't follow them).

Try not to cancel, miss, or be late for appointments. Doctors are busier than ever today, and oncologists are often forced to squeeze in emergen-

Tip: If medication isn't taken as prescribed, be sure to inform the doctor. Often, the reason the patient doesn't take medication properly—usually because it causes a side effect—can be addressed and resolved.

cies. Try not to get frustrated if the waiting time for an appointment seems unreasonable, even if the appointment is for cancer—more than likely the doctor is treating an urgent case, and families should be able to put themselves in another's shoes and consider that if it were their emergency, they would be grateful to the doctor for giving their loved one the necessary time. If the family is very bothered by delays, it is okay to express that frustration, but realize that it may be beyond the doctor's control.

Document and keep track of all aspects of treatment. The doctor has many patients, and paperwork may fall behind. When you visit a specialist who may be unfamiliar with your records, conserve valuable time for the discussion of pressing matters and difficulties by bringing a list of your medications with you.

Determine the degree to which the doctor would like the family to stay in touch with the office between visits, and within this context keep the staff informed of the patient's progress.

Know Your Patient Rights

Having cancer or helping a loved one with cancer is extraordinarily stressful and may be coupled with anger and frustration. Times will be trying, and doctors may be rushed. Since patients and their families are eager to discuss potentially curative treatments, they need to be careful that in their efforts to be "good patients," they do not neglect to explore questions related to pain, and to advocate for aggressive pain management.

Even though most doctors are very caring people, sometimes they may just seem not to understand what the patient and family are going through. Try to help the doctor understand, but don't be too frustrated if he seems distracted. No matter how caring a doctor is, no one can really know what another is feeling. In fact, many doctors pride themselves on their "objectivity"—maintaining a distance from their patients so they can be more scientific. This style may suit some, while others may prefer a doctor with a more humanistic style who has time for an occasional hug.

Ironically, with all the information available on how to be better health care consumers, many of us fail at this most fundamental task. We often invest much more energy in buying a new car. That's because tradition-ally, the doctor-patient relationship has been paternal; patients have his-torically been expected to blindly accept the recommendations of authoritarian doctors without question. This dynamic is steadily giving way to a more equal relationship that acknowledges that despite doctors' expertise, patients' rights should be respected. Indeed, today's hospitals typically require that a patient's bill of rights be posted in prominent loca-tions such as elevators, usually in English and Spanish. Medical ethics seeks to preserve and prioritize the rights of patients in the midst of in-creasingly complex scenarios. Many states require that physicians take continuing education in ethics as a prerequisite for license renewal, and most hospitals have a medical ethics committee that establishes policy and reviews cases in which someone has voiced an ethical concern. Among the many patient rights that have been proposed are the right to fully understand treatment choices, including the potential benefits and risks of each alternative, and freedom from discrimination arising from the choice of treatments, including the option of ceasing treatment and seek-ing a second opinion.

Being a Medical Partner and Advocate

Being an active partner in health care decisions helps the patient feel he has some control over the treatment, which may diminish feelings of helpless-ness triggered by illness. Exerting control, for example, over the time of day of a radiation treatment so that it is convenient can be very important psy-chologically at a time when psychological rewards are badly needed.

Families that keep track of the many aspects of care may also partici-pate in preventing errors that can occur in even the best of systems. For example, if a doctor overlooks a previously existing ulcer and prescribes medication that may aggravate it, a family member who makes the effort to check the library's copy of the *Physician's Desk Reference*, a standard ref-erence book of medications that lists contraindications or drug warnings, can bring this to the doctor's attention. (Information on medications is also available online at sites such as www.rxlist.com.)

In addition, with health care now so decentralized, a new medication or changed dose may be communicated over the telephone but not be entered in the patient's chart. A patient or caregiver who can accurately recite the current medications and doses, rather than describing "a pink pill in the morning and a blue one at night," is invaluable during any consultation, especially in case of an emergency. Likewise, when a doctor is unavailable, patients and families can be extremely useful in briefing the doctor's substitute.

What to Expect from Doctors

In the best of all worlds, all doctors would welcome informed patients who ask good questions. Unfortunately, this is not always so. Doctors are pressed for time, and regrettably, unconsciously or not, some may come to dread the inquisitive, informed patient, simply because answering questions takes precious time.

Although it may be difficult for a patient or caregiver to take the active role endorsed here, especially if it is discouraged by the doctor and staff's behavior, strongly consider it anyway. The well-being and survival of a loved one are at stake. Moreover, when appropriate areas of concern are approached directly but with sensitivity, not only is the issue usually resolved, but the process often will favorably shape future interactions, as the patient realizes he has earned the provider's additional respect.

Doctors may also sometimes avoid difficult discussions or convey an unrealistically cheerful forecast because they are uncomfortable giving unwelcome news or may feel that patients are unprepared for such discussions. Generally, doctors like to help people and make them feel better, and thus many find it difficult to deal with the daily drama of cancer, with its difficult choices, frequent disappointments, and compromises. Doctors should, though, welcome discussions about controlling the pain and symptoms because remedies are readily available for many such complaints. Doctors are increasingly becoming better informed about cancer pain and the need to control it. Remember, though, that if you fail to bring up pain problems, there is a good chance that the doctor will not ask, and as a result, pain will not be addressed.

What to Look for in a Doctor

One of the first things a cancer patient should do is to consult an oncologist, a doctor who specializes in treating cancer, with a list of questions and concerns. To find out the doctor's attitude and aggressiveness in treating cancer pain:

- Ask about the doctor's expectations for being able to relieve pain.
- Ask about the doctor's philosophy and strategies for treating pain.
- Ask the doctor if addiction or tolerance to narcotics will be a problem. (If he says yes, chances are the doctor is not well informed about modern cancer pain treatments.)
- Express the family's attitudes and expectations about treating pain aggressively.

- Ask about the doctor's team. Is there a nurse or other professional on the team who can take the time to talk more about the family's concerns about pain management if the doctor is busy?
- In case the pain persists despite treatments, does the doctor have any advanced pain training?
- Ask whether the doctor's philosophy for treatment with pain medications endorses as-needed or around-the-clock administration. If it is as-needed, the doctor may not be well informed about modern cancer pain treatments.
- In asking about possible treatments if pain medications don't work, if the physician does not mention the more liberal use of morphine (as much as is needed to counter the pain) or recommend a pain specialist, chances are the doctor is not up to date on the latest techniques and pain relief philosophies.

Checklist for Choosing a Doctor for Pain Management

Doctors have different training, biases, and attitudes about pain and its relief. Don't accept anything but complete satisfaction with your doctor's approach to relieving pain. Patients and their families can identify whether their doctor will treat the cancer pain adequately by exploring several issues. Be particularly wary if the doctor:

- Minimizes the importance of the pain or expresses doubts about the authenticity of the patient's pain
- Has low expectations for relieving severe pain
- Primarily relies on the prescription of analgesics as needed rather than around the clock
- Appears uncomfortable with an open environment that encourages patients to ask questions and express their needs, anger, and fears
- Discourages the family from bringing or presenting a prepared list of questions
- Doesn't seem to take pain complaints seriously or with full attention or interest
- Doesn't encourage the patient or family to get back to a member of the doctor's team as soon as possible if the current prescription is ineffective
- Is overly concerned about tolerance, addiction, or physical dependence
- Doesn't reassure the patient and family that many pain treatments are available
- Is unwilling to consider consultation with a pain specialist

When the Doctor Does Not Take Pain Seriously

If you discover that the primary doctor remains excessively concerned about the side effects of an aggressive pain management strategy or has a passive or unreceptive philosophy about treating pain, you might try discussing your concerns openly with the doctor. In the course of a busy day, the physician may just not have realized that the patient wasn't getting what he needed. In the best of situations, a calm but frank conversation can prompt both improved communication and pain control.

You can also ask about a pain specialist or a pain consulting service, such as at a teaching hospital or in a hospital's anesthesiology department (see Appendix 1 for more resources on finding a pain specialist). You might say: "We have full confidence in you to supervise the cancer treatments, but we'd like to take advantage of the recent developments in cancer pain management. Not every doctor can stay abreast of every development in all cancer-related fields, such as pain and symptom control. We'd like access to state-of-the-art pain management techniques." Express your hope that including a specialist for pain management will eliminate concerns about distracting the oncologist from treating the cancer and will help preserve your relationship with the doctor.

Asking for a second opinion for pain treatment is an equally valid alternative. You might say: "I hope you don't mind our asking, but since this illness is so important to us, we want as much information as possible about different strategies for treating pain. It's not that we doubt your recommendations, but we need reassurance that this is indeed the way to go. Would you mind giving us the name of a colleague with whom we could consult for a second opinion?" Referrals can also be obtained through the National Cancer Institute (see Appendix 1).

If the doctor's answers suggest that he may not be a proponent of aggressive pain management, is defensive about the subject, or is likely to talk the family out of seeking a second opinion, consider investigating other ways to gain access to information about more aggressive pain management . (Check Appendix 1 for other resources in obtaining a referral.)

Accept Nothing Less Than Satisfactory Relief

Dealing with cancer is bad enough without the additional burden of poorly controlled pain, especially when you become aware that unrelenting pain is not necessary. Rather than passively accepting persistent pain or disturbing side effects of medication, families must learn to be as assertive as necessary and should communicate frequently with their doctors until their goals are acknowledged and begin to be met. Although most consumers will spend countless hours choosing a car, they usually ignore the importance of being a good consumer when it comes to choosing doctors and seeking second opinions. Cancer can be a life-and-death situation, and families should recognize that they choose their physicians and need not accept anything less than the best, both for treating the cancer and for relieving the pain that often accompanies it.

It is the patient's and the family's responsibility to report the pain and its response to treatment, as well as to maintain expectations for the best relief that is possible. Ultimately, consumer demand will be the most powerful factor influencing doctors to take patients' pain seriously and to treat it aggressively. The goal is an illness that is as painless as possible, and, if the time should come, a painless death. We should accept nothing less.

Part II

THE PAINKILLERS

5

Understanding Medications Used to Treat Mild Pain

For mild to moderate pain, the first step in a typical treatment plan involves the use of a nonnarcotic pain reliever, according to the World Health Organization's analgesic ladder, a strategy universally endorsed by leading cancer pain specialists. The medications that constitute the first step of the ladder are the nonsteroidal anti-inflammatory drugs (NSAIDs), of which aspirin, ibuprofen (Advil), acetaminophen (such as Tylenol and Anacin-3), and the newer COX-2 inhibitors (a special kind of NSAID) are the best-known examples. Some of these products (especially acetaminophen) actually possess only weak anti-inflammatory effects but are still usually included in this category because they are nonnarcotic (nonopioid) analgesics. These analgesics do not cause many of the side effects commonly associated with the opioid analgesics (e.g., morphine), such as nausea and drowsiness, but, like all medications, they have potential side effects, and their use needs to be reviewed by a doctor or pharmacist to ensure that it is suitable.

If the doctor prescribes a common medicine, even one that is available over the counter (that is, without a prescription), don't be concerned that he is not taking the pain seriously. When taken in the right dose at the right time and for the appropriate circumstances (described here), these medications can be surprisingly effective for even severe pain, including pain that accompanies bone metastases and brain tumors. If the NSAIDs prove ineffective in quelling pain, stronger medications should be started, which are described in the two chapters that follow this one.

How NSAIDs Work

When a traumatic mechanical or chemical event injures body tissue, a substance called arachidonic acid is released from the injured cell walls and broken down into chemicals called prostaglandins (PGs), which help transmit pain and help regulate other essential activities, such as blood flow, sleep, and inflammation. This reaction—the production of prostaglandins (PG)—is governed by cyclooxygenase or COX enzymes (enzymes are chemicals that are necessary for a chemical reaction to take place).

NSAIDs, which relieve pain primarily by exerting actions in the body's peripheral tissues rather than by acting in the brain or central nervous system (as opioids do), work by blocking the COX enzymes (of which there are at least two types, COX-1 and COX-2), thereby disrupting PG production. The same process of arachidonic acid breakdown and PG formation regulates not just pain but also inflammation, which governs the sensitivity of pain receptors and is the same process that causes redness, local heat, swelling, and more pain. Thus NSAIDs help reduce not only pain but also inflammation.

Why NSAIDs Cause Gastrointestinal Distress

As noted, PG activity is by no means limited to regulating pain. Because PGs are involved in helping to regulate nearly every body function, reducing PG levels by taking NSAIDs exerts effects elsewhere as well. Whether an NSAID acts predominantly on one or the other COX enzyme is extremely important. For example, when PG production is reduced in the gastrointestinal (GI) tract (which is governed by the COX-1 enzyme), it can cause nausea, vomiting, diarrhea, and even ulcers, which, if they bleed or perforate, can be life-threatening. The older NSAIDs, such as ibuprofen, naproxen, and most others (with the exception of the newer COX-2 inhibitors, discussed below), interfere with *both* the COX-1 and COX-2 enzymes, thereby blocking the production of all prostaglandins, including those responsible for protecting the stomach, which is why taking the older NSAIDs increases the risk of gastrointestinal bleeding.

Unpleasant GI side effects occur in about 60 percent of patients taking NSAIDs and in 10 percent of patients are severe enough to warrant discontinuation. Patients taking NSAIDs are three to ten times more likely to develop ulcers, as well as ulcer complications (bleeding, perforation, and death). In fact, recent reports warn of potentially fatal gastrointestinal effects of aspirin and most other NSAIDs, as well as the risk of fatal liver failure from combining social drinking with even occasional acetaminophen use; these complications can occur with no warning. Indeed, experts estimate that about 16,500 deaths occur annually in the United States alone from ulcer-related complications associated with the use of these products. This very sobering data suggests that we should regard instructions related to the use of NSAIDs, even those available without a prescription, very seriously.

Why Newer NSAIDs May Not Cause As Much GI Distress

The newer, more specific NSAIDs (the COX-2 inhibitors or "super-aspirins"), which include Celebrex, Vioxx, and an even newer one, Mobic, appear to have a much smaller risk of producing serious GI problems. That's because they inhibit just the COX-2 enzyme, which is involved in inflammation, and have little or no effect on COX-1, the enzyme that influences gastrointestinal tract function.

Remember, though, these are very new drugs whose story is still unfolding. For example, even though the risk of serious GI-related events, such as perforated and bleeding ulcers, is reduced (not eliminated) with the COX-2-specific NSAIDs, the frequency of side effects from similar doses of both classes of drugs may still be similar. Also, COX-2-specific NSAIDs, while probably less damaging to the GI tract (especially in vulnerable patients), have recently been implicated in causing kidney problems and probably should be avoided in patients prone to them. Also, since the discovery of the importance of the COX-1 and COX-2 subenzymes is still new, experts don't know how much each contributes to pain relief, and it is not yet clear whether the newer NSAIDs, even if safer in some patients, will prove as effective as older NSAIDs. Also important is the fact that the newer, more selective NSAIDs may not provide the same heart-protective benefits as older drugs such as aspirin have been found to, at least in men.

But the COX-2 inhibitors, which are significantly more expensive, are rapidly replacing the older NSAIDs, and since cancer patients tend to be prone to side effects, they are a good choice, especially when their cost is covered by insurance. In the current cost-conscious environment, many insurers require that doctors justify their added cost by writing a special letter indicating that a particular patient is at high risk for an NSAID side effect—for example, because of a history of ulcer disease or gastroesophageal reflux disease (GERD).

Using NSAIDs with Opioids

While doses of opioids can be increased to very high (theoretically unlimited) levels if needed, NSAIDs have a ceiling dose beyond which there is no additional pain relief, only increased side effects. Although each NSAID is associated with a usual ceiling dose, there is still some variation among individuals, even for the same drug. As a result, the doctor may recommend a moderate increase in the initial dose of an NSAID, hoping for a corresponding improvement in comfort. Moreover, the side effect profile of the NSAIDs is very different from that of opioids. While opioids commonly cause constipation, nausea, drowsiness, and itchiness, the NSAIDs commonly cause GI problems (a risk that appears reduced though not absent with the newer COX-2 inhibitors), easy bruising, and bleeding.

Although NSAIDs are used frequently to soothe mild to moderate pain, they may also be very useful for more severe pain when prescribed in combination with the weak and strong opioids. The combination of an NSAID with an opioid provides an additive pain-relieving effect because, as we've seen, NSAIDs and opioids relieve pain through different mechanisms. By prescribing a nonopioid with a weak or strong opioid, the pain is attacked on two fronts—one cutting pain off on the peripheral level (in the tissue) and the other intercepting the pain message en route to the central nervous system (brain and spinal cord).

Such combinations are also used because the NSAIDs allow lower levels of opioids to be taken, which reduces the risk of side effects.

Although able to relieve many types of pain, the NSAIDs are particularly effective for bone pain and the pain resulting from inflammation; in addition, they help reduce stiffness, swelling, and tenderness.

General Dose Guidelines

Typically, doses should be started low and increased gradually every few days up to the usual ceiling dose. If a higher dose produces more pain relief, the ceiling dose has probably not been reached and the doctor is likely to continue increases until no further added effect is noted. To be sure that the ceiling dose is not exceeded, the dose may then be lowered to the previous level.

At higher doses, toxic effects of the NSAIDs are more common, so experts recommend avoiding doses totaling more than two times the standard dose. The goal of NSAID therapy is to find the lowest dose possible to achieve the greatest degree of relief. If you find relief with one of these drugs and stay on a higher-than-standard dose consistently, monthly or bimonthly tests of the stool, urine, and blood are recommended to identify potential GI, kidney, liver, or bone marrow problems.

Most people don't realize that NSAIDs possess more than one beneficial effect. In addition to their analgesic (painkilling) effects, they also reduce inflammation, which affects pain, but indirectly. Although simple pain relief may occur after just a few doses, up to two weeks may elapse before their full anti-inflammatory effects are realized. If pain is mild to moderate, be patient with a doctor's request to continue an NSAID, even if relief is uncertain. After a week or two, if there are no side effects, an ineffective dose can be boosted, or another NSAID can be substituted since patients' response to different NSAIDs often varies.

However, if pain is severe, ask about stronger medication (an opioid) rather than continuing ineffective therapy without complaint. Contemporary guidelines for treating severe pain recommend avoiding long intervals of frustration associated with lingering too long on each step of the analgesic ladder while progressing from NSAIDs to stronger opioids. Again, be sure to take the NSAIDs at scheduled, regular intervals—around the clock. Even over-the-counter medications taken on a regular basis can be powerful pain relievers, especially when their dose is adjusted to mimic the effects of physician-prescribed preparations. In fact, studies of cancer pain, as well as pain after surgery, childbirth, and oral surgery, have found that aspirin is just as effective as the weak opioids, such as codeine (discussed in the next chapter). And when used with weak opioids, NSAIDs are particularly useful.

Tip: Taking NSAIDs in scheduled, around-the-clock doses, without skipping any doses, makes these medication very effective pain relievers. Favorable results can be established in just a few days.

A few general precautions: For the elderly, those with impaired kidney or liver function, and those taking certain other medications, NSAIDs may have more side effects and so should be used cautiously, often at lower starting doses, or not at all. Also, these substances tend to mask fever, a problem that can be particularly important for patients who are actively taking chemotherapy or who have low white blood cell counts.

To be on the safe side, take all of these medications with a full glass of water and after food (if even only a cracker) to minimize gastrointestinal irritation. Do not take over-the-counter medications with aspirin in them in addition to these NSAIDs without the doctor's approval. In most cases, patients may continue to take a daily half tablet of aspirin for heart disease protection if recommended by their physician.

When Alternative NSAIDs Should Be Considered

In general, NSAIDs have very similar pain-relieving effects. Which drug is chosen will depend on:

- *The patient's prior history or experience with specific drugs.* For example, whatever might have worked well with no side effects for a sprained ankle a few years ago will probably be a good choice and should be mentioned to the doctor.
- *Whether the patient is particularly vulnerable to gastrointestinal irritation, kidney, or liver problems.* Trilisate, Disalcid, or the newer COX-2 inhibitors (Vioxx, Celebrex, Mobic) are more expensive but may be gentler on the stomach than aspirin, ibuprofen, and other older NSAIDs.
- *Whether the patient has a blood clotting problem such as hemophilia, has recently had chemotherapy, or is already taking a blood thinner such as heparin or Coumadin.* Although a weak anti-inflammatory, acetaminophen is the least likely to cause problems. Trilisate does not usually thin the blood as much as other NSAIDs, and the COX-2 inhibitors have minimal effects on blood thinning.
- *The doctor's experience with the drug.* New drugs are released all the time. It is hard to keep up, so the doctor might not yet be knowledgeable about newer ones, just as younger doctors may lack experience with some older drugs of proven value. Remember, however, that newer drugs are not necessarily better. They usually cost much more than their well-established counterparts, and despite FDA approval, their use should be regarded as somewhat more risky until years of accumulated experience are assessed.
- *Scheduling considerations.* In patients who are already taking multiple medications, it can be beneficial to prescribe an NSAID that needs to be taken only once or twice a day, such as piroxicam (Feldene), nabumetone (Relafen), or oxaprozin (Daypro). They seem to work just as well.
- *Cost.* In the absence of other factors, the least expensive NSAID should usually be selected, which in most communities is ibuprofen.

Nonsteroidal Anti-Inflammatory Drugs Used in Cancer Pain

The following NSAIDs are commonly prescribed for treating cancer pain and may be used alone or in combination with a weak or strong opioid. These medications are especially useful for pain due to bone metastases

Choosing NSAIDs		
	Good Choices	*Bad Choices*
For those with GI problems, a history of ulcers or bleeding	COX-2 inhibitor (Celebrex, Vioxx) Acetaminophen Choline/magnesium trisalicylate (Trilisate) Salsalate (Disalcid) Nabumetone (Relafen) Diflunisal (Dolobid)	Suppositories of any of the NSAIDs Aspirin Indomethacin (Indocin, Indocid, Indomethine) Flurbiprofen (Ansaid) Meclofenamate (Meclomen, Meclofen, Meclodium)
For severe kidney problems	Acetaminophen Sulindac (Clinoril)	Most NSAIDs
For those taking blood-thinning medication (anticoagulants)	COX-2 inhibitor (Celebrex, Vioxx)	Aspirin Phenylbutazone (Butazolidin, Antadol, Phebuzine) Diclofenac (Voltaren) Most NSAIDs, with the exception of those noted
For those with brain tumors		Most NSAIDs
For children	Ibuprofen (Advil, Motrin, Nuprin) Naproxen (Naprosyn, Naprosine, Proxen)	Aspirin

and when pain is associated with signs of inflammation, such as redness and local swelling. These are general guidelines and are not a suitable substitute for a doctor's judgment and collaborative care.

ASPIRIN

Brand Name
Available over the counter; many brands, too numerous to mention.

Dose Range
650 mg four times a day is the standard dose, although a few studies suggest that 900 or 1,000 mg may lengthen the duration of relief or improve pain relief. If doses are 1,000 mg or higher, GI problems are common.

How Long It Takes to Reach Peak Effect
About two hours.

Equivalent Pain Relief
A standard dose of aspirin is equivalent to 2 mg of morphine when injected into muscle (that is, intramuscularly or IM). A dose of 600 mg of aspirin is about equivalent to 60 mg of codeine.

Comments
- Used as the standard against which other NSAIDs are compared. The NSAIDs constitute the first rung of the WHO ladder, and aspirin is designated as the prototype for this drug class. This is in part because the ladder is intended for worldwide use and aspirin is both widely available and inexpensive.
- Inexpensive and available over the counter (doesn't require a prescription).
- Ceiling dose reached very quickly.
- Often prescribed as a preparation that includes a fixed dose of an opioid analgesic (e.g., Percodan).
- Rectal suppositories available.
- Enteric-coated preparations (e.g., Ecotrin) available to minimize GI side effects.
- The other NSAIDs are usually better tolerated; while both may thin the blood and thus promote bleeding, these effects last just a few days with most NSAIDs, but persist for 120 days after just a few doses of aspirin.
- To minimize side effects, take with a glass of milk, after meals, or with antacids, or take the specially coated (enteric) tablets.
- Like other NSAIDs, regularly scheduled use for several days is required to evaluate maximum effectiveness.

Precautions
- Can irritate GI tract, causing bleeding and other symptoms. In fact, a single dose may double an individual's bleeding time (the time required for a bleeding wound to clot or dry up), an effect that can last up to three weeks; antacids and other prescribed medications can help prevent and reduce GI symptoms.
- Can also cause nausea, diarrhea, and generalized GI discomfort.
- Often avoided during chemotherapy and radiation because of increased risks of bleeding and infection.
- Avoid with use of steroids to prevent acid reflux, ulcers, and stomach bleeding.
- Avoid if severe kidney problems are present.

- Avoid during pregnancy.
- Ringing in the ears (tinnitus) is an early warning sign of a toxic response from too much aspirin.
- Taken with alcohol, the risks of GI bleeding increase.
- If taken with Dilantin, becomes more toxic.
- If taken with Coumadin (a blood thinner), the risk of abnormal bleeding and clotting increases.
- Aspirin-sensitive asthma can occur.

The Story of Aspirin

One of the most commonly used drugs in the world, aspirin—known as acetylsalicylic acid to chemists—is so ordinary, readily available, and inexpensive that its potential value is often underestimated. In fact, it is one of the most powerful substances in the medicine cabinet.

Aspirin has been available since just before the beginning of the twentieth century, but crude preparations made from willow bark were used by Hippocrates as early as 450 BC. Rediscovered in the mid-1700s and synthesized by the Bayer Company in Germany in the 1800s, aspirin has been gaining popularity ever since. Some 80 million tablets are taken daily in the United States alone, and worldwide, over 1,200 tons are consumed annually.

Among Its Powerful Benefits
- Reduction of fever.
- Regular low doses can reduce the risk of heart attack, at least in men.
- Relieves aches, stiffness, and inflammation.
- Regular use in low doses reduces the risk of certain kinds of strokes.

Among Its Potential Benefits
- May help prevent colon, stomach, esophageal, and rectal cancer. May help prevent migraines from recurring.
- May help prevent gallstones and cataracts.
- May even help boost immunity to infection.

COX-2 INHIBITORS

Brand Name
Celecoxib (Celebrex), rofecoxib (Vioox), meloxicam (Mobic); new preparations are under development.

Dose Range
Celebrex: 100 to 200 mg twice a day.

Vioxx: Starting dose is 12.5 mg once daily but can be increased to 50 mg daily. Use of Vioxx for more than five days has not been studied.

Mobic: Starting dose is 7.5 mg once a day but can be increased to 15 mg.

How Long It Takes to Reach Peak Effect
About an hour.

Comments
- This new class of NSAIDs is at least as effective for pain, stiffness, and inflammation as the other NSAIDs, but is associated with reduced risks of stomach upset, ulcers, and bleeding side effects.
- Even though these medications are expensive, because they have no effect on blood clotting and a minimal effect on the GI system, yet have a strong anti-inflammatory effect, they are a good choice for those prone to stomach upset or with a history of ulcer or stomach bleeding.
- Preliminary research suggests that these medications may have potential cancer-fighting properties.
- They do not need to be taken with food.
- Mobic, used for several years in several million patients in other countries, was approved in the United States in 2002. It has been shown to be associated with considerably fewer GI side effects (dyspepsia, nausea and vomiting, abdominal pain, and diarrhea) as well as GI events (ulcers, GI bleeding, and perforation) than the older, more routine non-COX-2-selective NSAIDs.

Precautions
- Although these medications have been tested extensively for arthritic pain, they have not been tested for cancer pain.
- People who are pregnant, allergic to sulfa drugs, or have a history of asthma, hives, kidney, or liver problems or other allergic-type reactions to aspirin or NSAIDs should not take Vioxx.
- Side effects include upper respiratory tract infection, diarrhea, nausea, heartburn, swelling of the lower legs or feet, and high blood pressure.
- In rare cases, stomach ulcers and other gastrointestinal problems, similar to those caused by other NSAIDs, may occur.
- Recent reports suggest that Vioxx may increase the risk of heart attack and kidney problems, but many experts are divided about the risk; more research is needed. Extra caution may be taken in the meantime for those with a history of heart disease.

CHOLINE AND MAGNESIUM TRISALICYLATE

Brand Name
Trilisate.

Dose Range
Usually 1,000 to 1,500 mg twice a day; available as a pill and as an elixir (in liquid form), especially useful if swallowing is difficult.

In children, a typical dose is 25 mg/kg twice a day (usually prescribed by child's weight).

How Long It Takes to Reach Peak Effect
One to two hours; longer when suppository.

Equivalent Pain Relief
Uncertain.

Comments
- Unique among the NSAIDs in that effects on bleeding, blood clotting, and the GI tract are minimal, yet analgesic and anti-inflammatory effects are significant—making this a particularly good choice when an NSAID is needed even though there is a history of ulcers or stomach bleeding.
- May be particularly beneficial for bone pain.

Precautions
- May cause problems in patients who have severe kidney problems or severe gastric ulcers or gastritis.

ACETAMINOPHEN (PARACETAMOL IN THE UNITED KINGDOM)

Brand Name
Tylenol, Tempra, Anacin-3, Datril, Panadol, and others.

Dose Range
Usually 650 mg is the standard dose, every four hours.

In children, a typical dose is 10 to 15 mg/kg (usually prescribed by child's weight).

Equivalent Pain Relief
The equivalent doses of morphine and codeine are about the same as those for aspirin. The standard dose of acetaminophen (650 mg) is about equivalent to 60 mg of codeine or 2 mg of morphine.

Comments
- Has proven as effective as aspirin in relieving many types of pain but is generally a safer drug, although problems still can arise when excessive doses are used and, in some circumstances, even with routine dosing.
- Does not require a prescription.
- Although usually considered along with the NSAIDs, it is not generally considered an anti-inflammatory drug because its anti-inflammatory effects are very weak. However, new animal data suggest that its anti-inflammatory action may be stronger than previously thought.

- Does not cause typical NSAID-related GI problems, such as bleeding, ulcers, cramping, diarrhea, thinning of blood, or asthma.
- Rectal suppositories available for children and adults; also available as an elixir, syrup, or solution.
- Good alternative to aspirin when allergy or sensitivity to aspirin exists, or in the presence of concerns about blood-thinning (anticoagulant) effects or GI tract irritation, including most patients with peptic ulcers and many patients taking chemotherapy.
- Not a first choice for bone pain because its anti-inflammatory activity is very weak.

Precautions
- Large overdoses can cause serious or fatal liver damage. Normal dosing is usually not a problem, except with heavy alcohol use and, rarely, even modest alcohol use; should be avoided with hepatitis, cirrhosis, and active liver disease, although it can be safely used in the presence of small liver metastases.

IBUPROFEN

Brand Name
Motrin, Rufen, Advil, Haltran, Ibuprin, Medipren, Midol 200, Nuprin, Trendar, Aches-N-Pain, Dolgesic, Genpril, Ibren, Ibumed, Ibupro-600, Ibutex, Ifen, Pamprin, Profen, and others.

Dose Range
From 1,200 to 3,200 mg a day or up to 800 mg four times a day, although added benefit should usually be observed in order to justify maintenance of maximum doses.

In children, it is usually prescribed based on the child's weight, with typical doses of 5 to 10 mg/kg, generally not to exceed a total of 40 mg/kg per day.

How Long It Takes to Reach Peak Effect
One to two hours (more quickly for ibuprofen oral suspension, which is usually used in children).

Equivalent Pain Relief
Uncertain, though many studies suggest greater effectiveness than propoxyphene (Darvon).

Comments
- Usually provides more pain relief than aspirin, with fewer GI problems.
- The incidence and severity of side effects (especially GI) is very low compared to the other traditional (COX-1- and COX-2-inhibiting) NSAIDs.

- Available over the counter in low doses (200 mg).
- Like most other NSAIDs, this medication may increase bleeding by thinning blood (though less so than aspirin) and may cause gastrointestinal upset. It should be taken with food and used with caution in patients with kidney or liver problems.
- Recently available (by prescription) combined with hydrocodone as Vicoprofen (ibuprofen 200 mg/hydrocodone 7.5 mg), as described in Chapter 6.

DIFLUNISAL

Brand Name
Dolobid.

Dose Range
Usually 500 to 1,000 mg as the initial dose, then 500 mg two or three times a day.

How Long It Takes to Reach Peak Effect
Effects noticeable in one hour but peak at two to three hours.

Equivalent Pain Relief
Uncertain, although 500 mg of diflunisal usually provides at least comparable pain relief as standard doses of aspirin, acetaminophen, and propoxyphene and lasts considerably longer. A dose of 1,000 mg has been shown to produce comparable but longer pain relief than acetaminophen and codeine (650 mg/60 mg). When effective, relief persists for eight and even twelve hours in most patients.

Comments
- Less irritating to stomach than aspirin.
- Can take doses just twice a day.
- Lasts longer than ibuprofen and is stronger than aspirin.
- Not recommended as treatment for fever.

Precautions
- Like other NSAIDs, can irritate gastrointestinal tract and even cause bleeding, particularly when taken for long intervals (more than six months).
- Abdominal complaints, tinnitus (ringing in the ear), and thinning of the blood less common than with aspirin
- If eye complaints occur, patient should consult an ophthalmologist.
- Other occasional side effects include drowsiness in some but insomnia in others, dizziness, ringing of the ears (tinnitus), rash, headache, and fatigue.
- Should be taken with food.

SALSALATE

Brand Name
Disalcid, Amigesic, Diagen, Mono-Gesic, Salflex, Salgesic, Salsitab.

Dose Range
Usual dose is 3,000 mg a day in two or three doses. Pain relief may build up gradually over the first four days of use.

Comments
- Same as choline magnesium trisalicylate (see previous listing).
- Often recommended when NSAIDs are desirable despite a history of ulcer or stomach bleeding, because of minimal effects on blood thinning and gastrointestinal irritation.

Precautions
- Avoid taking with aspirin or blood thinners (e.g., Coumadin)
- Extra caution should be taken with patients having kidney or ulcer problems.
- Occasional side effects include ringing in the ears, nausea, hearing impairment, rash, and dizziness.
- Should be taken with food.

PIROXICAM

Brand Name
Feldene.

Dose Range
Usually 20 mg a day.

How Long It Takes to Reach Peak Effect
Despite nearly immediate benefit, may take five to seven days to reach its peak effect.

Comments
- Very convenient: only has to be taken once a day.

Precautions
- Higher doses (above 20 mg a day) for longer than three weeks are linked to higher rates of ulcers, especially in the elderly.
- Like most other NSAIDs, this medication may increase bleeding by thinning the blood (though less so than aspirin) and may cause gastrointestinal upset. May also cause fluid retention.
- Should be taken with food.
- Should be used cautiously in patients with kidney or liver problems, as it accumulates in the system.
- If eye complaints occur, patient should consult an ophthalmologist.

NABUMETONE

Brand Name
Relafen.

Dose Range
Usually 1,000 to 2,000 mg per day, in either one or two doses during the day.

How Long It Takes to Reach Peak Effect
Response is usually noted within the first day of starting treatment.

Comments
- Appears to produce less GI irritation and ulcerations than aspirin and other older NSAIDs (e.g., indomethacin, naproxen, ibuprofen).
- Has only recently been released in the United States.
- The potential for once-daily use is convenient, especially in patients taking multiple medications.

Precautions
- Like most other NSAIDs, this medication may increase bleeding by thinning blood (though less so than aspirin) and may cause gastrointestinal upset, but ulcers and gastrointestinal bleeding are less common.
- Should be taken with food.
- Should be used with caution in patients with kidney or liver problems.
- Fluid retention and skin reactions to sunlight occur occasionally.

ETODOLAC

Brand Name
Lodine, Lodine XL.

Dose Range
More recent introduction of a prolonged-release preparation (Lodine XL) makes once or twice daily administration possible in a wide usual dose range totaling 400 to 1,000 mg a day, and sometimes up to 1,200 mg a day. Plain Lodine is usually prescribed for acute pain as 200 to 400 mg every six to eight hours and for chronic pain as 300 mg every eight to twelve hours or 400 to 500 mg every twelve hours. Lodine XL is usually prescribed as 400 to 1,000 mg once daily, and sometimes as high as 1,200 mg once per day.

How Long It Takes to Reach Peak Effect
The onset of relief of acute pain after a single dose is about thirty minutes, after which pain relief peaks at one to two hours and lasts for four to six hours. Unlike most other NSAIDs, a therapeutic response for chronic pain is usually not achieved until one to two weeks of regular use have elapsed.

Comments

- A dose of 200 mg is about equal in potency to two regular aspirin (650 mg), and 400 mg provides similar relief to codeine and acetaminophen combined (60 mg of codeine and 650 mg of acetaminophen, or two Tylenol #3).
- Although a relatively long interval must elapse before effectiveness can be determined, once daily dosing is established, this drug affords considerable convenience.
- Loss of blood in the stool (from GI irritation) is generally minimal, especially compared to ibuprofen, indomethacin, and naproxen.
- Relatively recently released in the United States.

Precautions

- Like most other NSAIDs, this medication may increase bleeding by thinning blood (though less so than aspirin) and may cause gastrointestinal upset.
- Should be taken with food.
- Should be used with caution in patients with kidney or liver problems.

DICLOFENAC

Brand Name

Voltaren delayed-release (enteric-coated) tablets, Voltaren XR extended-release tablets, Cataflam immediate-release tablets. Also available as Arthrotec (combined with misoprostol, an antiacid drug).

Dose Range

For acute pain, Cataflam (immediate-release diclofenac) is usually administered in a starting dose of 100 mg, followed by 50 mg doses three times per day for a maximum daily dose of up to 200 mg on the first day, and then followed by no more than 150 mg a day thereafter.

For chronic pain, delayed- or extended-release tablets are recommended in total daily doses ranging from 100 to 200 mg. Delayed-release tablets can be used two to four times a day, while extended-release tablets are administered one to two times a day.

How Long It Takes to Reach Peak Effect

Immediate-release (Cataflam) preparations are typically associated with a thirty-minute onset of pain relief. Peak effects are delayed to one to six hours for delayed- and extended-release preparations.

Comments

- Of the available preparations, only Cataflam (an immediate-release formulation) is indicated for the rapid resolution of acute pain, while Voltaren delayed-release and Voltaren XR extended-release tablets are preferred for the management of chronic pain.

- Voltaren XR tablets are enteric-coated to minimize gastrointestinal problems, although such problems still sometimes occur, and when prescribed once daily are especially convenient.

Precautions

- Like most other NSAIDs, this medication may increase bleeding by thinning blood (though less so than aspirin) and may cause gastrointestinal upset. Although minor GI side effects occur in about 20 percent of patients using diclofenac, only about 3 percent of patients discontinued its use for this reason, and bleeding or ulcers were observed in just 0.6 percent of patients during three-month trials.
- The next most frequent side effects involved the central nervous system, consisting of headache in 7 percent and dizziness in 3 percent.
- Fluid retention and edema may occur.
- Should be taken with food.
- Should be used with caution in patients with kidney or liver problems.
- Drug interactions: blood levels of several drugs may be altered when used concomitantly with diclofenac. As a result, your physician may choose to check blood levels if you are also taking the heart drug digoxin, the transplant drug cyclosporin, the cancer and arthritis drug methotrexate, the psychotherapeutic drug lithium, and insulin and some oral antidiabetic drugs.
- Rarely, elevations in liver function tests, with or without liver injury, have been observed, and so periodic testing of liver enzymes is advised.

FLURBIPROFEN

Brand Name
Ansaid.

Dose Range
Dose range is 100 to 300 mg per day, usually in doses every six to twelve hours.

Comments
Similar to other NSAIDs (including aspirin, ibuprofen, and indomethacin) in its analgesic effect.

Precautions

- Like most other NSAIDs, this medication may increase bleeding by thinning blood (though less so than aspirin) and may cause gastrointestinal upset, and thus is usually best avoided with a history of ulcers or ulcer symptoms.

- Should be taken with food.
- Should be used with caution in patients with kidney or liver problems.
- Use may reduce the effectiveness of cardiac beta-blocker drugs—propanolol (Inderal), atenolol (Tenormin), labetalol (Trandate, Normodyne)—in patients with hypertension.

KETOPROFEN

Brand Name
Orudis, Orudis KT, Oruvail (extended release), Actron.

Dose Range
Usually from 200 to 300 mg per day, with extended-release preparations usually limited to 200 mg a day, and lower starting doses in elderly and fragile patients. Doses are taken every six to eight hours, except for the extended-release preparation, Oruvail, which is administered once per day.

Although convenient for chronic pain, because its extended-release properties are associated with a delayed onset of effect, Oruvail is not recommended for acute pain.

Comments
- Similar to other NSAIDs in analgesic effect. Although somewhat slower in onset, pain relief may be similar to that observed with acetaminophen (650 mg) combined with codeine (60 mg) and even oxycodone (10 mg).

Precautions
- Like most other NSAIDs, this medication may increase bleeding by thinning blood (though less so than aspirin) and may cause gastrointestinal upset. The rate of gastrointestinal side effects and headache may be slightly greater with ketoprofen than some other NSAIDs, and side effects may be somewhat more common in women than men.
- Should be taken with food.
- Increased caution and dosage reductions are advised for patients with kidney or liver problems, for patients with albumin levels of less than 3.5 g/L, and in those over the age of seventy-five.

FENOPROFEN

Brand Name
Nalfon, Fenopran, Nalgesic, and Progesic.

Dose Range
Usually 300 to 600 mg four times a day.

Comments
- Similar to other NSAIDs in analgesic effect.

Precautions
- Like most other NSAIDs, this medication may increase bleeding by thinning blood (though less so than aspirin) and may cause gastrointestinal upset.
- Should be taken with food.
- Increased caution and dosage reductions are advised for patients with kidney or liver problems.

MECLOFENAMATE

Brand Name
Meclomen, Meclofen.

Dose Range
Usually 200 to 400 mg per day split up into doses to be taken every four to six hours. The smallest beneficial dosage should be employed.

Precautions
- Although improvement may be seen in some patients in a few days, two to three weeks of treatment may be required for optimal benefit, after which doses can often be reduced.
- Somewhat higher rate of gastrointestinal problems (especially diarrhea) than other NSAIDs.
- Should be taken with food, and used with caution in patients with kidney or liver problems.

KETOROLAC

Brand Name
Toradol.

Dose Range
Intramuscular injection and occasionally through intravenous injection, either as a single 60 mg injection or repeatedly, up to 30 mg every six hours, not to exceed 120 mg per day or five consecutive days of use. By mouth, 20 mg for the first dose, then 10 mg up to every four to six hours, not to exceed 40 mg per day or five consecutive days of use.

How Long It Takes to Reach Effect
Pain relief is usually noted within thirty minutes of injection, peaks after one to two hours, and lasts four to six hours.

Equivalent Pain Relief

After surgery, the potency of a 30 mg intramuscular injection is similar to that of a 6 to 12 mg intramuscular morphine injection, and the potency of a 3 mg intravenous injection is about the same as 4 mg intravenous morphine, although ketorolac causes less drowsiness, nausea, and vomiting and lasts a little longer.

Comments

- A relatively recently introduced NSAID, initially available as an injection, ketorolac (Toradol) became extremely popular. Although a very strong NSAID, because of increased risks of bleeding, GI, and kidney problems, its use is usually limited to no more than five days, so it is typically reserved for acute pain, severe pain, or the short-term treatment of pain in patients who cannot swallow pills.
- Available both as tablets and for intramuscular or intravenous injection.
- Oral ketorolac is recommended *only* as a continuation of treatment that has been initiated by injection.

Precautions

- Initially overused because of enthusiasm over the availability of an injectable NSAID, the importance of avoiding extended use or excessive doses is now recognized. The incidence of stomach upset, bleeding and perforated ulcers increases with use in patients over age sixty-five, when higher than recommended doses are used, and when treatment is extended beyond five days. Kidney problems are more common in patients who are dehydrated.
- Like most other NSAIDs, this medication may increase bleeding by thinning blood (though less so than aspirin) and may cause gastrointestinal upset.
- Should be taken with food and used with caution in patients with kidney or liver problems.
- Oral form recommended only for short-term use (less than three weeks).
- Additional caution is warranted in patients with dehydration, hypertension, heart failure, and concomitant use of blood thinners of any kind; use with other NSAIDs, including aspirin and acetaminophen, is okay.
- Swelling (fluid retention), headache, constipation, diarrhea, drowsiness, confusion, itchiness, pain or bruising at the injection site, and postoperative bleeding from wound sites may occur.

TOLMETIN

Brand Name
Tolectin, Tolectin DS.

Dose Range
Usually 600 to 1,800 mg per day, split up into doses to be taken every six to eight hours.

Precautions
- Like most other NSAIDs, this medication may increase bleeding by thinning blood (though less so than aspirin) and may cause gastrointestinal upset. May also cause fluid retention.
- Should be taken with food.
- Should be used with caution in patients with kidney or liver problems.
- Use cautiously in conjunction with lithium, Coumadin, and cyclosporin, due to the potential for toxicity.

SULINDAC

Brand Name
Clinoril, Arthrobid.

Dose Range
Usually 300 to 400 mg per day, split up into two doses to be taken every twelve hours.

Comments
- Apparent reduced likelihood of kidney problems makes this one of the preferred NSAIDs in patients at increased risk for kidney problems.
- One to two weeks of use may be required before maximum benefit is established.
- At least as effective and at least as well tolerated as most other NSAIDs, including aspirin, indomethacin, phenylbutazone, and oxyphenbutazone.

Precautions
- Like most other NSAIDs, this medication may increase bleeding by thinning blood (though less so than aspirin) and may cause gastrointestinal upset.
- Should be taken with food and used with caution in patients with kidney (though less so than other NSAIDs) or liver problems.
- Observe for fluid retention and signs and symptoms of pancreatitis.

The Most Common Nonsteroidal Anti-inflammatory Drugs Used for Cancer Pain

Generic Name & Class a	Trade Name	Usual Dosing Schedule	Usual Recommended Starting Dose (mg/day)	Usual Maximum Recommended Dose mg/day)	Comments
Acetaminophen	Tylenol, Datril, Panadol, Tempra, Anacin-3, among others	4–6 hr	2,600	6,000	1
Salicylates					
Acetylsalicylic acid	Aspirin	4–6 hr	2,600	6,000	2
Choline magnesium trisalicylate	Trilisate	8–12 hr	1,500	4,000	3
Salsalate	Disalcid	8–12 hr	3,000	4,000	3
Diflunisal	Dolobid, Dolobis	8–12 hr	1,500	1,500	4
COX-2 Inhibitors					
Celecoxib	Celebrex	12 hr	100	600	5
Rofecoxib	Vioxx	24 hr	12.5	50	
Meloxicam	Mobic	24 hr	7.5	15	
Propionic Acid Derivatives					
Ibuprofen	Motrin, Rufen, Advil, Haltran, Ibuprin, Medipren, Midol 200, Nuprin, Trendar, and others	4–8 hr	1,200	4,200	6
Naproxen	Naprosyn, Naprosin, Proxen	12 hr	500	1,000	7
Fenoprofen	Nalfon, Fenopran, Nalgesic, Progesic	6 hr	800	3,200	
Ketoprofen	Orudis, Orudis KT, Oruvail (ER) [24 hr], Actron	6–8 hr	150	300	
Flurbiprofen	Ansaid	6 hr	200	300	
Diclofenac	Voltaren, Cataflam, Voltaren XR	6–24 hr		200	

Other

Drug	Brand names				Note
Pirocam	Feldene	24 hr	20	40	8
Etodolac	Lodine	6–8 hr	800	1,200	9
	Lodine XL	12–24 hr	400	1,200	
Nabumetone	Relafen	12–24 hr	1,000	2,000	9
Mefenamic acid	Ponstel, Ponstan, Ponstil, Namphen	6 hr	400	1,000	10
Meclofenamate	Meclomen, Meclofen	4–6 hr	200	400	11
Ketorolac	Toradol	4–6 hr	40	40	12
Tolmetin	Tolectin, Tolectin DS	6–8 hr	600	1,800	
Sulindac	Clinoril, Arthrobid	12 hr	300	400	13

Notes

1. Available over the counter in various preparations. Possess weak anti-inflammatory activity and is therefore not a first drug of choice for bone pain or pain that is accompanied by inflammation. For patients at greater risk for gastrointestinal problems (such as ulcers) or bleeding complications (for example, the patient is on a blood-thinning medication), this drug is an excellent choice. Taken in large quantities, this drug can be fatal due to liver failure. When used continuously at high doses, doctors will often wish to check kidney, liver, and bone function periodically.

2. Standard to which other medications in this category are compared; available over the counter in various preparations. May not be well tolerated as other alternatives.

3. May be particularly useful in some cancer patients due to its minimal effect on thinning blood or irritating the gastrointestinal tract. Available in liquid formulations.

4. Causes less gastrointestinal irritation than aspirin.

5. Has no effect on blood clotting and minimal effect on GI system, yet has a strong anti-inflammatory effect. Has not been tested for cancer pain. Expensive.

6. Available over the counter in low-dose formations; relatively economical and well tolerated for long-term use.

7. Relatively well tolerated and rapidly absorbed.

8. Convenient once-a-day dosing is an advantage for many patients with cancer. Higher doses (more than 20 mg) are associated with increased risks of ulcers, especially in the elderly. May take 5 to 7 days to reach maximum effectiveness. When patients has liver or kidney impairment, the drug may accumulate in the body.

9. May be administered 1 to 2 times a day.

10. Since this medication is often associated with gastrointestinal problems after one week of use, it is usually not recommended for cancer pain.

11. This medication is associated with a relatively high incidence of gastrointestinal irritation.

12. In low dose ranges, seems to be effective as morphine, but like other NSAIDs, has a ceiling dose above which no further pain relief is achieved.

13. Seems to be associated with fewer kidney problems than other NSAIDs.

For a variety of reasons, the doctor may choose to prescribe any of these NSAIDs, or a number of others too numerous to mention. We have listed the most common NSAIDs here, as well as the most common brand names.

Adding Weak Opioids to NSAIDs

If more pain relief is needed than can be offered by the NSAIDs alone, or if the use of an NSAID is not advised because of a medical condition such as an ulcer or kidney failure, the next step is usually to add a weak opioid to the current therapy. There is a growing trend, however, to proceed directly to a low dose of a stronger opioid analgesic, such as morphine, much earlier than doctors used to.

6

Understanding Medications
Used to Treat Moderate Pain

When pain is moderate and can't be adequately controlled with nonopioid (nonnarcotic) drugs, usually the next step (as dictated by the World Health Organization's analgesic ladder; see Chapter 1) is the addition or substitution of a weak opioid, of which codeine is the most well known. These codeine-like drugs, referred to in the past simply as the "weak" or "mild" opioids (in contrast to the "strong" or "potent" opioids such as morphine), are today referred to as "opioids conventionally used to treat moderate pain" (versus "opioids conventionally used to treat severe pain").

The opioids conventionally used to treat moderate pain are not really weak, but their dosages are limited by the other compounds with which they are formulated, such as acetaminophen (Tylenol) or aspirin. Although new terminology is more accurate, it is also more awkward, so we will still refer to the opioids conventionally used to treat moderate pain as "weak opioids" and those conventionally used to treat severe pain as "strong opioids." Because the dosing guidelines and side effects are so different for the weak (codeine-like) and strong (morphine-like) opioids, a fuller discussion of the medications for severe pain is in the next chapter.

Weak Opioids (Opioids Conventionally Used to Treat Moderate Pain)

As mentioned, most of these agents come combined with aspirin or acetaminophen (most commonly abbreviated as APAP), which limits how much can be taken (usually no more than an average of two tablets every three or four hours)—not because of their opioid content, but because too much aspirin or acetaminophen can cause serious, sometimes even life-threatening problems. Some experts suggest that the importance of these medicines stems from the fact that our society is so drug-phobic and overconcerned about using morphine, which is on the next step of the analgesic ladder. The weak opioids are a step between the NSAIDs and the strong opioids and are more socially and culturally acceptable than the use of stronger drugs. The use of stronger drugs is still often postponed despite their greater effectiveness, because their use has regrettably come to be associated with drug abuse. For these reasons, doctors and patients would generally rather use weaker drugs, even though they are not as effective and cannot be prescribed with as much flexibility.

In fact, one of the most common mistakes that doctors make is to keep patients on these weaker medications when stronger ones would better relieve the pain and truly are no riskier.

Side Effects

CONSTIPATION

Like the strong opioids, these weaker opioids relieve pain but also usually cause constipation, which can be minimized by diet (especially fruits, other sources of fiber, and lots of water) and increased activity (especially walking). However, to prevent constipation, other products are commonly used, including laxatives (such as Senokot-S, Metamucil, milk of magnesia, Dulcolax tablets or suppositories), stool softeners (such as Colace), or enemas as needed (see Chapter 10).

NAUSEA AND VOMITING

Nausea and vomiting are also common side effects of these weaker opioids (as is true of the stronger opioids as well), although they usually resolve after a few days of consistent use of these medications. The nausea is usually transient, which makes it more tolerable to put up with it briefly. Unless nausea is extremely severe, the temptation to stop opioid use should be resisted, since its regular use allows the body to become tolerant or used to these very useful medications. If nausea or vomiting is troublesome, calmly inform your physician, who may recommend the short-term use of an antinausea (antiemetic) medication, which can usually be tapered and stopped over a few days to a week.

DROWSINESS AND BREATHING PROBLEMS

Likewise, some degree of drowsiness is common when an opioid is first started (or its dose is increased), but this is another side effect that, with regular medication use, usually resolves on its own in a few days. Medication-induced drowsiness is often confused with "catch-up sleep," a term commonly used to describe the onset of otherwise needed sleep in a patient who has been sleep-deprived from unrelenting pain. If left undisturbed, patients commonly sleep soundly for a day or two once their pain is relieved, and this should not provoke worry as long as breathing is regular and in excess of about ten breaths per minute. When drowsiness is excessive or is associated with confusion, disorientation, or hallucinations, the treating physician should be informed. If these changes are manageable, treatment may be continued with the expectation that they will resolve in a few days, or the physician may wish to substitute another opioid analgesic that may be less likely to produce these effects.

PHYSICAL DEPENDENCE

Physical dependence (which means that withdrawal symptoms would occur if the drug were stopped suddenly) and tolerance (which means that as the body adapts to a dose, more is needed to achieve the same pain-relieving effect) are rarely seen with the use of the weak (as opposed to the strong) opioids, and on the infrequent occasions that they do arise, only rarely do they interfere with treatment or cause important problems.

As with other drugs discussed, when pain is chronic and relatively constant, these medications should usually be taken on schedule, around the clock—not waiting for the pain to flare but to prevent pain episodes.

Weak Opioid Medications for Cancer Pain

The following drugs are most commonly prescribed for moderate cancer pain when nonopioid drugs (NSAIDs) are no longer sufficiently effective. However, doctors often will maintain the use of a nonopioid medication to be used in combination with a weak (or strong) opioid because they relieve pain by different mechanisms; thus, when used together pain-relieving effects are typically enhanced. As a result, lower doses of the opioid may be used with fewer concerns about side effects. Many of the medications listed here may require triplicate prescription forms in the states that require such forms. An allergy (very rare) or side effect to one does not predict that another will be poorly tolerated.

Again, the following information is to be used as a guide only, and should not be used as a substitute for a physician's care and judgment.

CODEINE

Brand Name
Codeine is usually available in combination products; see the next section.

Combination Products
Although technically available as a single-entity drug (both in pill form and by intramuscular injection), by convention codeine is almost always prescribed in combination with acetaminophen (Tylenol or APAP) or aspirin, available under a variety of brand names, including those listed below. As indicated in the discussion of hydrocodone (below), the relative effectiveness, safety, and preferred dose for each combination product depends on how much of each medication is contained in a tablet or capsule.

Probably the most common means of prescribing codeine are as Tylenol #2, Tylenol #3, or Tylenol #4. One tablet of each of these products contains 300 mg acetaminophen (or APAP) combined with 15 mg, 30 mg, or 60 mg of codeine, respectively, with one or two tablets of Tylenol #3 every four hours usually being considered the standard adult dose. Another common brand is Phenaphen with Codeine, also available as #2, #3, and #4, each of which contains similar doses (each tablet of Phenaphen with codeine has 325 mg acetaminophen, and the #2, #3, and #4 preparations contain 15 mg, 30 mg, and 60 mg codeine, respectively). Empirin with Codeine, one of the commonest preparations of aspirin and codeine, uses a similar system, in which each tablet containing 325 mg aspirin, and Empirin with Codeine #2, #3, and #4 contain 15 mg, 30 mg, and 60 mg codeine, respectively.

Other preparations of codeine combined with acetaminophen include Atasol, Capital with Codeine, Cosutone, Medocodene, Parake, Pyregesic-C, Solpadeine, Sunetheton, and Tricoton.

A typical elixir formulation contains 12 mg codeine phosphate and 120 mg APAP per 5 ml (7% alcohol) and is favored in children or adults who find it difficult to swallow pills.

Dose Range
Although infrequently prescribed alone, standard doses of plain codeine range from 30 to 80 mg every four hours, which may be supplemented with 250 to 500 mg aspirin or 325 to 500 mg of acetaminophen every four to six hours, as long as maximum daily doses of aspirin and acetaminophen (3,000 to 4,000 mg) are respected.

In children, prescriptions are based on the child's weight and are usually provided as a liquid in a typical dose range of 0.5 to 1.0 mg/kg, to be taken every four to six hours.

How Long It Takes to Reach Peak Effect

Initial effects are usually first noted within thirty to forty-five minutes, with peak effects usually occurring at about one hour, with a duration of three to six hours.

Equivalent Pain Relief

A standard dose of codeine typically provides only somewhat greater pain relief than a standard dose of aspirin or acetaminophen. A 130 mg dose of codeine IM (intramuscularly) or 200 mg of codeine by mouth (about seven standard tablets) is about equivalent to 10 mg morphine IM or IV (intravenously).

Comments

- Even though codeine is probably the most commonly prescribed weak opioid, usually in combination with aspirin or acetaminophen, some doctors feel that it is more constipating and nauseating than some of its alternatives. If constipation or nausea are persistent problems on codeine, ask the doctor to select a related compound.
- Take codeine medications with milk or water, never on an empty stomach.
- Not available for IV use, but occasionally given IM.
- Almost always used in combination with aspirin or acetaminophen, which enhances its pain-relieving effect but also limits how much can be taken safely.
- These combination products do not require special or triplicate prescriptions in states that require such forms. This is one reason why doctors try to stick to these medications rather than more readily switching to a more powerful medication for more severe pain.
- Recent research on a controlled-release preparation of codeine (preliminarily called Codeine-Contin) shows that its effects persist for twelve hours; this product may be available in the near future. In addition, a controlled-release rectal suppository is under investigation.
- Can use up to three tablets every three to six hours to relieve pain.
- Although most opioids have no ceiling dose (above which there are just more side effects and no additional relief), codeine is thought to have a maximum dose of 300 mg. Most often, though, since codeine is usually prescribed only with aspirin or acetaminophen, doses are limited due to the dangers of taking excessive doses of aspirin or acetaminophen.

Precautions

- Constipation is extremely common with codeine, and preventive measures are almost always required. And, as with most opioids, the higher the dose of codeine, the more laxative is needed.

- As the dose is increased, nausea and sedation may occur, but these effects usually do not last. Drowsiness may represent catch-up sleep, and nausea may require brief treatment until it resolves. Codeine may also cause dry mouth, light-headedness, headache, and itchiness.

- Extra care should be taken with patients having breathing difficulties, increased brain pressure, or liver failure.

PROPOXYPHENE

Propoxyphene comes in two chemical forms, propoxyphene hydrochloride (HCl) and propoxyphene napsylate. Only the HCl form is available as a single entity (unmixed with other drugs). The two compounds have different potencies, with 65 mg of propoxyphene HCl about equal to 100 mg of propoxyphene napsylate. The most commonly prescribed formulation of propoxyphene products is Darvocet N-100, which contains 325 mg of acetaminophen (APAP).

Brand Name

Darvon available in tablets containing 32 and 65 mg propoxyphene HCl.

Combination Products

Genagesic, E-Lor, Cosalgesic, Distalgesic, Dolene Ap-65, and Wygesic (containing propoxyphene HCl 65 mg and APAP 650 mg); Darvon Compound (containing 65 mg of propoxyphene HCl, 389 mg of aspirin, and 32.4 mg of caffeine); Darvon N-50 (50 mg of propoxyphene napsylate, 325 mg of APAP); Darvon N-100 (100 mg of propoxyphene napsylate, 650 mg of APAP); Darvocet N-100 (100 mg of propoxyphene napsylate, 325 mg of aspirin).

Dose Range

For products containing propoxyphene HCl, the standard dose is usually considered to be 65 to 130 mg, and for those containing propoxyphene napsylate, standard doses are 100 to 200 mg, usually up to every four to six hours. Due both to the potential for propoxyphene to accumulate in the body and to the inclusion of aspirin or acetaminophen in many products, daily doses should be limited. Avoid more than 390 mg per day of propoxyphene HCl, more than 600 mg a day of propoxyphene napsylate, and a daily dose of acetaminophen or aspirin greater than 3,000 to 4,000 mg.

This drug is not recommended for children.

How Long It Takes to Reach Peak Effect

Initial effects are usually noted within about thirty minutes and peak in one to one and a half hours, with a duration of three to six hours. Two to three days of regular use may be required before full effectiveness is realized.

Equivalent Pain Relief

A 65 mg dose of propoxyphene by mouth provides similar pain relief to 600 mg of aspirin when single doses are compared. New data suggest that propoxyphene may be somewhat more effective than we once thought when used steadily around the clock.

Comments

- As the weakest of the opioids conventionally used to treat moderate pain, it is in fact not much more effective than standard doses of aspirin or acetaminophen, especially with intermittent use. Once considered vastly overprescribed because of doctors' unwarranted fears of using stronger drugs, many patients, especially the elderly, still clung to its use. Newer studies demonstrate that effectiveness may improve with regular use, especially in the elderly both because of some accumulation and due to new ideas about its mechanisms of action. Like another opioid, methadone, propoxyphene now appears not only to work at the conventional opioid receptor, but also to produce analgesia by a separate mechanism involving antagonism of an amino acid, N-methyl-D-aspartate (NMDA), which appears to be especially important when pain stems from nerve injury.
- There appears to be a ceiling effect that prevents safely increasing the dose of propoxyphene beyond the doses described above.
- Despite some renewed interest in propoxyphene, in general its use in cancer pain should be discouraged except for cases of very mild pain or in patients in whom its effectiveness and safety have already been demonstrated.
- Although relatively weak, indiscriminate use of propoxyphene compounds can cause problems.
- Effects of propoxyphene may be cumulative over time.
- Side effects will limit increasing doses.
- Combined use with alcohol markedly reduces safety.
- Should be avoided if kidney problems exist.

Precautions

- Can cause hallucinations, confusion, and even convulsions at high doses.
- Can become toxic when used over time at high doses.

HYDROCODONE

Brand Name

Not available in its pure form (as a single-entity drug) but only in combination with other drugs (aspirin, acetaminophen, ibuprofen, various cough and cold medications).

Combination Products

Anexsia, Co-Gesic, Hydrocet, Lorcet, Lortab, Oncet, Panacet, Vicodin, Zydon, Damason P, and many others (see below).

Hydrocodone is most commonly prescribed in tablets containing 5 to 10 mg hydrocodone and 325 to 650 mg of acetaminophen. Although confusion may arise because it is available under such a large variety of trade names, the most important distinction relates to the two numbers that follow the hydrocodone and APAP, which indicate the dose of each drug contained in a single pill or capsule. The first number refers to the amount of hydrocodone (5 to 10 mg) and is important because it correlates with the preparation's potency or strength, while the second number is important because it describes the dose of APAP or acetaminophen and indicates how many tablets can be safely taken each day without excessive risks of liver injury.

Brand names for hydrocodone/APAP change constantly but currently include the following (tablets, unless indicated otherwise): Vicodin (5/500), Vicodin ES (7.5/750), Vicodin HP (10/660), Bancap HC (5/500) capsule, Hydrocet (5/500) capsule, Hy-phen (5/500), Co-Gesic (5/500) capsule, Lorcet (10/650), Lorcet Plus (7.5/650), Lorcet-HD (5/500) capsule, Lortab (2.5/500), Lortab (5/500), Lortab (7.5/500),Lortab (10/500), Panacet (5/500), Anexsia (5/500, 7.5/650, 10/660), Anodynos-DHC (5/500), Dolacet (5/500) capsule, DuoCet (5/500) capsule, Margesic H (5/500) capsule, Medipain 5 (5/500), Norco (10/325), Stagesic (5/500) capsule, T-Gesic (5/500) capsule, Zydone (5/500) capsule, Ceta-Plus (5/500) capsule, Azdone (5/500), Damason-P (5/500).

Other combination products with ibuprofen, aspirin, and so on are also available, such as Vicoprofen, Alor 5/500, Azdone, Damason-P, Lortab ASA, Panasal 5/500, Hycodan, Hydromet, Oncet, and Tussigon.

Dose Range

The usual dose is 5 to 20 mg (one or two pills of one of the above preparations) by mouth every three to six hours. The maximum daily dose depends on the acetaminophen or aspirin content of the prescribed preparation and should not exceed a total of 3,000 mg of acetaminophen, 3,600 mg of aspirin, or 5,200 mg of enteric-coated aspirin per day.

Equivalent Pain Relief

It depends on the dose, but in general hydrocodone combination products are slightly weaker than oxycodone combination products (see next section) but stronger than codeine products.

Comments

- Hydrocodone, as well as the very similar drug dihydrocodeine (Synalgos-DC, which comes with aspirin and caffeine), is similar to codeine but is about one-third stronger. Its combination products are used commonly, because (like codeine combination products) not all states with restrictive prescribing practices require a special or triplicate prescription for them. Most experts feel that one of the most common mistakes doctors make is to overprescribe these drugs to avoid the hassle of triplicate prescribing.
- Available in the United States only as a combination product.
- Also a good cough suppressant.

Precautions

- Because several of the combination products have relatively high levels of acetaminophen (Anexia, Lorcet, Lorcet Plus, Vicodin ES, and Vicodin HP), taking them too often or taking too many may cause the toxic effects of acetaminophen. Patients should therefore be switched to a stronger drug rather than be prescribed large doses of this medication, especially preparations that contain high doses of acetaminophen or aspirin.

OXYCODONE

Combination Products

Percodan (5 mg oxycodone, 325 mg aspirin), Percocet (2.5 to 10 mg oxycodone, 325 to 650 mg acetaminophen), Roxicet (5 mg oxycodone, 325 mg acetaminophen), Tylox (5 mg oxycodone, 500 mg acetaminophen), Roxicet Oral Solution (5 mg oxycodone, 325 mg acetaminophen per 5 ml).

Dose Range

One or two tablets or capsule usually every four hours; children six to twelve years start at 1.25 mg every six hours, children over twelve start at 2.5 mg every six hours.

How Long It Takes to Reach Peak Effect

Onset of effect is usually within fifteen to thirty minutes, with peak effectiveness at sixty to ninety minutes, and a duration of three to six hours.

Equivalent Pain Relief

This is the strongest of the available opioids conventionally used for moderate pain and in many states requires a special (triplicate) prescription form. Twenty to 30 mg of oxycodone is about as effective as 200 mg of codeine given orally or 10 mg of IM morphine.

Comments

- Once available only as a combination product mixed with acetaminophen (APAP) or aspirin (Percodan, Percocet, etc.), oxycodone has recently become available as a sole entity (unmixed with other drugs), both as a relatively short-acting drug (Roxicodone, Oxy-IR, etc.) and in a long-acting controlled-release formulation (OxyContin). These new preparations allow doses to be raised when needed without fear of toxicity from too much aspirin or acetaminophen. New formulations of oxycodone taken as single medications are discussed further in the next chapter.
- Still considered the strongest of the opioids conventionally used to treat moderate pain when a combination product is prescribed, but when prescribed alone (plain oxycodone), it is now considered an opioid conventionally used to treat severe pain (strong or potent opioid).
- Similar to codeine and hydrocodone, but significantly stronger. Even though a triplicate prescription is required in some states, most experts prefer this alternative over the previously mentioned drugs.
- Not available for IM or IV injection in the United States.

Precautions

- Same as codeine.
- Try not to take it on an empty stomach.

TRAMADOL

Brand Name
Ultram.

Dose Range
Fifty to 100 mg every four to six hours. The maximum dosage under any circumstances is 400 mg (eight tablets) a day (300 mg or six tablets for those over age seventy-five).

How Long It Takes to Reach Peak Effect
Initial effects are usually noted in forty-five to sixty minutes and usually peak at two to three hours, with a usual duration of six to seven hours. May take up to two days of regular use before maximum effectiveness is realized.

Equivalent Pain Relief
About as effective as acetaminophen-hydrocodone combination products.

Comments

- Although tramadol (Ultram) has been used in Europe for decades, it has only been available in the United States for a few years. Its mechanism of action (how it relieves pain) is somewhat unique and is still not completely understood. It appears to work by several routes, in that it has some activity at the opioid receptor, which produces a partial narcotic effect, but it also boosts levels of several neurotransmitters (norepinephrine and serotonin) within the nerve synapse, which further promotes pain relief, especially when there is nerve damage.
- Has no anti-inflammatory effect.
- Abuse potential is probably lower than for more routine opioids (narcotics) but still exists. Seizures have been reported in abusers who have taken overdoses seeking a high.
- Tends to be more expensive than equivalent drugs.

Precautions

- Doses should be reduced for patients with liver or kidney failure.
- Potential side effects include constipation, nausea, dizziness, dry mouth, sedation, and headache.
- Doses may need to be increased in patients taking carbamazepine (Tegretol) and lowered in those on quinidine.
- The effects of digoxin and Coumadin may be amplified if Ultram is added.
- Exceeding the usual recommended dose is associated with the risk of seizure. This risk, which is small, is slightly increased in patients taking antidepressants and other opioids.
- Allergic reactions occasionally occur; avoid if a true allergy has followed the use of another narcotic.

Agonist-Antagonists and Partial Agonists

The opioids mentioned so far are those that are considered pure agonists, meaning that they reduce pain by the same mechanism, by binding to opioid receptors. Two other related classes of opioids, the agonist-antagonists and the partial agonists, are available, but their use is generally discouraged for treating cancer pain. These agents are also attracted to opioid receptors, but once bound have mixed effects, turning some on and others off. They tend to produce more mind-altering side effects than the weak opioids already described, and they have maximum (ceiling) doses above which they are no longer more effective. In addition, they can cause withdrawal symptoms

Common Medications Used to Treat Moderate Cancer Pain

Generic Name	Trade Name[a]	Route	Equianalgesic Dose[b]	Recommended Schedule[c]	Formulations	Comments[d]
Codeine	Tylenol #2 Tylenol #3 Tylenol #4	Oral	200 mg 130 mg	3–6 hr same	15, 30, or 60 mg 30 mg/ml	1
Codeine		IM	65–130 mg —	3–6 hr 3–6 hr	32 or 65 mg —	2 3
Propoxyphene	Darvon	Oral	20 mg	3–6 hr		4
Hydrocodone	Vicodin, Lortab, Lorcet, Norco, many others	Oral				
Oxycodone	Percodan Percocet OxyIR, Oxy-Alone, Roxycodone, others	Oral		3—6 hr	5 mg, 15, mg, 30 mg 50 mg	5
Tramadol	Ultram		100 mg			

NOT RECOMMENDED FOR CANCER PAIN
Buprenorphine, Dezocine, Temgesic, Buprenex, Dalgan, Butorphanol, Pentazocine, Nalbuphine, Meperidine, Stadol, Talwin, Talacen, Nubian, Demerol, Pethedine

Notes

[a]Listing is partial, comprised mostly of formulations available in the United States.

[b]Equianalgesic dose refers to the dose that provides the equivalent pain relief as 10 mg of IM morphine. These doses are based on values most frequently cited in the medical literature and on clinical experience, although these sometimes conflict. They are approximate and are intended to serve as guidelines only.

[c]This is a rough guideline only; physicians may deviate from these schedules as they tailor medication schedules to particular patients.

[d]Side effects for all the opioid medications include constipation, sedation, dysphoria (unpleasant moods or feelings), confusion, hallucinations, nausea, vomiting, respiratory depression (which is rare in patients who have developed a tolerance to opioids), urinary retention (difficulty urinating), and itching. How patients react to opioids differs from patient to patient and medication to medication, often even in the same patient.

Comments

1. For mild to moderate pain, traditionally marketed as combination product with aspirin or acetaminophen. Recently made available without aspirin or acetaminophen for mild to severe pain.

2. Weakest opioid, traditionally used for mild pain, often combined with aspirin or acetaminophen. Usually not appropriate for cancer pain except for very mild pain or when its safety has been demonstrated.

3. For mild to moderate pain, only administered with aspirin or acetaminophen, ibuprofen, etc.

4. Considered the strongest of the opioids conventionally used to treat moderate pain (mild or weak opioid) when a combination product is prescribed, but when prescribed alone (plain oxycodone), it is now considered an opioid conventionally used to treat severe pain (strong or potent opioid) (see Ch. 7).

5. Works by several mechanisms of action, so also good for nerve pain; lower abuse potential than other opioids but expensive.

in patients who have been using routine (agonist) opioids regularly. The use of this entire class of drugs is *strongly discouraged in cancer patients*, especially if they are taking an agonist opioid at the same time. Although their use is relatively outmoded, they are still favored by some doctors who still worry about addiction. The only one of these drugs available as an oral medication in the United States is pentazocine (Talwin, Talacen, Talwin NX, Talwin Compound). Because of the problems mentioned above, if it is prescribed for cancer pain, you may wish to seek a second opinion.

Buprenorphine (Temgesic) is a partial agonist, and although some of the above problems may exist with its use, it is a relatively strong opioid (see Chapter 7) that is available in the United States by injection and as an under-the-tongue medication in Canada and parts of Europe; it has been tested as a long-acting controlled-release preparation for future release in the United States. Butorphanol (Stadol, Stadol NS) is available in an injectable form and as a nasal spray that is sometimes used for migraine headache. Neither form is recommended for the treatment of cancer pain because their effectiveness is limited, they may reverse the effects of other painkillers, and they may add to confusion.

Note: Although meperidine (Demerol, Pethedine) is an effective pain reliever after surgery, it is also not recommended for cancer pain because of its short duration and potentially toxic side effects.

When pain is severe or these weak opioids are not controlling pain adequately, doctors turn to the opioids conventionally used to treat severe pain, the strong or potent opioids, which we'll explore in the next chapter.

7

Understanding Medications
Used to Treat Severe Pain

Misconceptions about the effects and side effects of morphine, the most well known of the strong opioids, and similar drugs are the primary reasons why people with cancer around the world are undermedicated. Yet with a proper understanding of these drugs, pain can be adequately relieved with a minimum of side effects in nearly all patients.

When pain is moderate to severe and mild opioids are inadequate, the next course of action is to try morphine or a similar opioid. Most of what we say about morphine, the standard strong opioid against which all others are compared, is true of about the other strong opioids mentioned in this chapter, unless otherwise noted. Within this family of medications, one or another may work slightly better, longer, or quicker for a given patient.

General Guidelines for the Use of Opioids

Although many patients don't need morphine until they are very ill or close to death, that doesn't mean that this is morphine's only use or that taking it necessarily signals the beginning of the end. In fact, probably the biggest change in contemporary pain management is the earlier use of strong pain medicines (in lower doses). Some patients do not have severe pain until their illness is very advanced and so do not need morphine earlier. Others may take morphine for weeks, months, even years. Many cancer patients need treatment with morphine even though their cancer is under good control for a long time. Taking morphine does not have any kind of negative effect on the course of the disease. In fact, many doctors believe that patients on morphine live longer because they are better able to rest, eat, and sleep, are more interested and active in the life around them, and therefore are able to use their natural ability to fight the disease more rigorously.

Once pain becomes a consistent problem, most patients will take not one but two opioids. One (the basal analgesic) is prescribed on an around-the-clock schedule to try to prevent severe pain, and one is taken when pain flares up (breakthrough pain) between regular scheduled doses. With cancer pain, which tends to be relatively constant, it makes good sense to keep a steady level of medication in the bloodstream by giving most of it around the clock—that is, on schedule, regardless of whether the pain has become bad again or not.

Starting Doses

Starting doses often vary by age and depend on effectiveness and side effects.

Although the dose needed to relieve pain varies widely among patients, doctors usually start with a low dose (such as 20–30 mg by mouth or a 5–10 mg injection of morphine), assuming the patient has been on weak opioids already. The dose is then increased as needed, often as soon as the evening of the first day and certainly during the second day, if pain is not relieved. The limiting factor is if the patient cannot tolerate a higher dose of the drug because of side effects that can't be controlled. If these side effects are persistent, another opioid can be tried. Sensitivity to one drug's side effects does not mean the patient will be sensitive to a similar drug's side effects.

AGE AND DOSES

Children's doses are calculated by body weight.

Patients forty and younger often need more frequent doses than older patients because they may metabolize morphine more quickly and so the pain-relieving effect doesn't last as long.

Older or malnourished patients or those with kidney or liver disease usually need about 25 percent less than the standard doses to start.

Expect that the dose of opioid will have to be increased periodically because of tolerance, pain escalation, disease progression, rehabilitation, or increases in psychological distress.

Myths about Narcotics (Opioids) and Other Painkillers

False	True
If you start taking morphine, it means that options are running out and health care providers are giving up on you.	Options do not run out. Opioids are appropriate for pain that is intensifying. If morphine's a problem, other strong medications are effective options.
Morphine and other narcotics will cause addiction.	Cancer pain patients almost never become addicted.
If morphine or another narcotic is used now, they won't work as well later. Waiting as long as possible is best.	Morphine and other narcotics do not lose their effectiveness. If pain gets worse, the dose may be gradually increased as much as needed (almost indefinitely) with good results.
Morphine and other narcotics cause delirium and other serious side effects.	Drowsiness usually fades in a few days, and the other side effects, such as nausea and constipation (if they occur) can be easily treated.
The doctor will view complaining about pain negatively.	Pain is bad for health. Doctors need to be well informed about pain to do their best.
Talking about pain will distract the doctor from cancer treatment.	Treating pain is part of treatment. Good pain control means better rest, which helps the body fight the disease.
Pain means the cancer is worsening.	Pain can be unrelated to the progress of cancer and is often caused by aggressive cancer treatments.
It's better to endure the pain than to have to have shots.	More than 90 percent of cancer pain treatments can be taken by mouth, skin patch, or lozenge. Injections are rarely absolutely necessary.
Morphine use leads to loss of control.	Very few cancer patients feel high or lose control when they take pain medication properly, although drowsiness is normal for the first few days. In fact, if you leave your pain untreated, you may find control slipping through your fingers, along with quality of life.

Means of Administration

In the past, morphine and other strong opioids were viewed as less effective in pill or liquid form, which is why some doctors still begin with injected morphine even though this is not usually needed. Opioids given orally, via a skin patch, or (most recently) even in lollipop-like form, however, work extremely well as long as higher doses are used to make up for some of the drug being lost in the gastrointestinal tract. So, in general, strong opioids should be delivered, whenever possible, by these convenient methods. This avoids the need for injections, allowing people to remain more independent and able to focus on their wellness.

Doses and Switching Medications

Patients on high doses of potent opioids who must switch to another narcotic should not receive a low dose to start. Each opioid has a different inherent strength or potency, so different doses of the various opioids are required to achieve equivalent pain-relieving effects. This is called the equianalgesic dose. When switching, patients should start with one-half or more of the predicted equianalgesic dose of the new medication. This is because tolerance to one drug helps your tolerance for another, but not completely. Incorrectly calculating the equianalgesic dose is a leading cause of undermedication. (See the table on page 154.) It shouldn't persist, though, since your doctor should be constantly adjusting your medication to achieve the best balance between pain relief and any low-grade side effects.

Scheduling of Doses

Most cancer patients will use two kinds of strong medications for pain—one is around the clock (on schedule), and one is on hand in case pain breaks through (rescue or escape dose).

AROUND-THE-CLOCK MEDICATION

Fixed doses should be prescribed around the clock so that doses are taken before pain intensifies. By keeping pain under control early on, patients can stay stronger to deal with the other problems associated with cancer. (Such use of analgesics is also known as time-contingent dosing, fixed dosing, or basal dosing.)

The ATC medication is usually a relatively long-acting opioid such as controlled-release morphine (MS Contin, Oramorph, or Kadian), controlled-release oxycodone (OxyContin), transdermal fentanyl (Duragesic), or sometimes even methadone (Dolophine). A regularly scheduled dose helps keep medication levels from becoming erratic—either too low (which would promote pain) or too high (which could trigger side effects). Imagine a hole in a bucket that produces a slow but steady leak. To keep that bucket consistently level, you would have to dribble in a fixed amount of water constantly.

AS-NEEDED MEDICATION (RESCUE DOSES)

In addition to the ATC medication, most cancer patients with moderate to severe pain also need extra medication on hand in case pain breaks through between the regularly scheduled doses, such as when there's increased activity. These are called rescue doses, escape doses, or boluses. They are prescribed to be taken whenever needed, and may be taken as often as every two to four hours. If more than three or so rescue doses are needed a day, it is probably time for the doctor to increase the fixed ATC dose. As-needed (PRN) dosing may also be necessary when the patient's pain status is rapidly changing—for example, during radiation treatments for a tumor of the bone or when pain only occurs intermittently (the exception, not the rule).

For rescue doses, usually a short-acting opioid such as the new formulation of fentanyl that can be administered in a lozenge (Actiq), immediate-release morphine (such as MSIR or Roxanol), hydromorphone (Dilaudid), or oxycodone (Roxicodone, etc.) are prescribed because they begin to work relatively quickly (five to ten minutes for the Actiq lozenge and fifteen to forty-five minutes for most tablets and liquids) and don't build up in the system like long-acting or slow-release preparations.

Ideally, the doses for the around-the-clock medication is high enough that only occasional rescue doses (two or three a day) are needed.

Brompton's Cocktail

In the past, a drink called a Brompton's cocktail (developed at Brompton's Chest Hospital in England) was used to treat pain in cancer patients. A combination of heroin or morphine with cocaine, phenothiazine (a tranquilizer and antinausea medication), alcohol, and chloroform water, these drinks are no longer used. Instead, oral morphine (in the United States), heroin (in the United Kingdom), or other similar opioids, given alone or along with other needed medications, are used because they are more easily adjusted (or titrated) to the patient's needs and more effective. If a patient is prescribed a Brompton cocktail these days, consider a consultation with another doctor, since this approach is old-fashioned and less effective for pain than the more modern methods described in this book.

Drug Combinations

Expect that a combination of drugs will be prescribed, either another analgesic (a non-narcotic one) or an adjuvant (complementary) drug, which will enhance the pain-relieving effect of the opioids or help control side effects. (See Chapter 8 for details.)

Side Effects

Be prepared for side effects that may include nausea, vomiting, sedation, constipation, dry mouth, itchiness, twitching, and difficulty expelling urine. (See Chapters 10 and 11 for a discussion of these side effects.) Side effects are predictable as doses increase, though they are often temporary and can usually be easily managed.

Ceiling Doses

Don't worry that you need to save higher doses for "when it gets really bad." This very common "money-in-the-bank" syndrome inappropriately makes patients think they need to save the morphine for when they *really* need it. Morphine doesn't stop being effective; doses just need to be increased over time, although many people stay on the same dose for week, months, and even years. If pain worsens, the dose can be increased accordingly. Since there's no ceiling dose, there's no cause for concern when morphine is started early.

Treating Severe Pain

- The goal is to prevent severe pain. Around-the-clock dosing keeps pain from escalating.

- Addiction should not be a consideration, despite the use of the strongest opioids.

- Prevent constipation and nausea by asking for an over-the-counter recommendation or a prescription for a laxative and an antiemetic (antinausea medication).

- Expect at least minor sedation during the first few days of using a new painkiller or escalating its dose, but know that it usually resolves within three to five days. If pain has interfered with sleep for some time, expect some catch-up sleep.

- Expect that the dose may have to be increased periodically, because of tolerance, escalating pain, disease progression, or anxiety and psychological distress.

- Expect to be prescribed a combination of drugs that work by different mechanisms.

- Remember: if the pain gets worse, the dose can always be increased. There's no maximum dose for the strong opioids.

How Doses Are Determined

Painkillers aren't prescribed like antibiotics, in rigid, fixed doses, but are adjusted constantly from patient to patient, over time, and in response to the pain relief achieved and the side effects that occur. If the patient has moderate to severe pain and the doctor seems reluctant to increase the dose, or if the dose is increased only very slowly or by very small amounts, try discussing the pros and cons of adjusting the dose faster or in different increments. The pain of cancer may not be entirely relieved without any side effects: the goal of pain treatment is to achieve the best balance between comfort and any side effects so that the patient can go about his business. If you remain uncertain about how the pain is being handled, consider seeking a second opinion on pain management (see Appendix 1 for resources).

How Opioids Are Chosen for Each Patient

The potent opioids work by similar mechanisms and generally offer the same kind of relief and same range of potential side effects. Although morphine is the best-known of these medications, doctors may select from among the many strong narcotics for any of the following reasons:

- The doctor may be more familiar with one drug than another.
- Cost. Methadone, for example, is one-tenth the cost of many preparations of morphine.
- Whether a longer-acting drug or shorter-acting drug is needed.
- Whether the patient has shown particular sensitivity to one opioid (such as nausea, vomiting, hallucinations, or another side effect), but not to another, or whether certain expected effects of a drug are important. For example, constipation tends to be less of a problem with the fentanyl patch (Duragesic), and morphine sometimes causes persistent nausea or sedation due to a buildup of its breakdown products.
- Repetitive use of meperidine (Demerol) is avoided due to risk of seizures.
- Actiq (the fentanyl "lollipop"), though costly, works almost as fast as an intravenous injection.
- Kadian (a brand of controlled-release morphine) can be sprinkled on food yet produces relief for up to a full day.
- If the patient has become very tolerant to one narcotic, the doctor may switch to another because cross-tolerance between narcotics

is often not complete—that is, the patient won't be as tolerant to the alternative drug, and lower doses can be used.

- If oral medication causes nausea or other stomach problems, or so many pills are needed that it becomes inconvenient, a skin patch, rectal suppositories, or another route may be recommended (details later in this chapter).
- Neuropathic pain (pain due to nerve injury) may suggest a particular drug. Methadone, though tricky to adjust, is particularly effective for this type of pain. Despite its reputation for its use with drug abusers seeking respite from withdrawal, methadone is being used more frequently these days to treat chronic pain because it is especially effective, very inexpensive, and much less likely to accumulate in the body, making it less risky for the elderly, those with kidney problems, and those who require quick dose adjustments.
- Medical history is also a consideration. Whether a particular drug has worked well, or poorly, for a patient in the past, the doctor should strongly consider that history when choosing a pain medication.

Understanding Tolerance, Dependency, Addiction, and Withdrawal

As detailed in Chapter 1, many health care providers and consumers are overly concerned about the potential for opioid addiction in cancer patients. Once the differences among tolerance, physical dependence, and addiction are understood, it will be clear why these phenomena should not be allowed to limit our treatment of cancer pain.

Addiction is a psychological dependence, a craving for a drug for its euphoric effect. Addiction is extremely rare in cancer patients. Cancer patients using opioids rarely report getting a high from morphine; in fact, some feel just the opposite of euphoric, reporting dysphoria (an unpleasant state in which the patient doesn't feel like himself). Most patients with life-threatening disease value their mental clarity, tending to avoid the fuzziness associated with excessive medication, even to the point of tolerating unneeded pain.

Even though patients, family members, and health care providers still fear addiction, studies show that it occurs in no more than one-tenth of 1 percent of cancer patients. Very rarely will cancer patients try to get more pain medication if their pain ceases, say, because of successful treatment of a tumor. In fact, it is more common for cancer patients to stop their pain medication too quickly (it should usually be tapered, or decreased gradually) when the source of pain is well resolved.

The fear of narcotic addiction should not be a factor in treating cancer pain.

Tolerance means that over time larger doses of a medication (such as an opioid) may be required to achieve the previous pain-relieving effect. When a dose of an opioid painkiller doesn't last as long as it used to, it is safe to have the physician prescribe a larger dose, and there is no ceiling effect. And just as patients may become tolerant to the pain-relieving effects of a medication, they become tolerant to side effects as well. Thus doses can be continually increased gradually, as needed.

The fear of tolerance to opioids should not be a factor in treating cancer pain because once their safe use has been established, varying doses of these drugs are well tolerated and do not produce addiction.

Physical dependence and *withdrawal* occur with the chronic use of opioids, but they are not psychological phenomena and therefore are completely unrelated to addiction. Physical dependence means that withdrawal symptoms might occur if the drug is suddenly stopped. These symptoms include anxiety, irritability, alternating chills and hot flashes, excessive salivation, tearing eyes (lacrimation), runny nose, nausea, vomiting, abdominal cramps, insomnia, sweating (diaphoresis), and goose bumps (piloerection). Physical dependence is easily treated, thereby avoiding withdrawal, by gradually decreasing the daily doses of the opioid, for example, by 10 to 25 percent. Once a low daily dose of morphine (20 mg orally) is reached, the opioid can be discontinued without withdrawal symptoms occurring.

The fear of withdrawal from opioids should not be a factor in treating cancer pain, as long as doses are reduced gradually once the drug is no longer needed.

To sum up, most people who take a strong opioid for more than a few weeks will grow tolerant and physically dependent on the medication because that is how the body normally reacts to opioids. Tolerance and physical dependence are not real barriers to good pain management since they are expected and can be managed by the doctor just as other side effects are controlled (for example, nausea and constipation).

Tolerance and physical dependence are (to some degree) inevitable, and they have nothing to do with addiction (or psychological dependence), which is extremely rare in patients with pain. Although a person who is addicted almost always becomes tolerant and physically dependent on the narcotic, the opposite is not true: a person who is physically dependent or tolerant to a medication is by no means necessarily addicted, and in fact, addiction from pain treatment, even with strong medicines, is extremely uncommon in cancer patients.

However, pain patients who have struggled with addiction or alcoholism in the past are at higher risk of becoming addicted to opioids that are prescribed for pain relief.

See Chapter 1 for a more detailed discussion of addiction, tolerance, and physical dependence.

Ways to Take Opioids

Although taking opioids by mouth is preferred, patients can't always reliably swallow pills or liquids. This may be because too many pills are required, patients' mouths are too dry, they are nauseated, their intestines are blocked, or they are unable to swallow. Many patients with advanced cancer are likely to use, at one time or another, two or three different methods for receiving medication as their condition changes.

Oral Medication

Liquid, syrup, lozenges, or tablets are usually preferred because medication by mouth (abbreviated *PO*) is the most economical, convenient, and safe. Although doses may vary and typically require a little longer to take effect initially, they last about as long or longer than drugs given by other routes.

Although fentanyl is still unavailable as a tablet, Actiq, a sweetened fentanyl lozenge mounted on a stick (resembling a lollipop), is now used strictly for treating cancer patients' breakthrough pain (a jolt of increased pain superimposed on constant chronic pain). Although unquestionably very effective and nearly as quick to act as an injection, Actiq has caught on slowly, in part because its concept is so new and unique.

Rectal Medication

When patients are vomiting or can't swallow medication, suppositories of morphine, oxymorphone, or hydromorphone may be used (the indication "by rectum" is abbreviated *PR*). When suppositories aren't available, enemas using 10 to 20 mg of water with morphine or hydromorphone can also be effective. In special circumstances custom-made suppositories can be formulated by a compounding pharmacy. Once a common institution, the compounding pharmacy or apothecary has become increasingly rare, but is now dramatically on the rise. Some doctors are more liberal than others in considering therapies that are not yet approved by the Food and Drug Administration, a practice that is legal but which is best applied in moderation. For example, MS Contin, a controlled-release form of oral morphine, though not formally approved for rectal use, has been shown to be safe and effective. Also, sometimes special compounding is needed when desired rectal medications are not commercially available in preferred doses.

While rectal medications are popular among some European cultures, others shun it, as do adolescents, who may be too embarrassed to use them. They also are usually ruled out with diarrhea, hemorrhoids, or a colostomy, or if it's too painful to position the patient to insert a suppository. Usually rectal medications are used just for short periods, especially when doctors want to avoid injections. Vaginal suppositories and even placement of suppositories into colostomies are occasionally considered, and controlled-release rectal formulations of painkillers, although not yet available, are being researched to achieve longer duration of effect.

Transdermal Medications

The use of skin patches (Duragesic is currently the only trade name currently available) is becoming an increasingly common way to deliver medications for pain and other disorders because of its convenience. The Duragesic patch for pain contains a large reservoir of a strong opioid, fentanyl, which slowly diffuses through a rate-controlling membrane, so the medication is delivered in a steady, metered dose.

Injections

Injections are no more effective for pain than other routes, though doses are lower because no medication is lost in digestion. Although injections work more quickly than swallowed medicine, this is not a big advantage for chronic pain, especially when adequate doses are prescribed. The main advantages to injections for chronic pain are to bypass the mouth because of recent surgery, vomiting, intestinal blockage, dry mouth, painful swallowing, or coma and to provide urgent relief in a pain emergency.

INTRAMUSCULAR INJECTION

Getting a shot involves a swab with alcohol and a quick, deep injection into a bulky muscle in the upper arm or buttock. Although common for emergency room use or just before surgery, intramuscular injections (abbreviated *IM*) are not recommended for long-term pain management because they are painful, can induce fear, produce somewhat unpredictable results, and do not last long. Injections also can occasionally traumatize nerves, and repeated injections can lead to infections. If your doctor is using injections chronically to treat pain, consider consulting another physician.

INTRAVENOUS MEDICATION

With intravenous (IV) administration, medications are injected directly into a vein through a needle or plastic catheter. Such administration is reliable, is useful in adjusting doses quickly, and provides immediate pain relief. However, it is no more effective for chronic treatment than well-planned oral and transdermal therapies.

For routine use, IV medications are administered through peripheral lines, a plastic catheter in one of the small veins of the hand, forearm, or foot. With chronic illness, veins "blow" or become used up quickly, making repeated or continued access difficult. If the need for IV therapies is anticipated, a more reliable solution involves installing a central line. These may be surgically implanted ports, plugs, catheters, a PIC line, or larger versions of regular IVs placed under local anesthesia, usually at the bedside, and families can learn to maintain them.

If one of these more durable IV systems has already been placed for other reasons (chemotherapy, antibiotics, nutrition), for pragmatic reasons it is often relied on for pain treatment as well.

SUBCUTANEOUS ADMINISTRATION

Subcutaneous administration (abbreviated *sub-q, SC,* or *SQ*) has become more popular especially in hospices or at home when medications can't be taken orally and an IV isn't already installed. Medications are injected in the loose fatty tissue planes just below the skin but above the muscle, through a tiny needle, which is relatively painless and easy to administer. Recently, hospice care workers have championed continuous and repeated injections through a tiny butterfly needle (or catheter), named for its shape—the needle's tip is left in the subcutaneous tissue and the plastic "wings" that anchor the needle are taped to the skin for periods of a week or more. This avoids hunting for scarce veins or for the need for repeated IM injections. While slightly less accurate than IV injections or drips, families can easily maintain them outside the hospital when oral medications are unreliable. Medications can be gently injected by syringe into the butterfly needle or continuously dripped via a portable, battery-powered, computerized pump (about the size of a portable tape player).

PATIENT-CONTROLLED ANALGESIA

With limits preset by the doctor, patient-controlled analgesia (PCA) has become increasingly popular because it allows the patient to decide when to take extra pain medication without waiting for a nurse. The patient (or sometimes a loved one) pushes a button to trigger a preprogrammed dose of painkiller (by IV, subcutaneously, or with an epidural, as described below) as a rescue dose for breakthrough pain or as a preventive dose before a painful activity, such as bathing. It is provided either alone or, ideally, in addition to a long-acting opioid administered around the clock through a pump. Patients are trained to recognize low-battery alarms and to change cassettes or syringes, and an on-call service is required to deal with both technical and medical issues that may arise.

When first introduced, many doctors feared patients would abuse PCA. Studies show, however, that they rarely take more medication than is needed. Most pumps prevent overuse by rendering repeated pushes ineffective if taken too close together, and most are secured to prevent addicts from breaking into the system. Another built-in safety measure is that a patient who accidentally gets too much medication will usually fall asleep and stop pressing the button.

PCA pain relief also gives patients some control at a time in their life when they often feel helpless; another benefit is that patients don't have to inappropriately negotiate for more painkiller if they hurt. Since patients are the best authorities on their own pain, it makes sense that they should have some control in treating it.

When a patient is unable to communicate his or her pain, family members may find it difficult to determine whether to push the button for a rescue dose at every grimace. Is the family treating the patient's pain or their own anxiety? Discussing these issues with the doctor or nurse is useful, since these health care professionals are familiar with the condition of the patient, know the extent of the cancer, and have experience in understanding expressions of pain in those unable to indicate it.

Also available are implantable pumps that can be externally programmed and activated by an external control pad or computer to deliver medication near the spinal cord. These devices allow more freedom of movement for bathing, working, and exercise.

Transmucosal Administration

Medications placed on the mucous membranes that line the mouth, tongue, throat, and nose tend to be rapidly absorbed and so work quickly and effectively. Also, since such medications bypass digestion, as do IV medications, lower doses can be very effective. Until recently, few medications were available to take advantage of these benefits.

Some traditional oral medications, such as morphine, have been found to be effective when crushed and given under the tongue (sublingually) or against the cheek (buccal route), and their use has become common even though not specifically approved. Many hospices routinely use certain types of liquid morphine under the tongue in patients who can't swallow, rather than starting a pump. Morphine tablets called solutabs, for example, which are made to be easily dissolved for injection, are now routinely given sublingually in hospices.

More recently, a short-acting opioid (fentanyl) has been marketed under the trade name Actiq as a sweetened lozenge on a stick, like a lollipop, for breakthrough pain. At first, officials were concerned about child safety and having a strong drug look like candy; they worried that the lozenges might send the wrong message in the war to avoid childhood drug abuse. Later studies demonstrated relative safety and a low potential for abuse, combined with extensive childproof packaging and added educational materials, which quickly led to approval. (See page 165 for more details.)

Although intranasal drugs would be convenient, they are currently not widely considered because many drugs for cancer pain are irritating to the nasal passages. Intranasal butorphanol (Stadol), although used as an alternative treatment for migraine headache, is not recommended for the management of cancer pain.

Research on inhaled opioids yields highly variable results, and so far, no reliable way of delivering uniform doses have been developed. Although not approved by the FDA, inhaled aerosolized morphine is used in hospices and some intensive care units with moderate success for pain and breathlessness. Technically, rectal, vaginal, and stomal (through a colostomy) modes of administration also belong here, but these have already been discussed (see page 144).

Central Nervous System Administration: Spinal and Intraventricular Routes

As we've said, since injections by most routes (IV, IM, sub-q) are usually not more effective than oral medication, their use should be limited to urgent situations or when oral medications can't be taken. However, giving morphine and other opioids through special catheters placed near the spine provides more relief with lower doses because the drug is so close to the body's pain receptors.

Relief can last weeks, months, and even years by using these spinal routes (epidural, intrathecal, or subarachnoid), which range from a standard epidural catheter taped to the back to the use of more durable catheters tunneled under the skin and connected to an external pump that can be carried in a handbag or even to miniaturized programmable pumps surgically implanted under the skin.

Adding dilute local anesthetic to an epidural system can produce just enough numbness to relieve even truly unbearable pain, such as that of a broken bone. These treatments are particularly useful for patients with pain in the lower abdomen, back, or legs for whom systemwide dosing causes persistent side effects, and often can relieve pain at other levels. These advantages, however, must be balanced against the risk of infection, back pain, and the need for specialist care and minor surgery, as well as a resourceful care network.

Intraventricular administration involves delivering opioids directly into the fluid (cerebrospinal fluid or CSF) surrounding the brain. Such treatment is especially effective for complex pain involving the head and neck that is resistant to more conventional treatment. A neurosurgeon with special training must establish access to the CSF, a procedure that is similar to putting in a shunt to reduce the raised intracranial pressure that accompanies some brain tumors. Fortunately, the need for this type of treatment is infrequent. As with other aggressive therapies that are by their nature associated with some increased risk, careful patient selection is of paramount importance.

Tip: Get a laxative! Everyone who takes opioids needs to take laxatives, at least from time to time, and usually on a daily basis. If you are prescribed an opioid and not a laxative, ask for one! Dietary fiber and fiber supplements are not adequate.

We'll now look at the strong opioids in more detail. The following information, however, is intended as a guide only and should not be used as a substitute for a doctor's care and judgment.

The Strong Opioid Medications

MORPHINE
As probably the most widely used opioid drug, and the one that has been around the longest, morphine is the standard opioid to which others are compared. It is available in such a wide variety of forms and concentrations (immediate-release and controlled-release tablets, liquid solutions or elixirs, suppositories, standard injections, and preservative-free spinal

injections) that have such different characteristics that doctors practically consider them different medications.

Brand Name

Immediate-release (short-acting) morphine comes in several forms. MSIR and Roxanol are immediate-release oral formulations (in tablet and liquid forms). While their effects are not truly immediate, they have earned this name to distinguish them from the more recently developed controlled-release (also called sustained-, delayed-, or continuous-release) forms. A special kind of immediate-release tablet is the morphine solutab, which, in addition to regular oral use, can be easily dissolved for injection or can be put under the tongue or in the cheek for absorption.

Brand names of controlled-release (long-acting) morphine include MS Contin and Oramorph. These tablets *should never be cut, broken, chewed, or crushed* and are best taken every twelve hours (sometimes every eight hours, but never more frequently). A newer controlled-release capsule, Kadian (also called Kapanol), is ideally prescribed just once per day but is sometimes needed as often as twice daily. Each capsule contains around a hundred tiny controlled-release pellets, which can be sprinkled on applesauce, pudding, and other foods.

The Psychology of Larger-Dose Medications

Prescribing may be influenced not just by science but by perception, psychology, and the fear of regulatory scrutiny.

For example, the first controlled-release oral morphine product, MS Contin, was originally only available in a 30 mg tablet. It was very popular because its effects lasted up to twelve hours. It was so widely embraced that multiple tablets were commonly prescribed for severe pain. But when a 60 mg tablet was introduced, it was only moderately successful, because doctors were concerned that prescribing the higher dose would draw the attention of the authorities. The 60 mg tablet only became a big seller when a 100 mg tablet became available, which in turn didn't take off until a 200 mg tablet was developed. At each stage, the highest-dose tablet has been less popular. Even today, doctors are more likely to prescribe two 100 mg tablets then a single 200 mg tablet, despite cost savings.

Although doctors are usually quick to embrace new products, when it comes to highly regulated (and scrutinized) drugs, they are reluctant to use the highest available strength, even though they may prescribe the same dose by combining multiple lower-strength tablets. Why? Because they fear being profiled as overprescribers. As a result, new guidelines emphasize the importance of prescribing analgesics using rational scientific principles, and new legislative initiatives have been introduced to indemnify doctors who prescribe analgesics appropriately. Although current prescribing is less influenced by the fear factor than in the past, perceptions are slow to change, especially when they involve a threat to doctors, reputations, and livelihoods. We still have more work to do to further decriminalize appropriate pain management.

The Story of Morphine

Opium is the powder derived from the milky juice of split, unripe seed capsules of the oriental poppy. Long renowned for its powerful narcotic effects, opium has been used as a pain reliever for centuries.

As early as 6000 BC the Sumerians carved stone tablets with pictures of the poppy and were evidently aware of its mind-altering and pain-relieving effects. The ancient Greeks wrote of it, and its constipating effect warranted its use in the treatment of dysentery in the Middle East. Hippocrates, the "father of medicine," endorsed opium's medicinal effects in 460 BC, and over the ages the Chinese, Egyptians, and Romans all referred to opium as a remedy for a variety of maladies.

So calming were its effects that the painkiller was used recreationally in the 1600s, a trend that peaked in the 1800s, when hypodermic syringes became available by mail order. Widely available, opium was used freely, initially without social stigma. Occasional to frequent users included Lord Byron, Shelley, Keats, Coleridge, Elizabeth Barrett Browning, Dickens, Turner, Freud, Darwin—even Florence Nightingale and the fictional Sherlock Holmes.

In 1801 chemists synthesized a substance from opium that was ten times as potent. Dubbed morphine—for the god of sleep, Morpheus—it was hailed as "God's own medicine." During the Civil War, 10 million opium pills, over 2,840,000 ounces of other opioid preparations (such as laudanum or paregoric), and almost 30,000 ounces of morphine sulfate were dispensed to ailing Union soldiers alone. The resulting "addiction" prompted research into strong painkillers that would not be habit-forming. In the late 1800s the Bayer Company marketed a derivative that was twenty-five times stronger than opium resin; promoted as being as strong as a legendary hero, it was dubbed heroin. Originally viewed as a nonaddictive cough suppressant and painkiller that would cure morphine addicts, the highly addictive nature of heroin soon became evident, and the Harrison Narcotics Act in 1914 banned opioids, cocaine, and cannabis from over-the-counter medicines.

Despite the potential for abuse, the World Health Organization and other public health bodies have always recognized that most of these substances are indispensable for the medical treatment of pain and that when they are properly used addiction is rare. The WHO and others have launched an international campaign to eliminate the confusion and misconceptions that inappropriately inhibit the appropriate medical use of these substances.

Other forms of morphine include RMS (rectal morphine suppository), a waxy bullet-shaped suppository, and preservative-free morphine (Duramorph, Astramorph, Infumorph), which is used for intraspinal use. *Sterile morphine solution* is a generic term for preparations suited for intramuscular, subcutaneous, and intravenous uses.

Dose Range

Starting doses vary considerably but in general are 20 to 30 mg by mouth every three or four hours. If administered subcutaneously, intramuscularly, or intravenously, the starting dose is 5 to 15 mg every one to four hours until an adequate dose that lasts for four hours is achieved. Controlled-release morphine is usually started at a dose of 30 mg twice a day. Intraspinal doses vary.

When switching from injection to oral morphine or vice versa, the oral dose should be two to three times the injected dose. Conversely, the oral dose should be cut by one-half or two-thirds if the patient is being switched to an intramuscular, intravenous, or subcutaneous dose. This ratio, however, applies to patients who have already been taking morphine for some time. When new to morphine, the ratio may be closer to 1 to 6 rather than 1 to 3. When a patient is switched from IM to oral medication, or vice versa, families may find it helpful to refer to the equianalgesic doses in the table on p. 154.

How Long It Takes to Reach Peak Effect

If administered via a needle, morphine begins to work within five to ten minutes; its effects peak at fifteen to thirty minutes, and last about three hours when administered in an adequate dose.

Slow- or extended-release oral preparations of morphine (MS Contin, Oramorph, MS-ER, Kadian) become effective within about one and a half to three hours and, when given in adequate doses, may last from eight to twenty-four hours, depending on the brand and its release properties. *These tablets must not be broken, crushed, or chewed.* To minimize the roller-coaster effect, long-acting opioid preparations are ideally administered on an around-the-clock schedule, so relief is continuous. This sometimes leads to a false perception that the short-acting breakthrough pain agent (the effects of which are more noticeable) is what is really effective, when it is the steady blood levels achieved by the scheduled long-acting agent that allows the as-needed medication to work.

Equivalent Pain Relief

The effects of 2 mg of IM morphine are about equivalent to those of 650 mg of aspirin (though their mechanisms and quality of pain relief differ).

Comments

- Starting doses can be hard to calculate. If the patient becomes overly sedated with the first dose and has no pain, then the next dose should be cut by 50 percent. On the other hand, if pain relief is inadequate in the first twenty-four hours after consistent around-the-clock use, then the starting dose should usually be raised by up to 50 percent; if pain breaks through, the doctor may prescribe a dose every two or three hours, rather than every four hours, to achieve pain relief.
- Immediate-release morphine tablets work relatively quickly for a relatively short period, while controlled-release morphine tablets

take longer to work but are effective for up to twelve hours. Long-acting or controlled-release tablets must be swallowed whole (fortunately they are small) and not taken more than every eight hours.

- Morphine solutions should be stored in cool areas, away from direct sunlight. Solutions used in warm climates should have antimicrobial preservatives.

- Close contact with the doctor, pharmacist, or nurse who is monitoring the medication should be maintained, especially during the first twenty-four hours and then not more than seventy-two hours later. Ideally, the family should have regular contact with the health care provider, at least every few days or more frequently if conditions change. Patients need to be monitored for side effects, altered mental status, and psychological complications.

- Although most patients take between 5 and 30 mg every four hours, doses range enormously, with no ceiling dose. A few patients require as much as 1,000 mg an hour or more. A recent survey of those with advanced cancer found that the average daily opioid dose was equivalent to 400 to 600 mg of intramuscular morphine; about 10 percent of those surveyed needed more than 2,000 mg, and one patient required more than 35,000 mg per twenty-four hours. By the same token, many patients require lower-than-average doses.

Precautions
- Although most morphine-related side effects (except constipation) resolve within a few days of steady use, persistent sedation or nausea occasionally occurs, especially when used in high doses, with the elderly, or in those with kidney failure.

- Constipation is extremely common, so preventive measures should be taken, from adding fruits, vegetables, and bulk-forming grain to the diet to encouraging activity (especially walking). Most patients also need a daily mild laxative, preferably taken at night. Some doctors warn that preventing constipation may be more difficult than preventing pain (see Chapter 10) and so suggest that the same hand that prescribes for morphine should also prescribe a laxative.

- Nausea is initially common when starting morphine but usually does not persist beyond a few days. About one-third of patients need antiemetic medication to prevent nausea (see Chapter 10), but often for less than a week after starting an opioid, and sometimes after its dose is increased.

- Vomiting requires treatment with an antiemetic, to prevent both dehydration and loss of medication, but usually does not last longer than a few days.

Equivalent Dosing: How the Doctor Switches Between Drugs

Drug	Oral Dose	Ratio Between Oral and IM and Sub-q Injection	IM or Sub-q Dose	Comments
Morphine				
Repeated dose (after patient has been on medication for at least a week)	30 mg	3:1	10 mg	1
Single dose	60 mg	6:1	10 mg	
Hydromorphone (Dilaudid)	8 mg	5:1	1.6 mg	
Oxycodone	30 mg	—	—	1
Fentanyl	—		.1 mg	2
Oxymorphone	—		1 mg	
Methadone hydrochloride (Dolophine)	10 mg	2:1	10 mg	
Levorphanol (Levo-Dromoran)	2 mg	1:1	2 mg	
Meperidine hydrochloride (Demerol)	300 mg	4:1	75 mg	
Codeine	200 mg	1.5:1	130 mg	

Note: One of the leading causes of undermedication is that errors are made in dosing when patients are switched from one method of administration to another (e.g., from receiving injections to receiving pills) or from one drug to another. This table is the same guide the doctor would probably use when planning such a change. The "conversion ratios" are approximate and may differ somewhat between patients. The ratio is given between oral medication and intramuscular (IM) or subcutaneous (sub-q) injection.

The reference dose against which other drugs are measured is 10 mg of intramuscular morphine in the treatment of severe pain.

Comments
1. Also available in slow release.
2. Patch (transdermal): 100 mcg/hr, roughly equal to 4 mg/IM morphine.

- Drowsiness, confusion, dizziness, unsteadiness, and sedation are very common during the first five days after starting treatment or raising a dose, and usually clear up within a week. Persistent sedation can sometimes be alleviated with stimulants, such as strong coffee or medication (see Chapter 8).
- Respiratory depression (the slowing of breathing) is rare in cancer patients but often erroneously cited as a reason for not giving enough pain medication.
- Other, less frequently encountered side effects include severe sweating (diaphoresis), hallucinations, difficulty breathing (bronchoconstriction), urinary retention, and twitching.
- These problems are side effects, not signs of allergy, and can usually be either waited out until the patient becomes tolerant to the side effects or managed with another prescribed medication (laxa-

tive, antiemetic, or stimulant). True allergy to morphine is extremely rare.

- Side effects don't always occur, but if they do, inform the doctor so that they may be treated. If a side effect does not subside, the doctor may consider trying a different opioid, another type of medication, or a whole new approach to treatment (see Chapters 8 through 11).
- Remember: addiction is *not* a problem when treating cancer pain.

TRANSDERMAL FENTANYL

Brand Name
Duragesic.

Dose Range
Available in four sizes that deliver 25, 50, 75 or 100 mcg (mg) of fentanyl hourly. A microgram is a thousandth of a milligram (1,000 mcg = 1 mg). Fentanyl is administered in microgram doses because it is such a potent opioid—about a hundred times stronger than morphine. The recommended starting dose is 25 mcg/hour for those who have been taking little or no opioid medication on a steady basis. Most patients are managed with one or two patches (of varying sizes) that are changed every seventy-two hours (three days), making treatment extremely convenient. Although as many as sixteen of the largest patches could be safely used at once (an approach humorously referred to as "fentanyl long underwear"), so much skin would be covered that the convenience factor would be greatly reduced.

How Long It Takes to Reach Peak Effect
When treatment is initiated or when the dose is increased, expect a delay of four to eight hours before effects are first noted and around six to twelve hours before it is fully effective because it takes time for the drug to be absorbed through the skin. Like other long-acting, around-the-clock medications, an appropriate dose should provide steady and uninterrupted relief even though patches are changed every three days. If treatment is interrupted, it may take up to twenty-four hours before most of the medication's effect dissipates. Thus, if an inadvertent overdose or a side effect arises, patients need to be observed for up to a day after patch removal. If pain escalates well before a patch is scheduled to be replaced, the patient probably needs a higher dose, though 5 to 10 percent of patients may benefit from more frequent patch changes, such as every sixty hours or even every forty-eight hours. Often several patches of varying sizes (doses) are used at once to achieve the desired dose.

Equivalent Pain Relief

A single 25 mcg patch equals about 60 mg of oral morphine per day. Up to 50 percent of patients will require slightly higher doses than suggested in the equianalgesic chart included in the drug's package insert.

Comments

- This skin-patch form of medication is now widely used because it's so convenient; it reduces the need for pills, needles, and pumps; and its use is independent of most external factors such as height, weight, age, skin color, sex, and skin thickness.
- As with other opioids, the patch still needs to be supplemented with a short-acting drug (orally or rectally) for breakthrough and incident pain, especially during the six to twelve hours before the drug takes full effect.
- Constipation tends to be much less of a problem in people who use the patches.
- A electrophoretic delivery system may soon be available; it uses a low-voltage current to drive fentanyl more rapidly across the skin, as well as an imbedded microcomputer chip that will allow patients to apply pressure to trigger a rescue dose for prompt relief within ten minutes. The proposed patch will need to be changed every twenty-four hours or after eighty discharges.

Benefits of Skin Patch (Transdermal Fentanyl or Duragesic Therapy)

- Convenient, noninvasive, and may minimize the need for so many pills.
- When effective, relief is continuous and steady.
- Can stay ahead of or prevent severe pain.
- May cause fewer constipation problems.
- Especially useful for patients who try to hold out as long as possible before asking for pills.
- Especially useful when the ability to swallow pills is compromised (dry mouth, nausea, swallowing problems, blocked digestion).
- Well accepted by patients and doctors alike.
- Difficult to abuse, but if an addict tries to inject the patch's content, it can be extremely dangerous.

Precautions

- Side effects are similar to those for morphine (although constipation is much less of a problem).
- Heat (such as from a waterbed, heating pad, or even a persistently high fever) is the only factor that has been shown to significantly increase doses (occasionally even to dangerous levels). Thus prolonged or excessive heat should be avoided when using the patch.

Tips on Using Skin Patches (Transdermal Fentanyl or Duragesic Therapy)

- Keep patches in a secure (preferably locked) location, away from children and those with drug problems.

- Never cut patches before applying.

- Choose a flat, less hairy surface of the chest, back, flank, or upper arm where movement will not loosen or dislodge the patch. The site should have no irritation, cuts, or sores. Excess hair may be clipped (but not shaved) to avoid irritation.

- There is no advantage to placing the patch directly over or even near the painful area.

- Before application, clean the skin area with water and pat dry.

- Immediately after placement, apply firm pressure to the entire surface (especially edges) with the palm of the hand for a full two minutes.

- The patch's adherence may be reinforced with paper tape or an occlusive dressing (like Tegaderm).

- Expect a six-to-twelve-hour delay in relief when the patch is first started or the dose is raised. So be sure to have a short-acting painkiller on hand for breakthrough pain.

- Avoid ointments, alcohol, and cologne near the patch area.

- When replacing a patch, pick a different site.

- Redness, irritation, and occasionally even droplets of fluid appear where a patch has been placed. This does not indicate allergy or infection, just irritation, and usually resolves on its own.

- If skin reactions are persistent, spraying three or four puffs of a prescribed metered dose of steroid inhaler, such as Vanceril or Beclovent, on the site before applying the patch may be helpful.

- Because skin temperature can affect drug absorption, keep the area away from heating pads, heat lamps, electric blankets, heated waterbeds, and other sources of external heat.

- Persistent high fevers can also increase drug delivery (up to 25–33 percent with a 104°F fever), so be alert to more side effects.

- If the patch produces side effects, they may persist for up to a day after treatment is stopped.

- The patch appears to be less prone to produce constipation than most other opioid therapies, but at least a mild laxative is still commonly needed.

- Patches are usually changed every seventy-two hours (three days), but relief is still relatively continuous.

- If pain intensifies (or more breakthrough medications are needed) consistently on the day that the patch is to be changed, the doctor may need to prescribe a higher-dose patch. There is no maximum dose, and if necessary multiple patches can be combined. Rarely, the doctor may consider instructions to change patches every sixty hours or even every forty-eight hours.

- For disposal, ideally fold patch to stick to itself and flush down toilet.

CONTROLLED-RELEASE OXYCODONE

Brand Name
OxyContin.

Dose Range
Tablets containing 10, 20, 40, 80, and 160 mg of oxycodone in a controlled-release matrix have been widely used. Due to street abuse by drug addicts (not patients) and publicity about this abuse, the manufacturer voluntarily stopped shipping the 160 mg tablets in 2001, at least on a temporary basis. Although they should never be broken, crushed, or chewed, tablets may be combined to achieve the desired dose.

The OxyContin Story

Introduced in 1995, OxyContin tablets slowly release their powerful opioid to promote steady comfort and a good night's sleep. Hailed as a wonder drug by patients and physicians, sales skyrocketed to more than $1 billion, greater even than those of Viagra. Originally targeted for cancer pain, OxyContin is now used increasingly for chronic pain from other causes. In 2000, however, reports of abuse skyrocketed with sensationalistic articles full of grim details of high street values, violent robberies, and methods of abuse. These reports so terrified doctors, patients, pharmacists, and family members that legitimate OxyContin use (along with the proper use of other opioids) plummeted, signifying a major step backward in the war to decriminalize the legitimate treatment of authentic pain problems. An almost evangelical crusade to promote more aggressive treatment of pain has underestimated the determination of addicts to abuse drugs by any means. Once again, innocent sufferers with unremitting pain and their committed physicians have became casualties of a war on drugs that has nothing to do with medical treatment.

Although it was originally assumed that OxyContin's potential for abuse was minimal because the narcotic was released slowly and does not produce a high when used properly, newer reports suggest that no other prescription drug in the last two decades has been illegally abused as much as OxyContin. While initial reports claimed that OxyContin was responsible for more than one hundred deaths, it is now recognized that most of the deaths resulted from the very dangerous practice of combining various depressant drugs, often with alcohol. Instead of swallowing the pill whole, abusers seeking to experience a high ingest all twelve hours' worth of the drug at once by crushing the tablets and swallowing, sniffing, or injecting the resulting powder.

Tales of abuse should not scare off families or health care providers. OxyContin was first embraced because it lacked the stigma of morphine but was just as effective. It is illogical to now attack its therapeutic use because addicts have learned to "cheat" its slow-release system by crushing tablets. We don't stop writing and cashing checks just because crooks pass rubber checks, and by the same token, patients should not be deprived of a useful medication because others abuse it. As with many things, drugs are either useful or dangerous, depending on the intent of the users.

How Long It Takes to Reach Peak Effect

This product has a dual action: an initial rapid release of the drug that provides quick relief within an hour or so, followed by a protracted-release phase to provide steady relief over a twelve-hour period. While doses can usually be adjusted for twice-daily use (every twelve hours), some patients benefit from three times daily use (every eight hours).

Equivalent Pain Relief

While studies suggest that oral oxycodone is about twice as potent as oral morphine, many clinicians feel that these drugs are about equally potent, and in some cases, oral morphine may be even more potent. Based on this data, 30 mg of oral oxycodone provides the same relief as a 5 to 10 mg injection of morphine.

Comments

- Offers twelve hours of smooth and reliable pain control.
- Swallow tablets whole; do not break, chew, or crush, as doing so could lead to potentially toxic doses.

Precautions

- Same as morphine; side effects, except constipation, tend to diminish over time.

IMMEDIATE-RELEASE OXYCODONE

Brand Name

With acetaminophen: Oxycet, Percocet, Roxicet, Tylox, Roxilox, Oxycodone/ACE (capsule 5/500 and tablet 5/325). With aspirin: Percodan, Roxiprin Full, Endodan (5/325), Percodan-Demi (2.5/325)—see Chapter 6. Single-entity agent: Roxicodone (5 mg, 15 mg, 30 mg), Oxy-IR, M-Oxy, Percolone, Endocodone.

In liquid form: OxyFAST (liquid), oxycodone oral solution (5 mg/5 ml), Intensol oral solution (20 mg/ml), Roxicodone SR.

Dose Range

Most commonly, 5 mg tablets, with the more recent release of less readily available 15 and 30 mg tablets.

How Long It Takes to Reach Peak Effect

"Immediate release" is somewhat misleading in that it means that the oxycodone is *not* imbedded in a slow-release matrix. It is most commonly used as needed for severe intermittent pain or for breakthrough pain, along with a long-acting opioid taken on a fixed schedule. Again, if rescue doses are consistently needed more than a few times daily, the dose of the long-acting ATC drug usually needs to be raised.

Comments

For years oxycodone was only available in fixed combinations with aspirin (Percodan) or acetaminophen (Percocet). That's why it is still regarded by many as a weak opioid conventionally used to treat moderate pain. As such, patients taking oxycodone for moderate pain can keep using the same drug if the pain turns severe or for breakthrough pain. Another advantage is that its breakdown products (metabolites) appear to be much less of a problem than with other opioids.

Precautions

- Similar to morphine.

HYDROMORPHONE

Brand Name

Dilaudid.

Dose Range

Orally, usually 2 to 8 mg every three to four hours; by injection, 1 to 2 mg every three to four hours.

How Long It Takes to Reach Peak Effect

Oral: fifteen to thirty minutes, peaking within an hour and lasting from two to four hours depending on the dose. Injection: five minutes, peaking in fifteen minutes, and lasting three to four hours.

Equivalent Pain Relief

Orally, four to five times more potent than morphine (7 mg hydromorphone is equal to about 30 mg oral morphine). By injection, about six times more potent than morphine (1.5 mg of hydromorphone IM is equivalent to about 10 mg injected morphine).

Comments

- Hydromorphone is used quite commonly as an alternative to morphine.
- Hydromorphone is relatively inexpensive and is available in a variety of forms (oral, rectal, and by injection).
- It works relatively quickly, and because it doesn't accumulate in the system, it is safe for patients with liver or kidney problems.
- Hydromorphone doesn't last very long, so it usually needs to be administered frequently (as often as every three hours).
- It is particularly useful for subcutaneous injections (usually given by a portable pump) because it is so soluble (in other words, it is possible to dissolve a great deal of the drug in a small volume of fluid), which helps maintain sub-q sites for longer intervals.

- Especially under its trade name, Dilaudid, this drug has a reputation for abuse and high "street value," so doctors may be reluctant to prescribe it.
- Several companies have perfected slow-release preparations of hydromorphone, but as of this writing, none is available.

Precautions
- See under morphine.

METHADONE

Brand Name
Dolophine.

Dose Range
Although doses are highly variable and difficult to predict, the usual starting dose is 5 to 20 mg by mouth, at intervals varying from every four hours to every twelve hours. If given intravenously (IV) or as an intramuscular injection (IM), 5 to 10 mg every four to six hours is a usual starting dose.

How Long It Takes to Reach Peak Effect
After a single pill or injection, effects are evident within thirty minutes, peaking within an hour and lasting four to twelve hours. Several days (four to fourteen) may be required before a steady state is reached. The way the body breaks down and disposes of methadone is less predictable than for most opioids, so it may take one to two weeks of use before the best dose and schedule can be determined. Frequent dose changes or erratic use may be unsafe when treatment is first started, especially in the elderly and in those with altered renal function.

Equivalent Pain Relief
With single doses or initial use, 10 mg of methadone given by injection or 20 mg orally is usually equivalent to 10 mg injected morphine or 30 of mg oral morphine. When used regularly, potency increases, sometimes up to five to ten times that of morphine (see below).

Comments
- Methadone is associated almost exclusively with drug addiction because of its usefulness to recovering addicts. However, methadone is being rediscovered for pain relief. More doctors are finding it is appropriate as a second- or third-line treatment for pain; it is not a preferred drug because adjusting doses quickly yet safely is more difficult.
- Methadone, unlike other opioids, may be especially effective for neuropathic pain (due to nerve injury) and intractable cancer pain.

That's because, unlike other commonly used opioids, methadone can antagonize or block the receptors for an amino acid, N-methyl-D-aspartate (NMDA), in the central nervous system. These receptors, which are activated by painful stimuli, are thought to be responsible for hypersensitivity and an amplified pain effect (the "wind-up" phenomenon).

- Treatment with methadone is very inexpensive, usually a tenth to a hundredth of the cost of treating with other opioids.

- When given steadily and repeatedly, methadone appears to be five to ten times more potent than morphine and can stay effective for a relatively long time, about eight hours (ranging from four to twenty-four hours).

- Conventional equianalgesic conversion tables are outdated, and using them can result in severe toxicity and even death.

- Doctors must carefully monitor dosing for the first ten days of use, until the blood has a high enough steady level of methadone. After the first few days and weeks, the chances of serious side effects are minimal

- Although around-the-clock treatment is usually preferred to as-needed treatment with the strong opioids, methadone is different. Since methadone is needed as frequently as every four hours in some patients and as infrequently as every twelve or even twenty-four hours in others, many authorities start with as-needed administration and switch to an around-the-clock dose only when a given patient's best schedule is established.

- Administering methadone effectively and safely takes more skill and closer observation by a doctor than morphine and the other opioids. That's why methadone is *not* recommended as a first choice. However, doctors who are familiar with methadone may prefer it because it is much cheaper than alternatives such as controlled-release oxycodone, morphine, and transdermal fentanyl.

- Methadone is very commonly used in methadone maintenance programs as a method to manage addiction in street addicts. This alternative use should not be confused with its medical use as an analgesic. Just as with morphine and other opioids, when methadone is used to treat cancer pain addiction is extremely rare.

- Recently, as law enforcement officials have become more vigilant about the abuse of OxyContin, drug seekers are increasingly turning to methadone when other high-inducing drugs aren't available because methadone is easier to obtain. Drug abusers can easily overdose when methadone doesn't produce the effect they have come to expect from other street drugs.

Precautions

- See precautions listed for morphine.
- Methadone is not usually used in elderly or confused patients, or in those with respiratory, liver, or kidney problems, especially if these problems are progressive.
- Methadone can cause sedation as it accumulates in the body, especially during the first days of treatment or after a dose increase. Generally, it is best to wait for about one week before drawing conclusions about a new dose's effectiveness and side effects.

LEVORPHANOL

Brand Name
Levo-Dromoran, Levorphan.

Dose Range
Orally, usually 2 to 4 mg every four to eight hours (like methadone, dose interval is variable). By IM injection, 2 to 4 mg every four to six hours. Intravenously, 1 mg every four to six hours.

How Long It Takes to Reach Peak Effect
Oral: onset usually within thirty minutes, peak effect at sixty to ninety minutes, and duration of four to six hours. Injection and IV: onset usually within fifteen minutes, peak within thirty minutes, and duration of four to six hours.

Equivalent Pain Relief
Oral levorphanol is about seven times more potent than oral morphine (4 mg oral levorphanol equals 30 mg oral morphine). Injectable levorphanol is about five times more potent than injectable morphine (2 mg levorphanol equals 10 mg morphine).

Comments

- Levorphanol lasts longer than morphine, so patients usually need fewer doses per day.
- Levorphanol may be useful for patients who cannot tolerate morphine.
- Compared to similar opioids, which usually last two to four hours, oxymorphone is relatively long-acting, usually lasting from four to six hours.
- As with oxymorphone, despite having been available for decades, its use is not common, levorphanol is still relatively expensive, and shortages are common.

Precautions
- See under morphine and methadone.
- Like methadone, caution is recommended when adjusting doses to avoid toxicity due to accumulation, especially in the elderly and if renal function is compromised.

OXYMORPHONE

Brand Name
Numorphan.

Dose Range
By injection, 1 to 2 mg every four to six hours. By rectal suppository, 10 mg every four to six hours.

How Long It Takes to Reach Peak Effect
Injection: onset is five to ten minutes, peaking within thirty minutes for IV and thirty to ninety minutes for IM, and lasting three to six hours. Rectal: onset within thirty minutes, peaking within two hours, and lasting up to six hours.

Equivalent Pain Relief
A 1 mg injection or a 10 mg suppository is about equivalent to 10 mg of injectable morphine and 30 mg oral morphine.

Comments
- Oxymorphone is not currently available in oral forms, but only as an IV or IM injection or as a rectal suppository. New dose forms, including controlled-release and immediate-release oral preparations, are expected to be available in the near future.
- Compared to similar opioids, oxymorphone is relatively long-acting.
- Despite having been available for decades, oxymorphone use is not common. It is still relatively expensive, and shortages are common.

Precautions
- See under morphine.

DIACETYLMORPHINE (HEROIN)

Brand Name
None.

Dose Range
Five to 20 mg IM every four hours, 60 mg by mouth.

How Long It Takes to Reach Peak Effect
Oral: one to two hours. Injection: thirty minutes to one hour; relief should last three to four hours..

Equivalent Pain Relief
A 5 mg IM dose of heroin is equivalent to 10 mg morphine IM.

Comments
- Scheduled by the FDA as a Class I substance (use restricted to research), heroin is not legally available in the United States but is a common drug of abuse. However, heroin is well accepted and used as a standard analgesic in the United Kingdom, where it is often called diamorphine. Because of so much interest in heroin as a pain reliever, the U.S. government has sponsored several clinical research programs, but researchers consistently find it no more effective than morphine, and with similar side effects.
- Heroin has no effect until the body naturally converts it to morphine, at which time it works rapidly; that makes it a drug of choice for abusers. Scientifically, researchers suggest that medicating with heroin is simply an inefficient way to give morphine.
- The main clinical advantage of heroin is that a large amount can be dissolved in a small volume, making it very efficient for subcutaneous use. Its continued use in the United Kingdom relates largely to tradition and the relative unavailability of hydromorphone there. Although theoretically available in Canada, it is used there only rarely.

Precautions
- See under morphine.
- Heightened addiction liability and risk of diversion.

ORAL TRANSMUCOSAL FENTANYL CITRATE (OTFC)

Brand Name
Actiq.

Dose Range
The lozenges come in 200, 400, 600, 800, 1,200, and 1,600 mcg doses. Usually started at the lowest dose (200 mcg) and increased if needed, with another unit as soon as fifteen minutes later.

How Long It Takes to Reach Peak Effect
Within five to ten minutes, which is ideal to manage severe or rapid-onset breakthrough pain. It peaks within forty-five minutes and lasts three to six hours.

Comments

- Actiq is a sweetened fentanyl lozenge, the first medication available as a lozenge mounted on a handle. It resembles a lollipop, but this term is avoided in order not to link it to candy. Instead, it's called a lozenge, unit, or oralette.
- It is the only painkiller specifically approved for treating breakthrough pain in cancer patients. It should be used when a patient is already taking longer-acting opioids for relief of baseline pain.
- The medication works nearly as quickly as an IV injection and so is well suited for severe or rapid-onset breakthrough pain.
- By taking fifteen minutes to finish a lozenge, about half the medication is swallowed, which helps the drug last a lot longer than if all of it were absorbed in the mouth's mucous membranes. Never bite or chew it, since this results in more drug being swallowed and reduces efficiency.
- Consistent use of more than four units a day suggests that the dose of the long-acting analgesic used should be raised.
- Although the packaging for these lozenges is extremely childproof (and very bulky and space-consuming), partially consumed lozenges should be thrown out to avoid accidental consumption.
- Actiq has been slow to catch on even though most people are highly satisfied with its rapid onset and are reluctant to return to their old breakthrough pain medication. Insurers balk at the higher cost (all that childproof packaging) and pharmacies don't always have enough storage space.

Precautions

- Most common side effects are drowsiness, nausea, and dizziness.
- Actiq may produce dangerous, even fatal, respiratory depression in children and in adults not already accustomed to using narcotic analgesics.

Other Drugs

Although there are other classes of moderately strong opioid drugs known as mixed agonist-antagonists and partial agonists (more fully described in Chapter 6), these are generally not recommended for treating cancer pain because they may interfere with and even reverse the effects of morphine and morphinelike drugs, they have maximum doses above which they are not more effective (ceiling effect), and they are more likely to cause excitation, hallucinations, and confusion (psychotomimetic effects).

Another medication that's not appropriate for chronic cancer pain is meperidine (Demerol or Pethedine), an analgesic that is still frequently prescribed for pain after surgery and other acute pain. Ongoing use of meperidine is linked with muscle jerks, confusion, agitation, and seizures. These side effects and other complications are more common in patients with kidney problems and in the elderly, as well as when meperidine is prescribed orally.

Analgesic medications are big business, and on the forefront are "smarter," less abusable drugs and innovative routes of drug delivery, as well as new, more specific compounds associated with fewer side effects.

For additional information about the most common opioids, see table on following pages.

Most Common Opioids Used for Cancer Pain

Generic Name	Trade Name[a]	Route[b]	Equianalgesic Dose[c]	Recommended Schedule[d]	Formulations[a]	Comments[e]
Immediate-release morphine	MSIR	Oral	30–60 mg g	2–4 hr	10, 15, or 30 mg	1,2
	Roxanol	Oral			2mg/ml; 4 mg/ml; 20 mg/ml; 10 mg/2.5 ml; 10 mg/5 ml; 20 mg/5 ml; 100 mg/5ml	
Controlled-release morphine	MS Contin	Oral	30–60 mg	8–12 hr	15, 30, 60, 100, or 200 mg	2,3
	Oramorph				various	2
	Kadian			12–24 hr	10, 20, 50, or 100 mg	
	Avinza			12–24 hr	30, 60, 90, or 120 mg	2,4
Morphine		IM	10 mg	2–4 hr	various	—
Morphine	RMS	Rectal	15 mg	72 hr	5, 10, 20, or 30 mg	5
Fentanyl	Duragic	TM	25 mcg		25, 50, 75, or 100 mcg	
Controlled-release oxycodone	Oxy-Contin	Oral	30 mg	12 hr	10, 20, 40, or 80 mg	6
Immediate-release oxycodone (single entities, not combined with another medication)	Roxocodone Oxy-IR, M-Oxy, Percolone, Endocodone *Liquid:* OxyFast (liquid) Oxycodone Intensol Roxicodone SR Proladone (suppository)	Oral	20 mg	72–48 hr	5, 15, or 30 mg	7
Hydromorphone	Dilaudid	Oral		2–4 hr	1, 2, 3, or 4 mg	8
Hydromorphone	Dilaudid	IM	7.5 mg	2–4 hr	1, 2, 4, or 10 mg/ml	8
Hydromorphone	Dilaudid	Rectal	1.5 mg	3–6 hr	3 mg	8
Methadone	Dolophine	Oral	7.5 mg	4–12 hr	5, 10, or 40 mg	9
			20 mg		1, 2, or 10 mg/ml	

Methadone	Dolophine	IM	2–4 mg	4–12 hr	10 mg/ml	9
Levorphanol	Levo-Dromoran	Oral	4 mg	4–8 hr	2 mg	10
Levorphanol	Levo-Dromoran	IM	2 mg	4–8 hr	2 mg/ml	10
Oxymorphone	Numorphan	IM	1 mg	3–6 hr	1 or 1.5 mg/ml	11
Oxymorphone	Numorphan	Rectal	5–10 mg	3–6 hr	5 mg	11
Diamorphine	Heroin	Oral	60 mg	4 hr		12
Diamorphine	Heroin	IM	5 mg	4hr		12
Oral transmucosal fentanyl citrate	Actiq	Oral	200 mcg	3–6 hr	200, 400, 600, 800, 1200, or 1600 mg	13

Notes

[a]Listing is partial, comprised mostly of formulations available in the United States. Doses are in mg unless stated otherwise.

[b]For parenteral routes (those taken in ways that do not involve the digestive tract), only the most commonly used route is listed; most medications, however, can be administered intramuscularly (IM), subcutaneously (sub-q), or intravenously (IV). TD means transdermal (absorbed through the skin).

[c]Equianalgesic dose refers to the dose that provides the equivalent pain relief as 10 mg of IM morphine. These doses are based on values most frequently cited in the medical literature and on clinical experience, although these sometimes conflict. They are approximate and are intended to serve as guidelines only.

[d]This is a rough guideline only; physicians may deviate from these schedules as they tailor medication schedules to particular patients.

[e]Side effects and precautions for all the opioid medications include constipation, sedation, dysphoria (unpleasant moods or feelings), confusion, hallucinations, nausea, vomiting, respiratory depression (which is rare in patients who have developed a tolerance to opioids), urinary retention (difficulty urinating), and itching. How patients react to opioids differs from patient to patient and medication to medication, often even in the same patient.

Comments

1. Usually recommended as the first drug of choice for moderate to severe cancer pain.

2. Despite a few studies that suggest a conversion ratio of 1:6 for a switch from intramuscular (IM) administration to one by mouth, clinical experience suggests that a ratio of 1:3 with regular use is generally considered more applicable. In other words, if a patient is going from an intramuscular (or IV or sub-q) route with a dose, for example, of 10 mg to an oral route of morphine, the physician is likely to prescribe 30 mg by mouth to get equivalent pain relief.

3. Controlled release means that the medication is time-release; it provides slow absorption of the medication and, consequently, doses may be farther apart. Using controlled-release formulation may result in more consistent blood levels of medication and, therefore, more consistent pain relief with fewer episodes of breakthrough pain. Controlled-release medication is extremely useful in providing a basic level of pain relief and its infrequent dosing schedule is very convenient for the patient. Physicians will usually supplement these doses with rescue doses of shorter acting medications to relieve pain that breaks through despite the controlled-release medication being prescribed. *Controlled-release medications should not be broken, crushed, or chewed.*

(continues on next page)

4. Morphine is the standard against which other analgesics (pain relievers) are compared.
5. For fentanyl, once the blood has achieved a consistent level of medication (steady state), doses last about 72 hours. From the first dose, it will take usually about 12 to 24 hours to achieve a steady state. If side effects occur and medication is removed (patch removed), adverse effects may persist for 12 to 24 hours. Extremely useful for patients who do not want to take medication frequently or who cannot swallow.
6. OxyContin offers 8 to 12 hours of relief, but tablets should never be cut or crushed or chewed.
7. Immediate-release oxycodone is used mostly for breakthrough pain.
8. Hydromorphone becomes effective relatively rapidly and offers short-acting relief, so it is particularly effective for breakthrough pain.
9. Unlike other opioids, methadone may be especially effective for neuropathic pain (due to nerve injury) and intractable cancer pain. Very inexpensive and an increasingly popular second- or third-line treatment for pain. Unlike other opioids, it's often started as needed rather than around-the-clock. Due to long half-life, it has the potential to accumulate, and doses should be raised gradually and erratic use avoided.
10. For levorphanol, see comments on methadone, except for cost (which is higher for this drug).
11. Not available for oral administration.
12. Not legally available in the United States but popular in the United Kingdom for pain treatment. Useful for sub-q use but otherwise an inefficient medication, as it rapidly converts to morphine in the body.
13. Lozenges used for breakthrough pain. Works rapidly (most patients note meaningful pain relief within 6 to 10 minutes) but is expensive.

8

Understanding How Adjuvant Drugs
Relieve Pain and Suffering

In addition to the basic pain relievers, other medications are often prescribed to enhance patient comfort. Called adjuvant drugs or co-analgesics, these drugs are auxiliary medications, most of which were developed for conditions other than pain, but can play an important role in the relief of pain. *Adjuvant* simply means "helper"; these drugs may help counteract side effects of the primary pain reliever(s) or help relieve other distressing symptoms, such as nausea, constipation, or breathlessness. Adjuvant analgesics, however, actually relieve pain in their own right in specific circumstances. Unlike the opioids and anti-inflammatories (NSAIDs), which are all-purpose analgesics that relieve any type of pain to some extent, the adjuvants are *mechanism-specific,* meaning that they may help relieve a particular type of pain but aren't effective for other types.

For example, nerve pain that persists despite opioid treatment may respond well to specific antidepressants or anticonvulsants, even though there is no depression or seizures. It may sound odd to recommend an antidepressant or anticonvulsant for a cancer patient's pain, but experience and research show such usage can be enormously effective when even very strong painkillers have not been helpful. That's because medications work by different mechanisms, and combining medications may have additive or even synergistic effects (meaning that total relief may exceed the sum of relief if each medication were given alone). Also, drugs usually have multiple effects, sometimes up to a dozen different ones.

Overview of Medications Used for Cancer Pain and Other Symptoms

	When Used	Benefits
Nonsteroidal anti-inflammatory drugs (NSAIDs) A large group of pain relievers that reduce pain and swelling	Used alone for mild to moderate pain (1–3 on 0–10 scale) and combined with stronger meds for moderate to severe pain, especially pain associated with swelling or inflammation, bone pain, and soft tissue pain.	Increasingly available over the counter; newer, safer preparations increasingly available by prescription.
Opioids So-called weak opioids	For moderate pain, usually 3–6 on a 0–10 pain scale.	No blood clotting problems or bleeding, ulceration or stomach problems, except for combination products that contain
So-called strong opioids	For severe pain, usually 6–10 on a 0–10 pain sale; require special prescriptions that cannot be called in or refilled.	
Tricyclic antidepressants	To relieve the burning, itching, tingling, numbing, shooting pain associated with nerve injury; may improve sleep and reduce depression.	Can enhance pain-relieving effects of other medications.
Anticonvulsants	To relieve the burning, shooting, stabbing, itching, tingling, numbing pain of nerve injury, especially when sudden and intermittent.	Can enhance pain relieving effects of other medications.
Corticosteroids Very strong anti-inflammatories	To relieve chronic pain, bone pain, brain tumor pain, spinal cord tumor pain, and whenever pain may be due to swelling around a tumor.	May reduce nausea; may improve mood, appetite, weight, breathing and sense of well-being.
Oral local anesthetics/ sodium channel blockers/ local anesthetics	Orally to relieve tingling, burning-type pain from nerve injury; as an ointment or in a patch, may numb pain that is close to the surface of the skin. Also injected near nerves or into the spinal canal (nerve block).	Can relieve pain due to nerve injury when the antidepressants and anticonvulsants don't help.
Bisphosphonates	Bone pain when cancer has spread to the bones; also used to treat elevated calcium levels.	Prevents bone loss and weakness.
Radiopharmaceuticals	Bone pain when cancer has spread to multiple bones.	Noninvasive relief for three to six months; takes from one week to one month for results.
Psychostimulants	To help relieve drowsiness associated with opioid use; can enhance the pain relief of opioids.	May also have an antidepressant effect; can offset daytime drowsiness

Side Effects	Common Examples
Can affect the ability of blood to clot; may cause upset stomach, ulcers, diarrhea, and bleeding in the stomach, and kidney problems, sometimes with no warning.	Aspirin, ibuprofen, naproxen, acetaminophen, and the newer selective COX-2 inhibitors (Vioxx, Celebrex, Bextra)
May cause manageable problems with constipation, drowsiness, nausea and vomiting, itchiness, and urinary problems; at first, may slow down breathing, but not dangerously so in usual doses.	Codeine, hydrocodone, and dihydrocodeine, combined with acetaminophen or aspirin, tramadol
Physical dependence and tolerance may arise with chronic use, but addiction is rare.	Morphine, hydromorphone, oxycodone, fentanyl, methadone, levorphanol, oxymorphone
May cause dry mouth, urinary retention, drowsiness, constipation, and, rarely, dizziness on standing up suddenly.	Amitriptyline, nortriptyline, imipramine, doxepin, desipramine, trazodone; newer SSRI antidepressants are not usually used specifically to treat pain
Some may affect liver and blood counts or cause drowsiness and confusion.	Gabapentin, carbamazepine, phenytoin, clonazepam, valproate, topiramate, lamotrigine
May cause confusion, edema (swelling due to fluid retention), stomach irritation, and gastrointestinal bleeding. Pain relief may recede over several weeks. More serious side effects possible with long-term use.	Prednisone, dexamethasone, prednisolone, methylprednisolone
Orally: GI side effects such as nausea, vomiting and constipation are most common; drowsiness, nervousness, dizziness, confusion, stuttering, tremor, and light-headedness may also occur. Topical formulations have no side effects. Rarely, injections can cause seizures.	Mexiletine, tocainide, EMLA, Lidoderm, Lidocaine, bupivacaine
Nausea, redness, swelling, fatigue, flulike symptoms.	Pamidronate, clodronate
Temporary pain flare-up may occur.	Strontium-89 (Metastron) and samarium-153 (Quadramet)
Avoid in patients with seizure disorders, primary brain cancer, and brain metastases. May cause anxiety or agitation, sleep disturbance, and anorexia; slight risk of heart palpitations especially in vulnerable patients; liver failure observed with pemoline.	Dextroamphetamine (Dexedrine), methylphenidate (Ritalin), pemoline, modafinil

(continues on overleaf)

Overview of Medications Used for Cancer Pain and Other Symptoms (*continued*)

	When Used	Benefits
Antihistamines	Minimal effect on pain, if any; may help relieve itching and anxiety.	Enhanced pain relief when combined with opioids and has antiemetic and antianxiety effects. Sedative effect may be useful, too.
Major tranquilizers	Minimal effect on pain, if any, except methotrimeprazine, which may relieve pain as well as morphine; mostly used to counteract nausea or agitation. The sedation from tranquilizers can provide comfort in advanced illness when opioids are inadequate.	May relieve nausea and anxiety, confusion, psychosis, agitation; sometimes enhances effectiveness of opioids.
Minor tranquilizers (anti-anxiety medications)	No direct effects on pain, but relief of anxiety and panic, may lower pain threshold; may help relax muscle spasm.	May relieve acute anxiety, panic, muscle spasm.
Muscle relaxants	Nerve pain, especially around head and neck; muscle spasm.	May help relieve shooting, stabbing nerve pain that has not responded to other measures, as well as dull aching muscle tightness.

When drug companies test and market a new drug, they focus on whatever property they think will be needed most in the marketplace and concentrate their very costly research efforts on gaining Food and Drug Administration approval exclusively for that property. Yet doctors may still choose to prescribe the same drug for any of its other indications or properties, such as pain, at any time, although these off-label uses cannot be promoted by the manufacturer.

The management of side effects and of other symptoms is discussed in Chapters 10 and 11; the role of the adjuvant analgesics as painkillers is discussed in this chapter.

General Comments about Adjuvant Drugs

Adjuvant drugs are usually used in addition to the more standard opioid drugs (rather than as a substitute for them), but they may also be used alone. Unlike the opioids, which become effective within a few minutes or half an hour and wear off within a few hours, most adjuvant analgesics have to be used for one to three weeks before they become fully effective, and often their effectiveness may be subtle. While it is tempting to relate such gradual improvement to other factors, such as the weather, well-planned and consistent use of the adjuvants is one of the pain specialist's

Side Effects	Common Examples
Sedation.	Hydroxyzine (Vistaril, Atarax); diphenhydramine (Benadryl)
Side effects may include drowsiness, confusion, blurred vision, dry mouth.	Such as phenothiazines, methotrimeprazine, fluphenazine, chlorpromazine, promethazine, haloperidol, Phenergan, Compazine
Side effects include sedation; depression and dependence with prolonged use.	Diazepam, lorazepam, midazolam
Older agents (Soma, Parafon Forte, Skelaxin, Flexeril, Robaxin) act as sedatives and are generally avoided due to sedation and dependence; newer agents (baclofen, Zanaflex) are better tolerated and more effective.	Baclofen, Zanaflex; Soma, Parafon Forte, Skelaxin, Flexeril, Robaxin

most powerful strategies but requires the patient's understanding, cooperation, and patience. And while opioids provide dependable time-limited relief, they do little to change the underlying cause of the pain and its long-range course. A properly selected adjuvant analgesic may actually improve the conditions responsible for persistent pain, thus providing more of a long-term solution.

While not all of these adjuvant drugs have been proven effective for pain, a trial of some of these medications may be of great value. The following information is a guide to the most commonly used adjuvant analgesics, but it should not be used as a substitute for a doctor's care and judgment.

Antidepressants

Although a person with pain who is also depressed may benefit from an antidepressant, definitive research shows that the pain-relieving effect of antidepressants occurs entirely independent of any effect on mood. In fact, when antidepressants are prescribed for pain, they are usually in doses much too small to help with mood.

Like the other drugs discussed in this chapter, the antidepressants have more than one use. In cancer patients, they treat depression, pain, and insomnia. They can be helpful to a person who is depressed but does not complain of pain, who has nerve pain headaches or other pain syndromes but is not depressed, or who is suffering from both depression and pain. Since some of the antidepressants are more useful for one condition than another, patients with both mood and pain problems may find themselves on two separate antidepressants, one in a low dose for pain and the other in a more standard dose for mood.

These drugs are among the most misunderstood of the painkillers. When a doctor, especially one who is rushed, prescribes an antidepressant when a patient reports pain, the patient may feel that the doctor suspects the pain is not "real," is "all in the head," or is only a reflection of depressed mood. To the contrary, these medications control pain directly by mechanisms that are totally independent of any effects on mood. To treat depression, much higher doses would be needed. Also, the older antidepressants, the tricyclic antidepressants (TCAs) or heterocyclics, are most often prescribed for pain, but these days the newer selective serotonin reuptake inhibitors (SSRIs) are the first-line treatment for depression, especially in cancer patients.

Antidepressants for Pain When Depression Is Not a Problem

The TCAs alter the amount of certain neurotransmitters (serotonin and norepinephrine), which are the neurotransmitters involved in pain transmission; these drugs are particularly useful for pain due to nerve injury but have roles in other pain problems as well, such as headache. In fact, a prescription of an antidepressant (with or without other pain medications, such as the opioids) is the first choice for patients with nerve pain, such as that due to shingles, diabetes, and many postoperative conditions. It is particularly useful for painful skin or hypersensitivity, which patients describe as burning, itching, tingling, shooting, numbing, and other odd qualities. This kind of pain may be facial pain or postsurgical pain, may be due to shingles (herpes zoster), or may result from a tumor pressing near nerves. The tricyclic antidepressants tend to be more effective for relatively constant nerve pain, while the anticonvulsants (see below) are first considered for more intermittent or episodic nerve pain. Also, these and other medications are commonly used together to get the best effect possible.

When Depression Is a Problem

More than half of cancer patients who are depressed say that pain is their main problem. For obvious reasons, many cancer patients are both depressed and in pain. The symptoms are similar: people who are chronically depressed or in pain become easily tearful, suffer from poor sleeping and eating patterns, are irritable, lose interest in sex, and suffer from other mood problems. Pain and depression also exhibit some similar physiological characteristics with regard to brain chemistry, specifically changes in levels of neurotransmitters.

Although sadness and a low mood are natural responses to having cancer or chronic pain, for about one-quarter of cancer patients these feelings become overwhelming and represent a full-blown depression that requires medical attention. Such feelings are common, and cancer patients should not be ashamed to admit them. In fact, trying to conceal and suppress low mood may be the worst thing to do, because it not only takes energy needed for other purposes but doesn't solve the problem. If patients are afraid to talk about their feelings because they don't want to appear weak or to upset their loved ones, they should tell their doctor, who can recommend a counselor or other treatment.

Pain, especially when unrecognized or inefficiently treated, is usually the primary problem; however, this can lead to frustration, anger, depression, and even suicidal thoughts. Such depression often lifts dramatically and rapidly once the pain is resolved, or even with the news that a pain specialist has been assigned to the case and will finally accept accountability. Less commonly, the main problem may be depression rather than pain. Depression can lower one's pain threshold, however, and a depressed person may complain a great deal about pain. In some families, pain complaints may even represent a more acceptable or less upsetting way of getting necessary attention than admitting to depression or feelings of hopelessness and helplessness. In these cases, the depression usually needs to be resolved before the complaints of pain will improve. It's hard, though, to know which came first, the pain or the depression, and so it is difficult to know where most of the treatment should be directed.

Whenever possible, pain and depression should be considered separately. All pain should be assumed to be real (related to physical injury), and although pain always has psychological components, complaints should never be taken lightly nor considered psychosomatic or "merely" a mental process. It is clear that whether pain is primarily a reflection of physical or psychological problems, the suffering is just as real and the need for help is just as compelling. When depression seems to be a prominent part of the problem, treatment with an antidepressant may be warranted. As noted above, since a tricyclic is more commonly used to treat pain and a newer Prozac-like SSRI is almost always considered first for depression, patients with both pain and depression commonly take two different antidepressants: a low-dose tricyclic antidepressant (such as amitriptyline) for pain and an SSRI such as Prozac in a routine dose of 20 to 40 mg.

For a fuller discussion of depression, see Chapter 14.

How Antidepressants Are Used for Pain

A variety of antidepressants are commonly used to treat pain. Like other pain medications, several different (but usually related) medications may need to be tried before a given person finds the most suitable one. The tricyclic antidepressants—which include amitriptyline (Elavil, Endep), imipramine (Tofranil, Janimine, Presamine, SK-Pramine), doxepin (Sinequan, Adapin), desipramine (Norpramin, Pertofrane), and nortriptyline (Pamelor, Aventyl)—seem to be most effective in controlling pain. Because they all promote drowsiness to varying degrees, they are usually prescribed in a single low nighttime dose to promote sleep and avoid daytime fatigue. Low doses (usually 10 to 25 mg) are used to start, and may be gradually increased to a moderate (50 to 100 mg) dose as needed and as tolerated, but high doses (100 to 200 mg) are rarely required. Although insomnia may improve immediately, *patients need one to three weeks before they usually recognize improvements in pain.* This is important to know, because otherwise, disappointed patients may prematurely stop these potentially very helpful drugs. Also, before rejecting a trial of one of these medications because it didn't help or caused problems in the past, note that a previous prescription may have been for a different problem, at a different dose, combined with other drugs, and so on. While you should express your concerns, stay open-minded.

Most of these medications may cause dry mouth, constipation, difficulty urinating (urinary retention, especially in men), heartbeat irregularities, sweating, drowsiness, delirium, dizziness, low blood pressure upon standing up suddenly, and tremors. In the doses used for pain, these medications are almost always well tolerated, and with the exception of dry mouth, side effects are uncommon.

The newer group of antidepressants, the SSRIs, have revolutionized the medical management of depression but appear to have a relatively minor role in the treatment of pain, though studies at the Mayo Clinic suggest they may help with the hot flashes associated with hormonal treatments in breast and prostate cancer.

The tricyclic amitriptyline has been most consistently proven the most effective and is thus often selected first, though its side effects may be somewhat more prominent. If side effects are a special concern, an alternative agent may be tried first; despite the similarities among the tricyclics, patients may respond highly favorably to one of these agents and not another.

AMITRIPTYLINE

Brand Name
Elavil, Amitril, Endep, Emitrip, Enovil, Etrafon, Etrafon-A, Etrafon-Forte, PMS-Levazine, SK-Amitriptyline, Dohme, Sharpe.

Dose Range

For pain relief, starting doses range from 10 to 25 mg by mouth, taken at bedtime. While sometimes sufficient, once a starting dose is well tolerated, it is common to gradually raise the dose, usually to no more than 50 to 125 mg, to attempt further relief of pain and better sleep.

For the elderly, the starting dose is usually 10 mg.

If used to counter depression, daily doses are usually much higher (150 to 300 mg).

How Long It Takes to Reach Peak Effect

While sleep may improve immediately, allow one to four weeks at a given dose to achieve its full pain-relieving effect.

Comments

- Amitriptyline is the prototype antidepressant for pain relief and thus is the most thoroughly studied and well-documented remedy of this type. It is particularly good for the bizarre burning, numbing, tingling, and hypersensitivity associated with nerve pain. It may have more prominent side effects than some of its alternatives but is still often tried first because its use is so well supported. Since it takes time for the blood levels of neurotransmitters to change, the onset of pain relief is usually gradual, although better sleep and mild side effects may be noticeable right away.
- It is also recommended for treating anxiety.
- It can help ease depression.
- It may be effective in treating phantom limb pain.
- It may be effective in treating pain near a surgical scar.
- Children's doses are based on body weight.
- Available as IM injection or as rectal suppository.

Precautions

- The most common side effect of amitriptyline is dry mouth, which often diminishes within one to two weeks.
- Morning drowsiness is relatively common and also tends to subside within a few days to a week, once the dose is held constant; if it doesn't abate, the condition may be relieved by taking the evening dose even earlier in the evening.
- Sedation may occur but usually diminishes within several days.
- Other side effects may include constipation, difficulty urinating (urinary retention, particularly among elderly men), light-headedness, confusion, weight gain and craving of sweets, and temporary low blood pressure upon rapidly standing (orthostatic hypotension), but these are uncommon with low doses used for pain.

Guidelines for the Use of the Antidepressants in Patients with Chronic Cancer[a, b, c]

Generic Name	Trade Name[d]	Dose Range[e]	Anti-cholinergic[a]	Sedative Effects	Orthostatis[a]	Comments[c, f]
Amitriptyline[g]	Elavil, Endep, many other	10–300 mg	+++	+++	++	1, 2, 3, 4
Imipramine[g]	Tofranil, Janimine, Tipramine, Tofranil-PM	20–300 mg	+++	++	+++	1, 4
Doxepin[g]	Sinequan, Adapin	30–300 mg	+++	+++	+++	1, 5
Desipramine[g]	Norpramin, Pertofrane	75–300 mg	+	+	+	1
Nortriptyline[g]	Pamelor, Aventyl	50–100 mg	++	+	+	1, 5, 6
Trimiptramine[h]	Surmontil	50–225 mg	+++	+++	+++	—
Protriptyline	Vivactil	15–40 mg	+++	+	+	—
Amoxapine[h]	Asendin	200–300 mg	+	+	+++	7
Fluoxetine[h]	Prozac	20–60 mg	—	+	—	8
Trazodone[h]	Desyrel, Trialodine	50–600 mg	—	+++	+++	9
Maprotiline[h]	Ludiomil	75–300 mg	+	+++	+	—

Notes

[a]Doses and the rating of anticholinergic side effects (that is, dry mouth, urinary retention or difficulty in urinating, constipation, sweating), sedation, and orthostatis (low blood pressure upon standing up suddenly) listed here are only intended as rough guidelines. Plus signs indicates a greater tendency to cause the side effect when compared to other medications. Other than dry mouth, most of the effects are uncommon with the low doses usually used for pain.

[b]These antidepressants are most often used for managing pain associated with nerve damage, which is often felt as a burning sensation.

[c]These heterocyclic antidepressants may produce pain relief at low doses without affecting mood; these doses are usually too low to counter depression. Initial treatment is usually prescribed as a low nighttime dose. While sleep problems are usually resolved quickly with these doses, maximal pain relief often takes 1 to 3 weeks.

[d]In the United States.

eThese values listed reflect the range between minimum and maximum recommended doses. In general, the higher range of doses are intended to treat clinical depression, and even then, it is recommended that dosage be reduced for maintenance therapy. In general, when antidepressants are prescribed for nerve pain, they are prescribed in the low range of the dose spectrum, often initially at the lowest possible dose.

fAs a class, these antidepressants, known as the heterocyclic antidepressants, are generally associated with the anticholinergic side effects (see note a). Infrequently, they may cause high blood pressure (hypertension), rash, bone marrow depression, vision or sexual problems, enlarged breasts sometimes with milk secretion (gynecomastia), jaundice (yellowing skin), and hair loss (alopecia). Noteworthy side effects are listed.

gIn controlled studies, these medications have been shown to have pain-relieving effects that are independent of their antidepressant effects.

Comments

1. Preferred for managing nerve pain because of greater clinical experience with this drug.
2. Best-studied drug of this class for relieving nerve pain, and therefore thought to be most reliable. Its use, however, must be balanced against the relatively greater potential for anticholinergic side effects (see note a).
3. Available as an intramuscular (IM) medication.
4. May be associated with weight gain.
5. Available in liquid formation for oral use.
6. Is very similar to amitriptyline, and because of its lower incidence of side effects, many doctors favor its use.
7. Occasionally associated with side effects known as extrapyramidal side effects (sudden involuntary movements, such as jerking).
8. Unlike other heterocyclic antidepressants, this medication appears not to produce sedative effects and may even produce stimulation. Its use may be associated with weight loss..
9. A side effect that men should be aware of is that the drug occasionally causes unexpected or prolonged erections (priapism); should that occur, discontinue use and contact the physician.

- It is not to be used in patients with glaucoma.
- Rarely, the drug may trigger hyperexcitability in the patient.

Several alternatives are available that may be prescribed in place of amitriptyline.

DOXEPIN

Brand Name
Adapin, Sinequan.

Dose Range
The usual starting dose is 25 mg at night. This may be gradually increased to up to 300 mg at night (the lower dose range is for pain; the higher one is for depression). May take several weeks to reach full effect.

Comments
- Doxepin is similar to amitriptyline but causes less dry mouth and constipation.
- It is available in liquid form, unlike most of the other antidepressants.

Precautions
- See under amitriptyline.
- It should not be used with patients who have glaucoma or urinary retention problems, especially older patients with these conditions.
- Doxepin may cause drowsiness.

IMIPRAMINE

Brand Name
Tofranil, Janimine, Tipramine, Tofranil-PM.

Dose Range
Usually from 25 to 300 mg a day (the lower dose range is for pain; the higher dose range is for depression). May take several weeks to reach full effect.

Comments
- The major breakdown product of imipramine is desipramine.
- See under amitriptyline; causes less severe dry mouth and less sedation.
- Imipramine may be associated with weight gain.

DESIPRAMINE

Brand Name
Norpramin, Pertofrane.

Dose Range

Usually from 10 to 100 mg a day for pain (200 to 300 mg a day for depression). May take several weeks to reach full effect.

Comments

- Usually considered to be the least sedating of these agents. Side effects, including anticholinergic (blocking of parasympathetic nerves) and sedative effects as well as low blood pressure upon standing, are less severe than for the abovementioned medications. Otherwise, similar to amitriptyline.

NORTRIPTYLINE

Brand Name

Pamelor and Aventyl.

Dose Range

Usually from 10 to 100 mg a day for pain (200 to 300 mg a day for depression). May take several weeks to reach full effect.

Comments

- As one of the major breakdown products of amitriptyline, its effects are similar, but side effects are more infrequent and usually milder.

TRAZODONE

Brand Name

Desyrel, Trialodine.

Dose Range

Usually 50 to 600 mg per day (the lower dose range is for pain; the higher one is for depression). May take several weeks to reach full effect.

Comments

- Although its pain-relieving effects have not been as well substantiated, trazodone, one of the newer antidepressants, causes relatively few side effects except for drowsiness, which can be quite prominent. Thus when insomnia is a coexisting problem, trazodone may be selected early.

Precautions

- A side effect that men should be aware of is that the drug occasionally causes unexpected or prolonged erections. Should this occur, the patient should discontinue use and contact the physician.
- Trazodone should be taken with food.

Anticonvulsants

Anticonvulsants are particularly useful in treating nerve pain because, like seizures, pain is a sudden electrical phenomenon. By suppressing the spontaneous firing of neurons (nerve cells), anticonvulsants quiet their excitability and interfere with the generation of the pain message. Thus, although doctors may prescribe an anticonvulsant to help with pain, this has nothing to do with a patient's being suspected of having seizures. The anticonvulsants are particularly useful for nerve pain that is intermittent, shooting, burning, or stabbing in nature. They are either used with or without a tricyclic antidepressant to treat pain.

GABAPENTIN

Brand Name
Neurontin.

Dose Range
Available in 100 mg, 300 mg, 400 mg, 600 mg, and 800 mg capsules. Most adults usually start with 300 mg at bedtime during the first few days of therapy, which is usually well tolerated and can be advanced to 600 mg in two divided doses for a few more days until achieving a dose of 900 mg in three divided doses. If it helps and is well tolerated, it may then be increased to 300 to 400 mg three to four times per day per physician instructions. A small proportion of patients, especially if elderly, may feel drowsy from very low doses, in which case they can be restarted on 100 mg nightly and gradually raised to 100 mg three to four times per day until effective. This medication is usually extremely well tolerated, though, and total daily doses of 2,400 to 3,600 mg for nerve pain are common. Over time some patients may take in excess of 5,000 mg per day when warranted.

How Long It Takes to Reach Peak Effect
Beneficial effects are typically noted within a week of regular use, although two to three weeks may be needed to be sure, especially if doses have been raised gradually.

Comments
- One of the first of a newer generation of "atypical" anticonvulsants, gabapentin is currently considered a first-choice medication to treat sharp, shooting, or burning pain because it stabilizes nerves and prevents them from firing spontaneously. It is much safer and better tolerated than other anticonvulsants, it has few drug interactions, and its use does not require laboratory monitoring, although it is currently more expensive (up to $200 per month) than many other medications used for nerve pain.

Guidelines for the Use of Anticonvulsants in Patients with Chronic Cancer Pain

General Name	Trade Name	Usual Starting Dose	Dose Usual Dose Range	Comments[a]
Gabapentin	Neurontin	300 mg	2,400 to 5,000 mg per day	1
Zonisamide	Zonegran	100 mg	300 to 400 mg per day	2
Tiagabine	Gabitril	4 mg	Up to 56 mg per day	3
Carbamazepine	Tegretol, Epitol	100 to 200 mg	Up to 800 to 1,200 mg per day	4
Phenytoin	Dilantin, Diphenylan, Phenytex	100 mg	300 to 400 mg per day	5
Valproic acid, Valproate Sodium, Divalproex Sodium	Depakene, Depakote, Depa, Deproic	250 mg once or twice a day	Up to 1,500 mg per day	6
Clonazepam	Klonopin	.5 mg	Up to 2 mg per day	7
Topiramate	Topamax	12.5 to 25 mg once or twice a day	Up to 100 to 200 mg per day	8
Lamotrigine	Lamictal	25 mg once or twice a day	Up to 400 mg a day	9

Notes: When nerve pain is described as shooting, piercing, or intermittent, these medications are often prescribed. Also used for other types of nerve pain when antidepressants do not seem to help. Many of these medications (except gabapentin and zonisamide) have a relatively high incidence of side effects as doses are increased.

Comments:
1. A first-choice medication to treat sharp, shooting, or burning pain; much safer and better tolerated than other anticonvulsants, though expensive.
2. Despite few studies on its use in pain, this medication appears to provide relief at times when other more routine medications do not.
3. As with zonisamide (above), although pain studies are lacking, this new antiepileptic medication is now being used enthusiastically for chronic nerve pain, and appears to provide relief for some patients when other medications do not.
4. Well-studied and the traditional drug of choice for shooting, shock-like (lancinating) nerve pain, though its high incidence of bothersome side effects and the possibilities of life-threatening liver and bone marrow complications makes it a less attractive choice (especially in cancer patients) given the newer alternatives above. Tegretol may produce life-threatening liver dysfunction and depression of blood counts, and thus its continued use requires regular blood tests.
5. Good choice when patients are unresponsive to other drugs in this category.
6. Available in various forms, including a syrup, a capsule that can be opened and its contents sprinkled on food for those with swallowing difficulties, and extended-release tablets. Capsules should not be broken, chewed, or crushed, both for safety reasons and to avoid irritation of the mouth and throat. An overgrowth of gum tissue (gingival hyperplasia) may occur but may be prevented or managed with regular oral hygiene measures (see Chapter 11). Other side effects may include acne or excessive hair growth.
7. Very effective in controlling pain due to nerve irritation, in addition to helping with anxiety and insomnia. The only medication that helps quell muscle jerking (myoclonus), which is harmless but can be bothersome in patients taking opioids. May cause pancreatitis, nausea and vomiting, insomnia, headache, tremor, hair loss, weight gain, and (rarely) impaired liver function.
8. Available only orally, it also comes in sprinkles for children. Dizziness, sedation, and fatigue are relatively common; may also relieve anxiety. If used for a long time, withdrawal symptoms may occur if drug is stopped suddenly.
9. Can potentially cause a life-threatening skin rash, particularly for those who also take valproate (Depakote).Contact your physician if fever or swollen glands are noted.

Precautions

- Gabapentin typically has fewer side effects than other anticonvulsants; when they do occur, most common are sleepiness and dizziness, but also fatigue, problems with balance, or unusual eye movements can be present.
- Do not take within at least two hours of any antacids.

ZONISAMIDE

Brand Name
Zonegran.

Dose Range
Starting dose is 100 mg once daily, to be taken at about the same time each day. After one to two weeks, the dose may be increased to 200 mg a day for at least two weeks and then to 300 mg a day and 400 mg a day, with the dose stable for at least two weeks to achieve a steady state at each level.

How Long It Takes to Reach Peak Effect
Within two weeks you should have a sense if it's working.

Comments

- Despite few studies on its use in pain, this new antiepileptic medication is already being used with enthusiasm for chronic nerve pain. Like other adjuvants, it appears to provide relief at times when other, more routine medications do not.

Precautions

- Side effects are infrequent and usually mild but may include drowsiness, nausea, dizziness, agitation, headache, or irritability
- Should not be taken by anyone who is allergic to sulfa drugs, such as Bactrim or Septra; by anyone with kidney disease; or by patients who use alcohol frequently.
- Should be taken with six to eight glasses of water a day to help prevent kidney stones from forming.

TIAGABINE

Brand Name
Gabitril.

Dose Range
Initiated at 4 mg once daily, which may be increased by 4 to 8 mg each week, up to 56 mg a day. The total daily dose should be given in divided doses, two to four times daily, and should be taken with food.

How Long It Takes to Reach Peak Effect
Depending on how fast the dose has been raised, within two weeks you should usually have a sense if it is working.

Comments
- As with zonisamide (above), although pain studies are lacking, this new antiepileptic medication is now being used enthusiastically for chronic nerve pain and appears to provide relief for some patients when other medications do not.

Precautions
- Side effects may include dizziness or light-headedness, lack of energy, sleepiness, nausea, nervousness or irritability, tremor, abdominal pain, and abnormal thinking or difficulty with concentration or attention.

CARBAMAZEPINE

Brand Name
Tegretol, Epitol.

Dose Range
The starting dose is 100 to 200 mg a day, with increases of 100 mg every three or four days if needed, up to 800 to 1,200 mg a day.

How Long It Takes to Reach Peak Effect
Carbamazepine usually takes two to four weeks of regular use to determine effectiveness for nerve pain.

Comments
- This anticonvulsant, commonly used for epilepsy, is by far the best-studied for nerve pain and is thus traditionally the drug of choice for shooting, shocklike (lancinating) nerve pain, exemplified by trigeminal neuralgia (tic douloureux), a type of facial pain that can occur with or without cancer. While it may relieve symptoms in up to 90 percent of cases of lancinating pain, it is less likely to be effective for aching, burning nerve pain that is constant.
- Despite its legacy of success, a high incidence of bothersome side effects and the possibilities of life-threatening liver and bone marrow complications makes it a less attractive choice (especially in cancer patients) given the newer alternatives discussed above.

Precautions
- Although still a commonly used anticonvulsant for the treatment of shooting nerve pain, because of its documented success, its use is approached cautiously. Unfortunately, side effects—nausea, vomiting, problems with gait and loss of muscle coordination

(ataxia), dizziness, lethargy, and confusion—are more common with this anticonvulsant, especially in the elderly. If administered in low doses and increased only gradually, such side effects can often be avoided.

- Very rarely (in fewer than one in twenty thousand patients) more major side effects, such as liver and bone marrow problems, may occur, and they may be persistent and devastating. If used for more than a few weeks, regular blood tests of liver and bone marrow function should be prescribed. Blood tests are carefully checked if carbamazepine is prescribed for patients who have recently undergone chemotherapy or radiation therapy because their bone marrow may already be depressed or especially vulnerable.

PHENYTOIN

Brand Name
Dilantin, Diphenylan, Phenytex.

Dose Range
Usually started at 100 mg a day and increased gradually by increments of 25 to 50 mg, with daily doses usually not exceeding 300 to 400 mg.

How Long It Takes to Reach Peak Effect
It normally takes one to three weeks to reach its full effect.

Comments
- This drug has been used for generations to help control seizures, and although it has not been studied as thoroughly as carbamazepine for controlling pain, it retains an important role for patients unresponsive to other drugs in this category.
- Phenytoin may increase or decrease the effectiveness of other medications being taken, a factor that should be discussed with your doctor or nurse.

Precautions
- Oral hygiene is very important to prevent gum problems, especially a condition referred to as *gingival hyperplasia*, which is an overgrowth of gum tissue. This can occur in up to 20 percent of patients, but it is usually only a problem in children and adolescents. (See Chapter 11 on side effects and other discomforts.)

VALPROIC ACID, VALPROATE SODIUM, DIVALPROEX SODIUM

Brand Name
Depakene, Depakote, Depa, Deproic.

Dose Range
Usually started at 250 mg once or twice per day. This dose can be increased gradually, usually to a range of about 500 mg three times a day, if well tolerated and associated with increasing relief of pain.

How Long It Takes to Reach Peak Effect
While each dose reaches its peak effect within one to four hours, like all adjuvants, it may take one to three weeks before pain is relieved.

Comments
- This drug is also used to prevent migraine headaches and to treat anxiety, bipolar disorders, rage, and urinary incontinence. Valproic acid can be used for nerve pain as an alternative to carbamazepine.
- Available in various forms, including a syrup and a capsule that can be sprinkled on food for those with swallowing difficulties, and as extended-release tablets. Capsules should not be broken, chewed, or crushed, both for safety reasons and to avoid irritation of the mouth and throat.

Precautions
- Possible side effects include headache, tremor, hair and weight loss, insomnia, and drowsiness. Most important, rare complications include liver damage (especially in children under the age of two) and severe inflammation of the pancreas (pancreatitis). Blood should be monitored if medication is used regularly; contact your doctor immediately if you experience indigestion, nausea and vomiting, stomach pain, loss of appetite, weakness, facial swelling, rash, dark urine, or yellow eyes or skin. These medications should be avoided during early pregnancy, breastfeeding, and with liver problems.

CLONAZEPAM

Brand Name
Klonopin.

Dose Range
Usually started and often maintained at 0.5 mg nightly. May be increased gradually to 1 or 2 mg nightly and occasionally higher doses, but daytime use is usually avoided due to the potential for drowsiness.

How Long It Takes to Reach Peak Effect
Drowsiness is noted within about thirty minutes and peak effects within one to two hours; nighttime sleep is usually restored immediately, but several weeks may elapse before pain relief is fully established.

Comments

- Also an antiseizure drug, clonazepam seems to be very effective in controlling pain due to nerve irritation, in addition to helping with anxiety, insomnia, and muscle jerking (myoclonus). Many patients taking opioids experience these total body jerks, which, although harmless, can be frightening and inconvenient, and while clonazepam is still not fully recognized by doctors, it is the only medication that acts as a rapid, reliable remedy for this condition.
- It is a benzodiazepine (minor tranquilizer), like diazepam (Valium), so in some states it requires a triplicate prescription.

Precautions

- Its most common side effect is drowsiness.
- Dizziness and fatigue are also relatively common.
- If used for a long time, withdrawal symptoms (anxiousness, irritability, sleeplessness, and occasionally seizures) may occur if the drug is stopped suddenly.

TOPIRAMATE

Brand Name

Topamax.

Dose Range

Started at 12.5 to 25 mg once or twice a day and increased by 12.5 to 25 mg every week, up to 100 to 200 mg per day in two divided doses.

Comments

- Available only orally. It also comes in sprinkles for children, and should be taken twice daily.
- Has few drug interactions with other medications or other anticonvulsants.

Precautions

- Major potential side effects include drowsiness, nausea, dizziness, and coordination problems.

LAMOTRIGINE

Brand Name

Lamictal.

Dose Range

Starting dose is 25 mg once or twice a day, increased by 25 or 50 mg every week or two, up to about 400 mg a day.

Precautions

- The most serious side effect is a potentially life-threatening skin rash, particularly for those who also take valproate (Depakote). Other side effects include headache, nausea, and dizziness. Contact your physician if fever or swollen glands are noted.

Steroids or Corticosteroids

There are two general types of steroids. The anabolic steroids are abused by some professional athletes; they have little medical use, especially in cancer patients. The glucocorticoids or corticosteroids, however, are used for many medical conditions, including problems related to breathing, arthritis, pain, and infection. Administered over a period of years, they often cause a multitude of side effects, some of which are serious, such as weight gain, diabetes, skin problems, osteoporosis, and fractures. Used for short periods of time, their benefits may strongly outweigh their risks. They are commonly used in patients with cancer, both as a part of chemotherapy and to control symptoms, especially with brain tumors and advancing disease.

General Use

Steroids are one of the body's fundamental hormones, and prescribed hormones are not foreign substances but serve to boost the effects of steroids produced constantly by the adrenal glands. Steroid therapy has many potentially useful roles in the treatment of patients with cancer, such as being very potent in reducing inflammation and its related swelling, and is used in some chemotherapy treatments to shrink tumors, to reduce excessive levels of calcium that are sometimes caused by tumors, and to forestall nausea. They may improve mood and appetite, thus helping to promote weight gain.

One of their most important roles is as a painkiller, traditionally used to relieve pain and other symptoms when a tumor is growing in a small enclosed space, like a brain tumor within the skull, or a spinal cord tumor within the spinal column. By reducing swelling (edema) and inflammation around the tumor and nerves, they may not only dramatically relieve headache and backache but can reverse evolving neurological changes (such as paralysis), although these effects often only last a few weeks. In addition, they may help relieve pain anytime it originates with pressure from a bulky or strategically located tumor, such as that caused by a swollen liver, a tumor near the nerves to the arm or leg (brachial or lumbosacral plexopathy), or cancer of the esophagus, rectum, or female pelvic organs (cervical, ovarian, or uterine cancer).

Steroids are also used to reduce breathlessness and swelling in the upper body (superior vena cava syndrome) and lower body swelling (inferior vena cava syndrome) when tumors or lymph nodes press on the large veins responsible for draining circulating blood. They may also reduce breathing difficulties when cancer has spread diffusely around the lungs' lymphatic drainage system (lymphangitic spread).

Until other, more specific treatments can be found, high doses of corticosteroids can sometimes provide quick, dramatic short-term relief when severe pain is caused by bone tumors or tumors that have spread near nerves. These drugs may also help by boosting a patient's mood, stimulating appetite, reducing nausea, increasing strength, and by just giving the patient an overall improved sense of well-being. If a patient has a serious illness with a short expected survival time, these drugs may be used more freely because the side effects from long-term use are less important. Yet even with short-term use side effects still occasionally occur, such as increased susceptibility to infection, diabetes, fluid retention, acne, depression, psychotic episodes, and delirium.

Unfortunately, the benefits of the corticosteroids often only last several weeks, either because effectiveness diminishes with time or because progression of the disease overrides the drug's benefits. Nevertheless, the use of corticosteroids is becoming more and more widespread. Studies have shown that half of all patients in some special cancer units are given corticosteroids for symptom control. Another benefit is that these drugs may allow opioid doses to be reduced, thereby alleviating opioid-induced side effects. And finally, as noted, depression, nausea, and breathlessness may be relieved in certain circumstances.

Thus steroids can improve the quality of life in some cancer patients. At least one study, conducted in Britain, has shown that selected patients on corticosteroids live longer as well. However, caution must be exercised with these medications. In particular, patients with peptic ulcers or poorly controlled high blood pressure are not good candidates for treatment with steroids.

The steroid of choice is usually dexamethasone.

DEXAMETHASONE

Brand Name
Decadron, Decaspray, Dexasone, Dexone, Hexadrol, Maxidex.

Dose Range
A common starting dose is 4 mg twice a day by mouth; depending on results and various circumstances, the dose may be reduced after a week or so to a lower maintenance dose, or alternatively may be increased progressively to maximize beneficial effects.

Comparison of Selected Corticosteroids*

Generic Name	Approximate Duration	Equivalent Dose	Relative Anti-inflammatory Action
Short Duration	12 hr		
Cortisone		25	0.8
Hydrocortisone		20	1
Intermediate Duration	12–36 hr		
Prednisone		5	4
Prednisolone		5	4
Methylprednisolone		4	5
Triamcinalone		4	5
Long Duration	48 hr		
Paramethasone		2	10
Dexamethasone		0.75	25
Betamethasone		0.6	25

* Based on oral administration. Steroidal anti-inflammatories (as opposed to the nonsteroidal anti-inflammatories, the NSAIDs) may relieve pain by reducing inflammation and swelling. They may also reduce nausea as well as boost mood and appetite.

Higher initial doses (up to 100 mg a day) are often used for pain, especially when due to pressure induced by brain or spinal tumors.

This medication can be given orally, intravenously, or subcutaneously.

Comments

- Dexamethasone is particularly useful for shooting or burning nerve pain, headache resulting from a brain tumor or brain metastasis, back pain resulting from nerve compression in the spinal cord (epidural spinal cord compression, or ESCC), and pain due to tumor invading bone. Also, pain from any large, bulky tumor may respond to the steroid's ability to reduce local swelling.

- Although patients on steroids may feel jittery and occasionally even confused (steroid psychosis), they more typically feel more energetic and less depressed, often eating better and enjoying an overall improved sense of well-being.

- Sometimes overlooked, steroids can be a good choice when large doses of opioids are ineffective and pain is caused by tumors growing in the nerves of the arm or leg (brachial or lumbosacral plexus) or by any large tumor.

Precautions
- Side effects include infection, weight gain (often a reassuring and comforting effect for the family), GI bleeding (especially when taken with NSAIDs), muscle weakness, insomnia, high blood sugar, and, rarely, hallucinations and other psychotic effects.
- Should not be taken with NSAIDs.
- This drug should not be stopped abruptly, but should be gradually withdrawn.
- Other corticosteroids that are sometimes used with cancer patients include prednisolone (Prelone), prednisone (Deltasone and Sterapred), and methylprednisolone (Medrol). For a more complete listing of selected corticosteroids used with cancer pain, see table on previous page.

Oral Local Anesthetics or Sodium Channel Blockers

For continuous or shooting nerve pain that has not responded to tricyclic antidepressants or anticonvulsants, a sodium channel blocker may be recommended to calm unstable nerve membranes and prevent them from firing erratically. These oral versions of numbing medications or local anesthetics were developed to treat the irregular heartbeat (arrhythmia) that occurs when the heart's electrical system is damaged, and likewise can help quell unrelieved pain due to injured nerves.

MEXILETINE

Brand Name
Mexitil.

Dose Range
Usually started at 150 mg once or twice a day, which can be increased to up to 800 to 1,200 mg per day.

How Long It Takes to Reach Peak Effect
One to two hours, but several weeks of treatment may be needed for full pain-relieving effect.

Comments
- Mexiletine works by calming and stabilizing nerve membranes, which may quiet other kinds of pain as well.
- It is usually prescribed for the burning, tingling, or jabbing pain that accompanies nerve injury when the antidepressants and anticonvulsants have not been helpful.

Precautions
- While GI side effects are most common, drowsiness, nervousness, dizziness, and light-headedness may also occur.

TOCAINIDE

Brand Name
Tonocard.

Dose Range
Usually 200 to 400 mg twice a day.

How Long It Takes to Reach Peak Effect
One to two hours; may take several weeks to reach full pain-relieving effect.

Comments
- When mexiletine does not work, this medication may be useful.

Precautions
- Side effects are similar to those of mexiletine but may be more severe.
- Breathing problems should be reported promptly.

Bisphosphonates

Originally developed to treat osteoporosis (bone loss due to aging, especially in postmenopausal women) and sometimes referred to as aminobisphosphonates, diphosphonates, or biphosphonates, this new class of medication can relieve pain from cancer that has invaded the bones under some circumstances. These drugs are also used urgently when widespread bone involvement releases excessive calcium into the bloodstream (hypercalcemia), a condition that can otherwise be fatal.

The bisphosphonates work by interfering with the activity of cells that cause cancer-ridden bones to break down abnormally, and they may even slow cancer spread and prolong survival. Although cancer originating in the bone (osteosarcoma) is rare, the skeletal system is the most common site for tumor spread (metastases) and also the most common cause of cancer pain. Pain from bone metastases is especially common in those with prostate, breast, and lung cancers, as well as multiple myeloma. In myeloma, a cancer originating in plasma cells, bisphosphonates can reduce the frequency of fractures.

These medications not only reduce bone pain and the need for as much pain medication but also tend to help prevent bone fractures and the need for splints and surgery to stabilize bone and treat fractures. The two most commonly used bisphosphonates for bone pain are pamidronate and clodronate, with newer agents such as ibandronate and zoledronate being enthusiastically tested. Pamidronate is generally given by IV drip in the office, the hospital, or an infusion center, but it causes reactions at the injection site and flulike symptoms in a number of patients. These side effects seem to be less prominent with newer IV drugs. Clodronate is given orally and must be followed by drinking up to 240 milliliters of water and remaining upright for thirty minutes to avoid abdominal pain and irritation (esophagitis). Although oral medication is more convenient, absorption is not as good and requires more tablets and higher doses; it also carries a greater risk of stomach upset.

Although not a bisphosphonate, calcitonin is a hormone released by the thyroid gland that also helps regulate calcium levels. A synthetic preparation made from salmon is now commonly used as a nasal spray (Miacalcin) to help control osteoporosis, and it may help control hypercalcemia and bone pain in cancer, taken either nasally or by injection. The spinal administration of calcitonin has powerful pain-relieving effects, but its use is still confined to the research stage in the United States.

Radiopharmaceuticals

Although often overlooked, these treatments (which are similar to a bone scan, a diagnostic test) are relatively noninvasive and in well-selected patients can dramatically reduce pain from widespread bone invasion by cancer, especially when the primary tumor originates in the breast or prostate gland.

The radiopharmaceuticals have two parts—a targeting molecule or "magic bullet" that is attracted to cancer sites in the body, and a radioactive tracer or tag that treats targeted cancer cells by delivering low-level doses of radiation. Because of radiation safety concerns, a radiologist usually administers the treatment. Although different intravenous injections or oral cocktails of these medications have been given for over half a century, adverse reactions have tended to outweigh benefits until the recent introduction of strontium-89 (Metastron) and samarium-153 injections (Quadramet). These newer agents are conveniently administered by IV injection in one session. Side effects are generally minor and infrequent. Although about 20 percent of patients experience a temporary flare-up about forty-eight hours after treatment, this pain is easily managed and may even predict that treatment will ultimately be helpful. Although significant relief usually doesn't occur for about ten days and sometimes not until as much as thirty days after treatment, about two-thirds of patients who are treated appropriately experience significant relief for three to six months, after which treatment is often repeated.

As with external radiation therapy and most chemotherapies, the main potential complication of radionuclide therapies is reduced blood cell counts, especially of platelets, the elements that are needed for normal clotting. Thus, this type of treatment is not used when platelet and white blood cell counts are below 60,000 and 2,400, respectively.

Despite a high up-front cost, savings may be realized over time.

Other Miscellaneous Drugs for Pain

Calcium Channel Blockers and Beta-Blockers

Medications called calcium channel blockers (such as nifedipine [Procardia]) and beta-blockers may be useful to treat certain types of headaches, as well as for reflex sympathetic dystrophy, a pain syndrome associated with re-duced blood flow. Prialt (ziconotide or SNX-111), a new calcium channel blocker for intraspinal administration, is being reviewed by the FDA and would be marketed for nerve pain.

GABA Agonists and NMDA Receptor Antagonists

Increasingly, medications are being developed as a result of recent research that suggests that the sensitization of certain sites on neurons, such as the GABA (gamma-aminobutyric acid) receptors and the NMDA (N-methyl-D-aspartate) receptors of the central nervous system, can cause chronic pain. Baclofen (Lioresal), for example, is a GABA agonist. Usually pre-scribed to treat muscle spasm in multiple sclerosis or spinal cord injuries, it may help shooting, stabbing nerve pain that has not responded to other measures. Usual doses are from 20 to 120 mg per day orally. Baclofen is approved for intrathecal (spinal) administration via implanted pumps to combat severe spasticity, although direct effects on pain seem minimal. Its most common side effects are sedation and confusion.

Some of the NMDA receptor antagonists, which include ketamine and dextromethorphan, are sometimes effective for chronic nerve pain as well. Many studies show that the NMDA receptors are involved in maintaining nerve pain that may be insensitive to opioids. By inhibiting the NMDA receptors, the NMDA receptor antagonists provide pain relief (especially in conjunction with an opioid receptor agonist, such as morphine). Ketamine, once used only to sedate animals or induce general anesthesia in children, has been used in cancer patients with nerve pain that persists despite high doses of IV morphine and may both relieve pain and reduce morphine requirements. However, in higher doses, ketamine produces adverse psychological effects and is a general anesthetic, so its use is usually restricted to terminal states.

Local Anesthetics

Also effective for treating burning, itching, tingling, numbing, or nerve pain is a skin patch impregnated with lidocaine (a local anesthetic used by dentists) called Lidoderm; side effects are infrequent, and it is easy to apply. Unlike Duragesic patches, these can be cut to fit.

Available in an over-the-counter strength and in a stronger concentration by prescription, a topical cream called Zostrix can be helpful for some patients. Made from capsaicin, the substance that makes peppers hot, Zostrix is usually prescribed for pain due to shingles (herpes zoster) but sometimes also for pain from arthritis and other conditions. Zostrix is believed to make skin and joints less sensitive by its actions on a body chemical known as substance P, which is thought to be involved in the pain transmission process. By depleting substance P from nerve endings and preventing its reaccumulation, the area may become less painful. It may also work by being a counterirritant, in that by exciting some nerves, it may block pain signals from others. When Zostrix is applied, patients initially feel a burning sensation that persists for one to four weeks, which is thought to represent the initial outpouring of substance P. The burning may be so severe that some patients will discontinue its use, although they might otherwise obtain relief if they could wait it out.

For superficial, localized pain, compounding pharmacists are increasingly mixing topical gels from a variety of substances, including ketamine, anti-inflammatory agents, and muscle relaxants, although data supporting their use are sparse and insurance companies may not extend coverage.

Adjuvant Drugs for Symptoms Other Than Pain

The rest of the drugs discussed in this chapter are predominantly used for symptoms other than pain, such as treating anxiety, nausea, and depression. While many of these medications produce drowsiness or calmness, there is little evidence that these medications influence pain directly. Although good for nausea and other problems, doctors who are uncomfortable prescribing pain medications may rely on them excessively, rather than simply starting a stronger pain medication or increasing the dose of pain medication.

Only one of these medications—methotrimeprazine (Levoprome)—not only helps restlessness, nausea, and agitation but also has direct pain-relieving properties. The others, fluphenazine, prochlorperazine (Compazine), chlorpromazine (Thorazine), and haloperidol (Haldol), help reduce restlessness, anxiety, and nausea and as a result can lower pain thresholds, but they should not be relied on as treatment for escalating pain.

Tranquilizers That Help Relieve Pain

METHOTRIMEPRAZINE

Brand Name
Levoprome.

Dose Range
Although oral (as well as IV) use has been reported, approved use is limited to subcutaneous or IM injections, so treatment is usually limited to hospice or hospitalized patients, and even so, its use is much less common in the United States than in Europe. The recommended starting dose is 5 to 10 mg, because it may cause oversedation (unless that is desirable in anxious patients who have not responded to more conventional analgesics or who are unable to take opioids), and then is increased.

How Long It Takes to Reach Peak Effect
One and a half hours.

Equivalent Pain Relief
Methotrimeprazine 15 mg by intramuscular or subcutaneous injection is equivalent to the pain-relieving effect of 10 mg of morphine IM.

Comments
- Methotrimeprazine is a sedative and antinausea drug and is best reserved for patients with pain and agitation, with or without nausea.
- This agent lacks the constipating effects of opioids.
- Methotrimeprazine's pain-relieving effect may be as strong as morphine, and it also treats agitation and nausea. But it's an injection and is not readily available by mouth.
- Because its mechanism for relieving pain is different from that of morphine, methotrimeprazine may be particularly useful in patients who have become tolerant to high doses of opioids or who can't take opioids. Can avoid the severe constipation or respiratory depression of opioid use.
- Sedation and sudden low blood pressure upon standing quickly (orthostatic hypotention) tend to diminish after the initial days of taking the drug, and so over time doses may be increased as needed.

- Methotrimeprazine is particularly useful in the advanced phase of cancer when the side effects associated with the drug (low blood pressure problems when standing, sedation, and antianxiety effects) are not a problem; in fact, they may be desirable.

Precautions
- Side effects include sedation, low blood pressure upon standing (orthostatic hypotension), and uncoordinated motor movement, such as uncontrollable twitching (tardive dyskinesia).

FLUPHENAZINE

Brand Name
Prolixin, Permitil.

Dose Range
Usually 1 to 3 mg a day by mouth.

Comments
- This drug helps prevent vomiting and is a major tranquilizer.
- It may help relieve nerve pain and is often prescribed with a tricyclic antidepressant (such as amitriptyline or imipramine) or with an opioid for pain relief.

Precautions
- Side effects include sedation, low blood pressure upon standing (orthostatic hypotension), and uncontrollable twitching jerky movement (tardive dyskinesia) similar to Parkinson's disease.

Tranquilizers Used to Prevent Nausea and Relieve Anxiety

Although often used in conjunction with painkillers, in general the following medications, referred to as major tranquilizers, are primarily used to manage nausea, delirium, agitation, or anxiety.

HALOPERIDOL

Brand Name
Haldol, Haloperon.

Dose Range
Starting dose is 1 to 2 mg by mouth every four to twelve hours.

    If given to treat psychiatric symptoms (agitation), doses may be adjusted up to 10 to 15 mg two or three times a day. Children's doses are based on weight.

Comments
- Although in the United States this drug is associated with emergency treatment for disturbing or violent mental illness, haloperidol is used the United Kingdom extensively to manage nausea and mild agitation. Used in low doses for nausea, vomiting, or agitation, it may produce less drowsiness than other antinausea medications such as Compazine and Phenergan.
- When extremely high doses of opioids are needed for pain, haloperidol often enhances their effect (permitting lower morphine doses), especially in cancer patients who are frightened, agitated, confused, or psychotic.

Precautions
- This drug may cause drowsiness, dry mouth, urinary retention, and twitching (tardive dyskinesia).

CHLORPROMAZINE

Brand Name
Promapar, Thorazine, Sonazine.

Dose Range
Usually 10 to 25 mg every four to eight hours by mouth.

Comments
- Although not a pain reliever, its antianxiety and antinausea properties are often useful when anxiety is aggravating the pain or agitation interferes with assessment and treatment.

Precautions
- Side effects include low blood pressure, blurred vision, dry mouth, difficulty in urinating, constipation, rapid heartbeat (tachycardia), and uncontrolled twitching (tardive dyskinesia).

PROCHLORPERAZINE

Brand Name
Compazine.

Dose Range
Usually 5 to 10 mg every four to eight hours by mouth.

Comments
- This drug is useful as an antinausea and antivomiting medication, but it also helps quell anxiety.
- Available in oral form, IM, and as a suppository.

Precautions

- It can cause dry mouth, drowsiness, dizziness, jerky movements, and blurred vision.
- May turn urine pink or purple.

TRIMETHOBENZAMIDE

Brand Name

Tigan, Arrestin, Benzacot, Bio-Gan, Stemetic, Tebamide, Tegamide, Ticon, Tiject-20, Triban, Tribenzagan, Trimazide.

Dose Range

Usually 250 mg three or four times a day.

Usual rectal suppository dose is one suppository (200 mg), three or four times a day.

For children, dose is calculated by weight: for 30-to-90-pound children, usually 100 to 200 mg (oral or rectal) three or four times a day is prescribed.

Comments

- Trimethobenzamide is helpful for relieving nausea and vomiting.
- It is available in capsules to be taken by mouth, as a suppository, or as an injection.

Precautions

- It can cause drowsiness, dizziness, jerky movements, and blurred vision.
- Trimethobenzamide and other antiemetics should not be used in children suspected of having or developing Reye's syndrome.

THIETHYLPERAZINE

Brand Name

Torecan, Norzine.

Dose Ranges

Usually one 10 mg tablet one to three times a day. In children, appropriate doses have not been determined.

Comments

- Thiethylperazine is helpful in relieving nausea and vomiting.
- It is available in tablets, as a suppository, or as an injection.

Precautions

- The medication contains a sulfite that may cause allergic reactions in sulfite-sensitive people, especially those with asthma.

- It may impair mental and physical abilities, and so the patient should avoid driving and other potentially dangerous activities.
- Occasionally this drug may cause jerky movements, convulsions (more common among young adults), dizziness, headache, and drowsiness with the initial dose.

Medications to Treat Anxiety

These antianxiety (anxiolytic) medications are called the minor tranquilizers, sedatives, or hypnotics. Anxiety is common among cancer patients and may range from feelings of nervousness to full-blown panic attacks that trigger hyperventilation and can mimic a heart attack. Minor symptoms are best treated with simple reassurance and loving contact. When anxiety persists, treatment usually includes some form of psychotherapy (with a psychologist, psychiatrist, counselor, or trained social worker) and antianxiety medication.

Antianxiety medications do not directly relieve pain and should not be used as a substitute for a strong painkiller. However, when pain and anxiety are both problems, it's hard to know which one is the cause of the other, but if significant anxiety persists, both may need to be treated at once. Someone who is characteristically nervous and high-strung may demonstrate a lower pain threshold, complaining of pain when it is really more a question of feeling ill at ease, frightened, or isolated. When complaints of pain seem to be based at least in part on anxiety, treatment with an antianxiety medication can be extremely helpful. Even when anxiety appears to be driving complaints of pain, this should be explored cautiously and with sensitivity to avoid invalidating the patient's suffering.

Psychological and physical dependency can develop with most of these medications, so doctors are often hesitant to prescribe them, especially on a frequent basis for chronic complaints. Moreover, in some states, a triplicate prescription is required. Nevertheless, cancer patients with a genuine need should not be denied them, but at the same time, they should be accompanied by efforts to bolster natural coping mechanisms. Taken over long periods of time, they may actually increase depression, and if they are stopped suddenly, patients may experience physical withdrawal and even seizures.

BENZODIAZEPINES

Diazepam (Valium) is the best-known of this class of drugs, although many new benzodiazepines have become available and are widely used, both to promote sleep and to counter anxiety.

DIAZEPAM

Brand Name
Valium, Vairelease, Vazepam, Diazepam Intensol.

Dose Range
Usually started at a dose of 2 to 10 mg. Can be taken once at night for insomnia or several times each day as needed for anxiety.

Comments
- Although not an all-purpose pain reliever, diazepam helps reduce pain that is associated with muscle spasms because it relaxes the muscles.
- It also is used to relieve anxiety.
- It is available in oral forms, as a rectal suppository, or as an injection.

Precautions
- The most common side effects are drowsiness and disorientation. It may increase depression if used on a frequent basis.

ALPRAZOLAM

Brand Name
Xanax.

Dose Range
For anxiety, 0.25 to 2 mg three times a day, or 0.125 to 1 mg every six hours.

Comments
- Recently introduced and commonly prescribed, it is relatively short-acting and so may be preferred in elderly patients in whom there could be a problem with a buildup of drugs in the body.

Precautions
- Not appropriate for women who are pregnant or for those whose primary diagnosis is psychosis or depression.

Newer Benzodiazepines

Many new benzodiazepines have become available and are widely used, both as sleeping pills and to counter anxiety. Ones that are usually used once at night to improve sleep include flurazepam (Dalmane; 15 to 30 mg), triazolam (Halcion; 0.125 to 0.5 mg), and temazepam (Restoril; 15 to 30 mg). A popular drug used to quell anxiety (and used during the day or night) is lorazepam (Ativan; 0.5 to 4 mg every six hours; this medication is sometimes administered sublingually [under the tongue] in hospice care settings). Midazolam (Versed), only available as an injection in the United

States, is extremely short-acting and may be used to provide sedation for hospitalized patients before stressful procedures and tests, as well as in the late stages of hospice care.

The barbiturate hypnotics (Seconal, Nembutal) are rarely used now because of their potential for abuse and the availability of better drugs. They are still sometimes helpful, however, in a single nighttime dose to enhance sleep. A newer drug, buspirone (BuSpar), also an antidepressant, seems to avoid the habituating effects of the more traditional medicines mentioned in this section.

A drug in this class that is also considered an antihistamine and is sometimes used for cancer pain is hydroxyzine (Vistaril), because it is a sedative and may help relieve pain, usually when administered in combination with an opioid.

HYDROXYZINE

Brand Name
Vistaril, Atarax, Anxanil, E-Vista, Hydroxacen, Hyzine-50, Quiess, Vistaject, Vistazine.

Dose Range
Usually 10 to 50 mg by mouth or 25 to 50 mg by intramuscular injection, three to six times a day.

Children's doses are based on weight.

Comments
- Also considered an antihistamine, hydroxyzine may help dry up secretions.
- This drug is particularly useful for the nauseated patient who is also anxious and in pain. It produces an additive pain-relieving effect when prescribed with morphine or another opioid.
- Its role in cancer pain is controversial because it is sometimes used to ease pain when larger doses of strong opioids would be more effective.

Precautions
- Hydroxyzine can cause sedation or hyperexcitability.

Stimulants

This class of drugs has traditionally been avoided by doctors because they were highly abused in the 1950s and 1960s to promote weight loss. Also, one of the stimulants, methylphenidate (Ritalin), is used to treat hyperactivity and behavior problems in children, creating another source of controversy. They require a triplicate prescription in many states. The research on their use in cancer patients is still relatively new, so some doctors may not be fully experienced with their important uses in patients with cancer. They are used mainly along with the opioids when the sedative effects of the painkilling drugs are compromising quality of life. Taken during the day, they are often very effective in reducing the sedation produced by the opioids. They may also enhance the effectiveness of stable doses of opioids, improve alertness, and boost mood. All of these drugs have the potential to make people jittery, and occasionally appetite may suffer. They should generally not be prescribed to patients with severe psychiatric problems, brain metastases, seizure disorders, or irregular heartbeat (arrhythmia).

METHYLPHENIDATE

Brand Name
Ritalin.

Dose Range
The usual starting dose is 10 mg on awakening and 5 mg with the noontime meal. Tolerance may occur and, as a result, dose increases to 80 mg a day or more may be needed to maintain a beneficial effect.

Comments
- To avoid interference with nighttime sleep, this medication should not be given at night.
- Its main effect is to enhance daytime arousal by minimizing or counteracting the sedation that sometimes persists when higher opioid doses are used. It may also be helpful for daytime fatigue, even when opioids or pain is not the cause. Often improves cognitive function and resolves confusion or delirium. It also can have an antidepressant effect; unlike classic antidepressants, improvement occurs promptly.
- It acts quickly, and if well tolerated initially, problems rarely arise later.
- It poses a low risk of serious problems but occasionally causes agitation and loss of appetite. Cardiac problems and increased confusion are rare.
- While methylphenidate has long been available in a controlled-release form, it does not always work reliably beyond six hours. Concerta (available in 18, 36, and 54 mg tablets) is a new extended-release form that is reliable over a twelve-hour interval and ap-

pears to boost energy more smoothly. Metadate CD (available in 10 and 20 mg doses) is another new sustained-release preparation of methylphenidate that appears to be quite reliable.

- Attenade is a new version of methylphenidate that may be advantageous because it contains just the active components of the two mirror-image compounds that usually make up Ritalin.

DEXTROAMPHETAMINE

Brand Name
Dexedrine, Oxydess II, Spancap No. 1.

Dose Range
Usually 5 to 20 mg by mouth, twice a day. In children, dose is based on weight.

Comments
- Known as "speed" in street language, Dexedrine can offset the drowsiness and sedating effects of the opioids, which is a legitimate medical use, especially when methylphenidate (Ritalin) has been ineffective or is poorly tolerated.
- It should not be given in the evening because the patient may have trouble sleeping.
- It may help enhance the pain-relieving effect of morphine and improve mood.
- Also available in a controlled-release form
- Adderall is a new admixture that may last longer and have a smoother effect than plain methylphenidate or dextroamphetamine. While its main use is for children with hyperactivity, it has been used successfully to boost energy in cancer patients.

Precautions
- An occasional side effect is agitation. Its use should be avoided in the presence of severe agitation or psychosis, brain metastases, heart arrhythmias, and seizure disorders.

PEMOLINE

Brand Name
Cylert.

Dose Range
The beginning dose is one 18.75 mg tablet taken in the morning and at noon, and the daily dose can be gradually increased to up to 75 mg.

Comments

- Unlike the other psychostimulants, pemoline is available in a chewable form as well as nonchewable tablets.
- It can often be used in offsetting opioid-induced sedation and was once considered a front-line choice, largely because its use does not require a special prescription.

Precautions

- Recently the FDA issued a "black box" warning (the FDA's most serious warning, and required to be printed on the label) against pemoline as a first-line treatment due to reports of a rare but very serious association with life-threatening liver failure.

MODAFINIL

Brand Name

Provigil.

Dose Range

The usual dose is 200 mg once a day in the morning, with additional success observed in some patients treated with 400 mg on awakening or 200 mg on awakening and 200 mg in the afternoon.

Comments

- Originally marketed to counteract the excessive daytime sleepiness of narcolepsy, Provigil can help maintain alertness in people with daytime sleepiness from other causes. That can be very useful for people who are sleepy from morphine or other opioids, as well as for the fatigue associated with cancer independent of pain or medication use.
- Modafinil appears to combat sleepiness without the same level of stimulation as other agents and so may be less likely to be associated with a high and thus less habit-forming and less subject to abuse. It does not require a special prescription.
- Although very helpful in chronic pain, the older psychostimulants may be preferred in cancer patients because they are more potent and doses are more easily adjustable.

Precautions

- Although headache is the most common symptom, other possible side effects include nervousness, nausea, dry mouth, diarrhea, anxiety, and insomnia.
- Provigil may reduce the effectiveness of birth control pills and implantable contraceptive devices. While taking Provigil (and for a month afterward), other birth control should be used.

COCAINE

Although used for a long time as part of Brompton's cocktail (a pain-relieving drink that was used before the 1980s and is described in Chapter 6), studies show that cocaine, in fact, has no pain-relieving effect. Although it can theoretically prevent opioid-induced sedation, the safer, legal, standardized psychostimulants described above are used instead.

CAFFEINE

Although not usually prescribed, caffeine may be useful for patients who are drowsy. Caffeine is included in many over-the-counter headache medications, and a strong cup of coffee or tea may help improve alertness.

Antibiotics

Antibiotics help fight infections. Sometimes tumors break through the skin, a process known as *ulceration,* and infection may set in. Antibiotics can help relieve the pain from these open sores, particularly ones on the head and neck. Occasionally tumors that do not break through the skin can get infected as well.

Infection is usually accompanied by fever and other symptoms, but it has recently been observed that pain from head and neck tumors often improves when antibiotics are given, even when there are no obvious signs of infection. Antibiotics can usually be administered orally, except when an infection is severe, in which case they must be given intravenously, usually in the hospital.

Even when the best of care is given, some ulcerated tumors may produce odors, fluid, and pus. This odor can be a source of tremendous embarrassment and suffering for patients, causing them to isolate themselves. Antibiotics such as metronidazole (Flagyl), either administered orally or placed directly on the open sore, may help control this unpleasant smell. Other treatments to help control odor are described in Chapter 11.

Muscle Relaxants

The traditional drugs used to treat muscle spasm (cyclobenzaprine or Flexeril, carisoprodol or Soma, methocarbamol or Robaxin, and chlorzoxazone or Parafon Forte), though often prescribed, are actually not very effective and are best avoided because they produce drowsiness. If muscle spasm is chronic and painful, the best choice may be treatment with diazepam (Valium), which is also an anticonvulsant and a sedative (see discussion above). More recently, baclofen (Lioresal; discussed above), a drug used to treat the severe muscle spasms associated with multiple sclerosis,

Adjuvant Drugs That May Help Particular Types of Conditions

Bone pain	Aspirin or NSAID, such as flurbiprofen (Ansaid) or naproxen (Naprosyn), among others; corticosteroids, such as dexamethasone (Decadron); bisphosphonates; radiopharmaceuticals
Pain from pressure on nerves	Anticonvulsants; antidepressants; mexiletine; corticosteroids such as Decadron or prednisone
Pain from brain tumor swelling	Corticosteroids such as dexamethasone; diuretics (to expel fluids); NSAIDs
Pain from nerve damage	Antidepressants; anticonvulsants; corticosteroids; sodium channel blockers; mexiletine; NMDA antagonists, including methadone (an opioid)
Shingles and other superficial, burning nerve pain	Antidepressants; anticonvulsants; mexiletine; Zostrix; Lidoderm
Intermittent stabbing pain	Anticonvulsants, such as carbamazepine (Tegretol) or valproate; antidepressants; mexiletine
Nerve pain after chemotherapy or radiation	Antidepressants; anticonvulsants; mexiletine
Pain from swollen stomach, hiccoughs	Metoclopramide; an antigas antacid
Pain due to muscle spasm	Antianxiety drug, such as diazepam; sometimes a muscle relaxant, such as baclofen (Lioresal), Zanaflex , or dantrolene may help
Rectal or bladder pain and spasms (tenesmus)	Chlorpromazine or other antianxiety drug; antispasmodic, such as bethanechol (Urecholine) or oxybutynin (Ditropan); suppositories (belladonna and opium)
Pain from swellings in lymph system and other tissues	Steroids; diuretics
Back pain due to spinal cord injury	Corticosteroid, such as dexamethasone (Decadron); diuretic; or both
Infected skin ulcer	Antibiotics such as metronidazole or clindamycin
Tension headaches	Antianxiety drug; calcium channel blocker; beta blocker
Pain and depression together	Any tricyclic antidepressant, such as amitriptyline, unless anxiety is present; caution with the long-term use of the benzodiazepines because these drugs may aggravate depression over time
Severe pain with anxiety and insomnia	Antianxiety drug, such as one of the benzodiazepines
Pain and anxiety together	Benzodiazepine; phenothiazine
Depression and insomnia	Antidepressant, especially the SSRIs (Prozac, Paxil, Zoloft, Celexa, etc.)
Daytime drowsiness	Stimulant, such as Provigil, methylphenidate, or an amphetamine

Note: This list presents only a guide to possible treatments and should in no way be used as a directive. Complete medical evaluations are necessary to determine the best treatment for a particular patient. Some of the listings in the table are also considered controversial and should be discussed thoroughly with your physician.

has been used successfully to help treat muscle spasms as well as nerve pain, especially around the head and neck.

Tizanidine (Zanaflex), an oral medication, helps treat muscle spasms and can be very effective for chronic pain, both as a muscle relaxant and because it can reduce pain by direct mechanisms with continued use.

Dantrolene (Dantrium) is another muscle relaxant that may be tried to relieve spasms, cramping, and tightness of muscles, although it often is poorly tolerated due to gastrointestinal or other vague but disturbing side effects. When none of these options works well, a nerve block (see next chapter) or, although results have not yet been reported in cancer patients, even an injection of botulinum toxin may be considered.

9

High-Tech Options

In recent years, important advances in pain management have dramatically contributed to our ability to provide comfort for today's cancer patient despite nearly any eventuality. Although some of these advances are still being tested, specialists at medical centers around the world have effectively integrated others into routine care. This chapter sorts out the various high-tech options available today, to help the reader balance the potential benefits and risks of each treatment.

Strategies to Relieve Pain

As described in Chapter 3, once a doctor has performed a complete medical workup to determine the source of pain (not all pain is related to the cancer or treatment), each of the many different available treatments falls under one of just three general strategies:

1. *Eliminate or modify the source of the problem* by removing or shrinking the cancer with either surgery, radiation treatment, or chemotherapy (including hormones). Like all therapies, each treatment has some risk. Unfortunately, not everyone is always a treatment candidate, and there are limits as to how much radiation and chemotherapy can be safely or effectively administered. These treat-

ments are discussed in greater detail in books dealing more specifically with cancer, rather than its pain.

2. *Interfere with the interpretation of the pain message,* which is the most common intervention. Here, altering how the brain interprets the information it receives controls pain. Analgesics, such as morphine, blunt pain by altering the brain's perception of it selectively and reversibly. These medication-based treatments can be given by routine routes (orally and by regular injections), as discussed previously, or can be given directly into the spinal cord, as discussed in this chapter.

3. *Interfere with the pain signal itself,* which is the most invasive strategy and thus the least common intervention. Here, the pain signal is interrupted somewhere between the tumor and the central nervous system (the spinal cord and brain) by effectively short-circuiting the pain transmission, like cutting an electrical wire to cause a limited power outage. Alternatives include neurosurgical procedures and anesthetic nerve blocks that interrupt pain transmission by cutting nerves, injecting chemicals, or applying extreme heat, cold, or electrical currents near nerves to disrupt their specific functions. We discuss these techniques below.

New Views of the Role of Opioid Drugs

By far, the most important contemporary advance is not a technical one but an attitudinal one: the refreshingly new appreciation that the pain of cancer is highly treatable with better assessments and a liberal use of tried-and-true analgesics that, although available for generations, were stigmatized and subjected to limited and often erratic and arbitrary medical use.

Among the most sobering of a physician's responsibilities is the imperative to achieve the greatest benefit possible with the least invasive form of treatment, to minimize risk in physically or psychologically demanding or disruptive procedures. It is especially important that patients and doctors don't use questionable innovative treatments simply to avoid using opioids because of lingering concerns about addiction or impairment. When feasible, sticking with oral or similarly noninvasive painkillers (including narcotics) is nearly always preferable, since their treatment effects (wanted and unwanted) are reversible, their risks are low, and treatment can be adjusted easily as needed. As we've said, with some educated trial and error, good comfort levels can usually be obtained by choosing the right dose of the right drug for the right individual at the right time. Only when pain cannot be relieved or side effects persist should the high-tech methods described in this chapter be considered to control pain. Being aware early on of the full spectrum of treatment approaches is comforting, and knowing there are many options available in the remote case they might be needed brings peace of mind.

Intraspinal Opioid Therapy

This way of relieving pain has gained tremendous popularity recently because of its high rate of success, predictability, and relative safety. Because it demands more attention than treatment with simple oral medications, it is only used when oral medications don't provide enough relief or cause unpleasant side effects. Many terms are used to describe what amounts to similar treatment, including epidural morphine, intrathecal or subarachnoid morphine, and spinal implants or spinal pumps.

The Basic Theory: Drug Receptors

As described earlier, morphine is a basic painkiller that traditionally is taken orally, rectally, or by an injection into a vein, muscle, or under the skin. In each case, relatively large doses must be given so that enough can eventually get to the specific locations in the body where morphine produces its effects. The key factors responsible for morphine's capacity to relieve pain are receptors, highly specialized microscopic protein structures that are wedged into cell walls. Receptors are scattered throughout the body but are concentrated in specific areas in the brain and spinal cord. These receptors can be compared to a lock that is opened only by a specific, correspondingly unique key (in this case, morphine and related drugs). Once the receptor is activated, a complex series of biochemical events relieves the pain.

The main advantages of this type of treatment are based on the more-bang-for-your-buck principle: by placing the painkiller directly where it is most effective, very tiny doses can bring dramatic relief with few, if any, side effects. Patients who may require doses of 100 to 1,000 mg of morphine by mouth or even by IV usually get the same or better relief with doses of only 1 to 10 mg given near the spinal cord.

Internal and External Pumps, Implants, and Catheters

The main disadvantage of spinal opioids is that for consistent, reliable pain relief medication must be delivered on an ongoing basis, often over long periods of time. This usually involves minor surgery for implanting a tiny catheter, which is placed with its tip near the spine, either outside the sac that holds the spinal cord and its surrounding fluid (in the epidural space) or within the sac where medications mix directly with spinal fluid (in the intradural, intrathecal, or subarachnoid space). A key advantage to treatment with intraspinal opioids is that simple, reliable methods can confirm whether treatment will be effective before undertaking surgery for the placement of a permanent catheter (implant). Typically, patients undergo either two trial spinal injections of morphine or have a temporary catheter taped to their back for a trial period. These test doses help determine that relief is sufficiently dramatic to warrant ongoing treatment and help rule out placebo effects in hopeful patients. When performed by a skilled anesthesiologist, these procedures are relatively painless and take only a few minutes. Temporary catheters are usually only used for several days or at the most a week or two to avoid the risk of infection and their falling out. However, when a patient is too sick to have a more durable catheter put in, a temporary one is sometimes used for longer periods.

More permanent spinal catheters, such as IV lines, are usually protected by tunneling them for a distance under the skin. This makes these catheters more convenient and safer, reduces the risk of infection and falling out, and allows bathing.

The spinal catheter still must be connected to a source or reservoir of medication, and the medication must be driven (pumped or injected) in a sterile, well-regulated manner. Initially patients and their family were taught to inject morphine syringes through the catheter hub or into a port using sterile techniques. Although relatively simple, inexpensive, and ultimately still acceptable, this approach is demanding of family members and has mostly been replaced with higher-tech approaches that minimize the risk of human error.

Using External Pumps

Now that home care nursing and home hospice care are more available and sophisticated, a portable external pump, which is usually covered by insurers, is frequently used. These battery-powered devices are about the size of a Sony Walkman and include alarms that are triggered if there is a block in the line, the battery power is low, or little medication is left in the reservoir. A home care nurse usually supervises its use and teaches patients and families how to change batteries, drug cassettes, or syringes, and when to call for help. This treatment requires that a nurse always be available to troubleshoot technical problems, with a physician for backup in case the dose needs to be changed or if other problems arise.

USING INTERNAL PUMPS

An even newer and more sophisticated way of administering drugs to the spinal area involves implanting a miniaturized pump (about the size of a hockey puck) under the skin of the patient's abdomen during surgery, a procedure much like that used to insert a pacemaker. This device is refilled with morphine or other medications every one to three months, and between refills the drug dose can be adjusted noninvasively in the doctor's office with a special laptop computer. An important advantage of this device is that patients need not carry cumbersome equipment and can more readily go about a normal life. However, such pumps can cost up to $10,000 and cannot be reused, so doctors are very selective about which patients should receive them. A similar, less expensive implantable device pumps medication at a fixed rate but needs to be refilled with a different strength of pain medication for dose changes.

Regardless of the system used, one end of the catheter goes into the epidural or subarachnoid space to deliver preservative-free morphine or another opioid near its spinal receptors. The other end is either left protruding from the patient's abdomen (externalized catheter) to be attached to an external pump or syringe or, for fully implantable systems, attached to the pump under the skin. Alternatively, the catheter may be connected to a port, a small plastic dome the size of a silver dollar implanted under the skin, which is pierced with a special noncoring needle and connected to a portable external infusion pump or syringe.

Problems and Alternatives

Although uncommon, implanted catheters can become plugged, may kink, or may even break. Infection is also a concern, although infrequent; if an infection occurs, it may spread near the spine, causing meningitis or an epidural abscess, serious conditions that require hospitalization. As with drugs taken by mouth, tolerance to spinal morphine may develop, requiring higher doses. If pain or side effects become difficult to control, other medications can be administered near the spine, such as strong opioids, like hydromorphone (Dilaudid), methadone (Dolophine), fentanyl (Sublimaze), and sufentanil (Sufenta), or weak solutions of anesthetics, such as bupivacaine (Marcaine). Strong local anesthetics are usually not used because they may produce weakness in the legs and bladder, but often a weak solution will produce just enough mild numbness to relieve even severe pain. Newer drugs, such as clonidine, a medication used for high blood pressure, are being used more commonly to relieve persistent pain. One of the advantages of intraspinal opioid treatment is that, unlike nerve blocks, treatment is reversible (no nerves are destroyed) and can be adjusted as needed.

"Cutting the Wires": Nerve Blocks and Neurosurgery

Temporary Nerve Blocks

Nerve blocks can be as simple as the shot of novocaine dentists use to numb a tooth. By injecting a drug near the path of a nerve, you can block the transmission of painful signals before they reach the spinal cord and brain. Such blocks are used for minor surgery and sometimes for chronic pain, such as from a back injury. An epidural nerve block, used commonly for labor pain, provides more extensive pain relief because the anesthetic (numbing medicine) is injected into the epidural space, a compartment that surrounds the spinal cord. These local anesthetic blocks are considered temporary nerve blocks because numbness lasts for only several hours. For cancer pain, which often is progressive and unrelenting, temporary or local anesthetic blocks are usually used for secondary pain that is only indirectly related to the cancer itself or to diagnose or test the use of a more lasting nerve block, rather than for therapeutic use.

The Role of Temporary Nerve Blocks in Cancer Patients

- Diagnostic block (to determine nerves involved in the pain mechanism)
- Prognostic block (as a test to determine whether a more lasting neurolytic block would be appropriate)
- Management of a pain emergency
- Management of pain immediately after surgery
- Management of pain during physical therapy or rehabilitation
- Treatment of muscle spasm, especially from prolonged bed rest
- Treatment of pain from shingles (herpes zoster)
- Management of pain from compression fracture of one or more of the spine's vertebral bodies
- Treatment of reflex sympathetic dystrophy (a form of nerve injury)
- Management of pain from cancer treatment (such as after radiation therapy, mastectomy, thoracotomy, or amputation)
- Management of chronic pain that was present long before cancer was diagnosed

---

Potential benefits of local anesthetic nerve blocks include the temporary or repeated disruption of an established vicious cycle of pain and spasm, the restoration of painless mobility during therapy, and enhancement of local blood flow.

Often, pain relief from a local anesthetic nerve block can be enhanced with a steroid, such as Depo Medrol or Kenalog (triamcinalone). Entirely unrelated to the steroids abused in competitive sports, these steroids mimic substances produced by our own adrenal glands and possess powerful anti-inflammatory effects. Commonly used orally or by intravenous injection for arthritic and respiratory disorders and to treat cancer and its symptoms, directly depositing steroids in a painful area with a nerve block may more effectively reduce local inflammation associated with injury and even tumor. While the local anesthetic provides immediate but short-term relief, the benefits of the steroid can last several weeks or more once they take effect (which may take up to three days). When these injections are used specifically to improve symptoms, they are also referred to as therapeutic nerve blocks.

A temporary or local anesthetic nerve block also may be used to help predict whether long-lasting pain relief is likely to occur from cutting a nerve or injecting a stronger substance to interfere with its function for a longer interval (months or more). This prognostic nerve block mimics the ultimate effect of a more permanent procedure and ideally helps predict any side effects that might result from a more enduring procedure. Unfortunately, the results of the temporary block are not always completely accurate in predicting the effects of a more permanent block.

Permanent Nerve Blocks

Although called permanent nerve blocks, it would be more accurate to call these procedures semipermanent blocks because their effects generally last, on average, from three to six months. These nerve blocks are usually intended to destroy a portion of a nerve to provide relatively lasting relief, which when successful can be a godsend in certain cases. Called a destructive or neurolytic block, or more generally neuroablation, 100 percent ethyl alcohol (absolute alcohol) or phenol is injected very close to the targeted nerve. Occasionally (especially for pain involving the head or neck), instead of an injection, a needle's tip is superheated with a form of insulated electricity (radiofrequency thermoablation) or is frozen with gas (cryoablation) to create the nerve block lesion.

More permanent (destructive) nerve blocks are usually reserved for cancer pain that is likely to persist over time and which is so localized that the patient can reliably point to it. Except for pain involving the abdomen and pelvis, destructive nerve blocks are usually best avoided when pain covers a wide area or is scattered over multiple areas distant from each other. Destructive blocks are also usually performed only when the cancer and its pain are unlikely to improve or be completely eliminated.

Destructive blocks require a great deal of skill to ensure safety and minimize risk (such as interfering with movement or dexterity) and thus are best performed only by specialists, usually anesthesiologists with specific training. To avoid the risk of injury to mixed nerves (combined sensory and

---

Semipermanent Nerve Blocks

Also called neurolytic, ablative, or destructive nerve blocks, semipermanent nerve blocks are used when tumor pain is:
- Severe
- Expected to persist
- Nonresponsive to treatment or cannot be treated with more conservative methods
- Well localized (easy to point to) and consistent (the same complaints persist)
- Predominantly in one area
- Present in patients for whom complete cure of cancer is unlikely

These nerve blocks carry some risks:
- Return of pain, usually beginning after three to six months
- New burning pain in 5 to 15 percent of patients due to nerve injury (neuritis)
- Incomplete relief if pain extends beyond the blocked area
- Rarely, unexpected and sometimes lasting numbness, weakness, or even paralysis if an injection spreads excessively
- New pain in other locations if a tumor progresses or metastasizes
- Apparent worsening of other, milder pains when attention shifts from the treated area

---

motor nerves) or neighboring nerves uninvolved in the pain problem, these procedures must be performed with the utmost accuracy, usually with help from X-rays, fluoroscopy, and occasionally CAT scans. Even in the most skilled hands, patients may occasionally experience muscle weakness of an arm or leg, or even bowel or bladder problems, which may persist for months or longer. Such problems are of particular concern if the patient is not confined to bed. Although these risks are small, they are the main reasons why neurolytic blocks are not performed more frequently.

Another consideration is that while successful nerve blocks eliminate or reduce pain, they numb the area somewhat. Most patients gratefully exchange pain for numbness, but occasionally the numb feeling is irritating (a condition called anesthesia dolorosa). Thus, a destructive nerve block may be preceded by a temporary prognostic block to assess whether long-lasting effects of the procedure are likely to be satisfying.

Unfortunately, no treatment has a perfect success rate, and even when done properly, pain may be only partially relieved or not relieved at all. Since many doctors would rather limit how much alcohol or phenol is injected, to minimize risk, repeated treatments are often needed. This approach is like carefully covering a fence with several thin coats of whitewash instead of applying one thick coat all at once with no drop cloth. To alleviate the discomfort involved in doing a nerve block, the doctor will often numb the area or administer a pain reliever intravenously. The doctor usually cannot put the patient out (general anesthesia) because he will need feedback about whether the temporary nerve block relieves the pain or not. Patients should also be prepared for a severe burning pain when the neurolytic drug (alcohol or phenol) is injected; this is difficult to blunt but lasts only about a minute.

TYPES OF NERVE BLOCKS BY BODY PART

The body's nervous system consists of hundreds of distinct branching nerves, large and small, each responsible for a different function. Any nerve in the body can be blocked, either temporarily or much longer. But with each different nerve block that is considered, the balance of potential benefits and risks varies not only from patient to patient but even in the same patient at different times. For example, a procedure that carries a tiny risk of a limp weighs heavily in an active person with a new pain but may count little if the same pain has persisted despite therapy and prevents activity. Despite the need for carefully individualized decision making, some general guidelines apply nearly universally.

PERIPHERAL NERVE BLOCKS

Treatments of this type involve injecting individual nerves or bunches of nerves (nerve plexuses) located outside the central nervous system (spinal cord and brain) in the periphery of the body. Many of these nerves are mixed nerves, meaning that in addition to sending information about touch and pain, they also send messages about movement and strength. As a result, neurolytic or destructive blocks are used very cautiously (if at all) to avoid the risk of adding limb weakness to the other burdens of being sick. Since there is some overlap in the areas covered by each nerve, sometimes more than one nerve must be blocked. Again, there is usually some numbness after a semipermanent block, which may be desirable but can be disturbing or even painful in some cases; thus a temporary (diagnostic or prognostic) block is often tried first.

For head, neck, or facial pain, a cranial nerve block, usually some form of a trigeminal block, may be recommended. This usually involves placing a needle beneath the skin of the face with its tip near the skull bone. These are technically difficult procedures requiring X-ray guidance and considerable skill. Because problems with swallowing, breathing, or vision occasionally develop, a temporary block is usually performed first.

When pain involves the chest wall, trunk, or abdominal wall, intercostal nerve blocks may be considered. In this case, nerves that run just above and below the ribs near the painful area are injected. Because of the small chance of a collapsed lung (pneumothorax) after this procedure, a chest X-ray is usually taken afterward. A small collapse can usually just be monitored, but more severe cases need to be hospitalized. In serious cases, a chest tube may be inserted for a few days. A spinal (subarachnoid or intrathecal) block may also be considered and is preferred by some physicians trained in its use.

Chronic pain involving the arm or leg is particularly difficult to treat with an injection because of the risk of weakening the limb. Temporary blocks can be performed quite safely, but neurolytic (destructive) blocks of the nerves to the arm or leg are rare unless the limb is already severely weakened or nonfunctional. Even then, an arm that is weakened and swollen from breast or lung cancer may still be needed for minor but important tasks, such as working with the good limb to button a shirt or pull on pants. Nerves sometimes blocked for shoulder, arm, or hand pain are the brachial plexus, a group of nerves that run near the collarbone (clavicle) and which can be injected just above it or in the armpit, and the suprascapular nerve, located near the shoulder. Sometimes the sacral nerves (near the tailbone) are blocked for leg pain, either individually or bunched together (sacral plexus block), but usually a spinal block (also called a subarachnoid or intrathecal block) or occasionally an epidural block is selected instead.

SPINAL AND EPIDURAL NERVE BLOCKS

Also called central blocks, these injections enter between two adjacent vertebrae near the nerve roots, just before the nerves become peripheral nerves. Temporary central blocks (with local anesthetic) are routinely performed every day in most hospitals for labor pain and minor surgery. The epidural injection of steroids mixed with local anesthetic, often used for common low back pain, may also help some cancer patients, especially after vertebral compression fractures, but as with all procedures in cancer patients, it must be undertaken with special vigilance. Spinal (or epidural) administrations of morphine and other opioids, which require continuous infusion, have already been discussed.

Neurolytic spinal blocks with alcohol or phenol, though used for years, are very specialized procedures. They are relatively safer when performed in the midback (thoracic spine) for chest or abdominal wall pain, because the nerves to the arms, legs, and bladder are so distant and shouldn't be affected. Riskier when undertaken near the neck (cervical spine) or lower back (lumbar spine), they should be reserved for special circumstances, although in experienced hands results are usually gratifying. While such blocks can be an excellent treatment for leg pain, they are best reserved for bedridden patients. Even then, bladder weakness (usually temporary) remains a concern, unless diapers or a urinary (Foley) catheter are already needed.

The treatment involves the patient adopting an uncomfortable, curled position for about fifteen minutes. However, the procedure usually relieves severe unrelenting pain and yields to feelings of warmth and numbness within moments, and ideally, relief will last for many months. To avoid complications such as a spreading numbness or weakness, patients must be selected carefully. Prudent physicians take care to avoid risk by not trying to do too much at once, so the treatment may need to be repeated to extend the relief. Impeccable attention to detail can render this and similar therapies invaluable and safe.

When excruciating pain occurs in the genitals or inner buttocks (sometimes occurring with gynecological and anorectal cancers) and a patient, for example, can't even sit, a phenol saddle block may be recommended to calm certain nerve roots. Relief can persist for months, and the procedure may be repeated if needed.

Although most of these procedures are best performed in a supervised institutional setting, they can be performed at the patient's own bedside under extreme circumstances when a patient is too weak or unstable to be moved from home.

SYMPATHETIC NERVE BLOCKS

The sympathetic nerves travel with and help regulate our internal organs, and so when they are injected, patients are not ordinarily bothered with numbness of the skin or risks of muscle weakness. Although a relatively difficult procedure, one of the most common and successful nerve blocks for cancer pain—especially for pancreatic and other cancers associated with abdominal and back pain—is the celiac plexus block or splanchnic nerve block. It involves an injection to the solar plexus, near where your ribs meet at the bottom of the chest cavity. Since this network of nerves is located deep in the abdomen, X-ray or CAT scan guidance is now used routinely along with other safety measures. Usually light sedation is used with the skin numbed before a long needle is introduced below the lowest ribs and on each side of the spine.

For this and other deep nerve blocks, once the skin and underlying muscles have been numbed, the needle's position can be adjusted relatively painlessly, usually with the aid of a radiology technologist and fluoroscope, which provides immediate X-ray feedback. Dye is usually injected to help confirm placement. If a temporary, diagnostic, or prognostic block is planned, a local anesthetic (with or without steroids) is injected.

After the initial local (diagnostic and prognostic) celiac block, the doctor may immediately follow it with a more permanent alcohol or phenol therapeutic neurolytic block, though the treatment may be performed in a series if the diagnosis is in doubt, if the patient is apprehensive, or if difficulties arise in the course of treatment. Once the dye has been visualized and a test dose of local anesthetic administered, the patient will be roused so that a brief neurological exam can be performed to confirm that the local anesthetic has spread predictably, with no compromise of muscle power or numbness. The patient may be lightly remedicated just before the alcohol injection, and despite the local anesthetic he may experience a few moments of severe discomfort, but it is so transient that it begins to fade nearly as soon as it is perceived.

Neurolytic celiac plexus blocks eliminate or reduce pain by more than half, beginning within twenty-four to seventy-two hours and lasting an average of three to six months, in about 80 to 90 percent of well-selected patients. Patients usually require less pain medication and experience fewer side effects after the procedure, which can be repeated if needed. Complications, which are rare, may include transient diarrhea or lowered blood pressure (which responds to IV fluid), a temporary backache, cough, or chest pain. The remote possibility that lower body paralysis may occur keeps this procedure in reserve for those with serious pain problems. If an extensive tumor has "sheltered" the targeted nerve, the procedure may be repeated using a different position or approach.

A celiac plexus block can relieve abdominal and radiating back pain, especially from cancers involving the pancreas, stomach, liver, gallbladder, biliary tree, intestine, spleen, or adrenal glands, as well as pelvic pain that is vague, diffuse, deep, pressing, pulling, dragging, heavy, tight, or full. Rectal pain, which may be sharp, burning, stabbing, or poking, can often be relieved by a similar neurolytic block.

These types of blocks can relieve pain from internal structures without bothersome numbness or motor weakness but are not considered for pain emanating from the body's surrounding somatic structures, such as bone, skin, muscle, or soft tissue. Less commonly, the sympathetic nerves pertaining to the blood vessels of the limbs and face are blocked to treat burning pain and hypersensitivity, a condition resembling reflex sympathetic dystrophy (also called causalgia or complex regional pain syndrome), which is more common after trauma but can occur in patients with lung cancer, breast cancer, lymphoma, or rectal or pelvic cancers, especially in association with edema (swelling), after radiation, and after some surgeries (especially thoracotomy, mastectomy, and amputation).

For burning pain and hypersensitivity in the arm or face, especially in patients with lung or breast cancer, the stellate ganglion, a star-shaped mass of nerve tissue located at the base of the neck near the voice box (larynx), is often injected with a local anesthetic. Lasting pain relief may occur after a series of local anesthetic injections, and for persistent pain, neurolysis is occasionally cautiously considered, with precautions to avoid complications. For burning pain in the lower limb, nerves running along the outside surfaces of the bony spine (lumbar sympathetic ganglia) can be injected safely under X-ray guidance with a local anesthetic or neurolytic drug.

Neurosurgery

With the exception of a few procedures performed at a limited number of centers, many complex neurosurgical pain management procedures have been abandoned in recent years since more liberal use of pain medications has finally been accepted. Also, their decline relates to the risks of neurosurgery, the need for a prolonged recovery from surgery, and a shortage of trained specialists.

However, a cordotomy, a specialized procedure that involves making a cut or burning a small hole in a specific spot in the upper spinal cord, is still occasionally extremely useful. Pain must be strictly limited to one side of the body, should ideally be confined to its lower half (below the waistline, trunk, or armpit), and should be resistant to treatment with simpler, safer methods. Whereas the procedure used to require major surgery, a newer and less invasive percutaneous (through the skin) cordotomy requires neither general anesthesia nor even a skin incision. With the patient sedated, a specialized probe is positioned between the first two cervical vertebrae near the targeted bundle of nerves (lateral spinothalamic tract). Confirmed by fluoroscopy or a CT scan and eliciting the partially awakened patient's responses to light shocks applied to the needle's shaft, radio-frequency electrical energy interrupts the pain fibers. In trained hands, this relatively simple, safe, and effective procedure does not require prolonged recovery. Patients occasionally experience minor balance or gait problems, but despite its admittedly frightening aspects, serious complications are uncommon.

Electrical Stimulation and the Gate Control Theory of Pain

The gate control theory of pain is a theoretical model suggested by pain specialists Drs. Ronald Melzack and Patrick Wall to explain why certain types of mild electrical shocks can relieve certain pains. They proposed that if many nonpainful messages are sent to the spine, there might be enough of a "traffic jam" to block out the painful messages. An example is a burned hand or a finger banged by a hammer; sometimes the pain is lessened if the hand or finger is held under cold water or sucked on—the nonpainful stimuli actually close the "pain gates" in the spinal cord. The use of the cream Zostrix (see Chapter 8) and skin stimulation (vibration, massage, and hot and cold packs; see Chapter 12) are other examples.

In practice, four types of electrical stimulation have been used with some success, although they are not commonly recommended to treat cancer pain.

Transcutaneous Electrical Nerve Stimulation (TENS)

TENS uses a mild electrical current applied to the skin to reduce pain. Like acupuncture, it may work by triggering the body's natural chemical painkillers, and also like acupuncture, there may be some placebo effect that harnesses the mind's powerful desire for treatment to work but which may cause benefits to decrease over time. Commonly used for low back and other musculoskeletal pain, it can be used for cancer pain, and although its effects alone are not usually strong enough to block severe pain, it can help some patients.

A small battery-powered box, about the size of a beeper, is connected with insulated wires to patches (like EKG stickers) that are placed on the skin over the area that hurts. When the unit is activated, a gentle tingling or buzzing sensation is felt that, in about half of patients, may interfere with the pain sensation.

The patient can adjust the unit's many controls, manipulating the current's amplitude (strength), frequency, and other features, much like the volume and tone knobs of a portable stereo. Its advantages include a sense of empowerment in that the patient can control the treatment, safety (although it should be avoided in patients with a cardiac pacemaker), almost no side effects, portability, ease of use, low cost (units can be leased), and coverage by most insurers. TENS is usually not effective for severe pain, however, and often pain relief deteriorates within a few months. Because relief varies so much between patients, it is best to ask for a unit that has at least a thirty-day trial.

Spinal Cord Stimulation

This more costly and complicated treatment involves hospitalization and minor surgery to place one or more miniature electrodes near the areas of the spinal cord that transmit a patient's pain. Although full-blown surgery is sometimes required, because the electrodes reside in the epidural space they can often be positioned through an epidural needle, much like the catheters described above. The electrode is tunneled under the skin and attached to a surgically implanted portable battery pack (like that for a pacemaker or intrathecal pump). A preoperative trial is required to try to predict effectiveness, but even when relief seems likely, permanent systems are hampered about half the time by technical problems.

This treatment has become more popular recently, but mostly for chronic low back pain, sciatica, and cervical spine problems, and even then it is controversial because of costs up to $20,000. It is rarely considered for cancer pain, although some suggest that it could have value in cancer survivors who have well-localized pain due to cancer treatments, such as shingles or pain after radiation, mastectomy, or thoracotomy. Tumor-related pain is usually too variable and requires a more reliable approach.

Brain Stimulation

Though still considered experimental by many, brain stimulation (also called deep brain stimulation and thalamic stimulation) has been used for cancer pain with good results and may be one of tomorrow's answers for the few pains that cannot be treated with standard methods. By activating the brain's opioid receptors, deep brain stimulation seems to release more of the body's natural painkillers (endogenous opioids or endorphins). Stimulation of the thalamus, one of the brain's relay centers, is currently being investigated for help with certain nerve pains, such as shingles and phantom limb pain. Under local anesthesia, a small electrode is guided to the correct spot in the brain through a small hole drilled in the skull and is then attached to a battery pack. Precise placement is increasingly possible using computer-boosted stereotactic methods. Brain stimulation is performed by neurosurgeons specializing in the procedure in only a few medical centers, and may not be fully covered by insurance.

Percutaneous Electrical Nerve Stimulation (PENS)

For chronic bone pain, a newer procedure involves temporarily inserting tiny acupuncture-like needles into the soft tissue near bones. As with TENS, a low-voltage electrical current is applied to the needles, which produce a tingling sensation that may provide temporary relief by interfering with the transmission of pain signals.

Miscellaneous Techniques

Other than cordotomy, most neurosurgical operations for pain are performed only rarely, although a few specialists have reported very good results, which is especially meaningful since most of these patients had difficult pain problems. These kinds of procedures include neurectomy (which involves cutting nerves), myelotomy or commissurotomy (which involves making an incision in the spinal cord to sever certain nerves), and many others that are even more technical.

Pituitary Ablation

The pituitary gland is centrally located at the very base of the skull, below the middle of the brain and behind the center of the face. Working with the hypothalamus, the pituitary helps regulate the body's most fundamental activities, including sleep, temperature, nocturnal and diurnal rhythms, growth, sexuality, and blood pressure. Regarded as a "master gland," its stimulatory and inhibitory hormones control the functions of secondary glands such as the thyroid, adrenals, ovaries, and testes. Despite its importance, damage or removal of the pituitary gland by disease, tumor, surgery, and radiation is well tolerated as long as hormone supplementation is provided afterward.

In years past, surgically removing the pituitary was found to eliminate severe bone pain. Today, this can be done by carefully inserting a needle through the nose into the pituitary gland (under anesthesia), where with X-ray guidance, a few drops of alcohol are injected. Despite some serious risks, the long duration of near complete pain relief in most treated patients initially led to increasing popularity. With the more liberal use of opioids, including spinal administration, this procedure is now performed in only a few medical centers, but it can still be very helpful for a relatively small number of patients with many different areas of persistent bone pain, especially when pain is due to metastatic breast or prostate cancer. More recently, there has been a renewed interest in using heat, radiofrequency, and now gamma knife radiosurgery (focused radiation therapy) in place of alcohol injection.

Psychosurgery: A Largely Outmoded Method

Psychosurgery, not a very likely treatment today, includes about a dozen procedures that deliberately injure brain tissue to treat mental illness and pain. Psychosurgery, such as lobotomy, has been inappropriately used over the years; because it causes irreversible personality changes and because of the advent of effective antipsychotic drugs and analgesics, it has mostly been abandoned. However, advanced technology, such as stereotactic radiosurgery, permits the generation of a precise, focused lesion without even an incision and has led to a cautious renewed interest at specialized centers that have investigated modified procedures that possess minimal risks of personality change, such as cingulotomy and capsulotomy, to treat intractable pain and psychiatric disorders.

Thermotherapy

A new image-guided treatment that is not yet widely used destroys tumors either by heat generated by a laser or radiofrequency unit or by extreme cold (cryotherapy) provided by compressed gas, often relieving associated pain. Tumors are pinpointed with either computer tomography or magnetic resonance imaging and must meet approved criteria to be considered treatable with these new therapies.

Part III

OTHER APPROACHES
AND CONCERNS

To cure sometimes
To relieve often
To comfort always

—Robert G. Twycross and Sylvia A. Lack

10

Dealing with Constipation, Diarrhea,
Nausea, and Vomiting

Pain is not the only factor that can take its toll on a patient's quality of life. Side effects from radiation, surgery, chemotherapy, and other medications, as well as other ailments resulting from cancer, can cause significant discomfort. Just as the pain of cancer can be well controlled when treated aggressively, most of these symptoms, such as nausea, vomiting, diarrhea, and constipation, can also be effectively managed.

As with pain, families shouldn't ever assume that these unpleasant symptoms are inevitable and must be tolerated. When a family reports these symptoms as problematic, few doctors will say, "I give up; there is nothing I can do." Time-tested remedies are available for many of these symptoms, as are new treatments for problems that persist. Effective treatment may be simple or complex, but regardless, cooperation and communication between patient and doctor are as important here as they are to achieve adequate pain control. To ensure a cancer patient the best quality of life possible, the same careful attention needed to control pain should be applied to address other symptoms and sources of discomfort.

Most Side Effects Can Be Treated

Cancer is typically a multisymptomatic disease. In other words, because of its potential to interfere with so many of the body's systems, cancer can be responsible for a tremendous variety of complaints. Problems may arise from substances the cancer produces, from the cancer's invading or pressing on normal structures, or from organ failure. Symptoms may also result from the treatment of the cancer with surgery, chemotherapy, radiotherapy, and analgesics. A person may suffer from problems that are caused indirectly by the cancer, such as those related to depression or being confined to bed for a long period. Finally, problems may arise that are completely unrelated to the cancer or its treatment. Some of the symptoms that can occur with cancer are listed below, along with their estimated frequency.

Symptoms in Patients with Advanced Disease

Common symptoms (occurring in more than half of patients)
Pain
Weight loss
Lack of appetite (anorexia)
Constipation
Weakness and fatigue
Drowsiness
Nausea/vomiting
Depression

Less common symptoms (occurring in less than half of patients)
Difficulty breathing (dyspnea)
Coughing

Swelling
Insomnia
Urinary problems
Difficulty swallowing (dysphagia)
Bedsores (decubitus ulcers)
Bleeding (hemorrhage)
Diarrhea

Rare symptoms (occurring in less than 10 percent of patients)
Paralysis
Jaundice
Colostomy
Dry skin (pruritus)
Mouth sores

It goes almost without saying that if the doctor is not aware of distressing symptoms that are plaguing the patient, he cannot help. That is why it is essential that the doctor be informed of any problem that arises, particularly if it is unusual, no matter how small. *Do not assume that these symptoms are too minor to warrant the doctor's attention or that they cannot be controlled and must be tolerated.*

Remedies for some of the common symptoms of cancer—especially nausea, vomiting, and constipation—have been well known for years, and most doctors will have recommendations readily available to treat them. Even symptoms that persist despite treatment or that used to be considered untreatable are now the subject of extensive research with many promising results. For example, difficult symptoms such as weight loss, fatigue, and shortness of breath have responded well to new treatments. Some of these approaches are so new that not every doctor will be familiar with every recent development, so if something in this chapter may be helpful for a loved one, share the information with the doctor. Most of these symptoms can be treated effectively by your family doctor or oncologist. If the condition persists despite aggressive treatment, the primary doctor may consult with a pain or palliative care specialist (for example, through the some of the organizations listed in Appendix 1).

Constipation

As emphasized by Cicely Saunders, one of the originators of the modern palliative care movement, nothing matters more than the bowels when it comes to helping a person who is ill with cancer. Constipation is exceedingly common among cancer patients because many of the drugs used to treat cancer or cancer-related symptoms (including opioids, anticonvulsants, antidepressants, tranquilizers, muscle relaxants, and chemotherapy agents, such as vincristine and vinblastine) can contribute to constipation. Constipation may also be triggered by lengthy stays in bed with no exercise, tumors in the gastrointestinal region, changes in the diet such as reduced food and liquid intake, low fiber intake, dehydration from fever and vomiting, and anxiety and depression. Patients who are weak, who have difficulty breathing, or are suffering from paralysis or leg weakness may have problems with constipation as well.

Sometimes constipation causes pain that patients do not suspect as being the result of constipation, because the pain can be perceived as being as high up as the ribs. If constipation is not addressed, the result can be extremely serious, even life-threatening. Patients should not feel embarrassed or ashamed to bring up problems with bowel movements. Nor should they assume that a doctor's help is not needed just because medication can be obtained without a prescription.

Probably because it involves a very private bodily function, constipation and bowel habits are not generally discussed fully enough. As a result, bowel problems may be overlooked when a preventive approach would forestall problems. Because many laxatives are available over the counter, without a prescription, patients are often left on their own to seek a remedy. This should be highly discouraged—it is important to put embarrassment aside and consult the doctor on how to manage constipation.

One of the problems with regulating bowel habit is that each of us defines regularity differently. Some individuals feel constipated if they do not have a bowel movement daily, while others are accustomed to waiting several days or even a week between normal bowel movements. Treatment should try to reestablish an individual's regular bowel habits as much as possible. Most authorities feel that a bowel movement at least every three days is an appropriate guideline.

If constipation is treated before it gets too bad (in other words, prophylactically), the problem can almost always be managed effectively. As noted, however, if constipation is allowed to become severe, it can produce extremely serious health problems, sometimes bad enough to require hospitalization and even surgery. Too, patients may mistakenly believe it is normal to require regular treatment with enemas or manual disimpaction, and may be pleasantly surprised to learn how easily their bowel habits can be regulated with a preventive approach.

Patients should never have to be afraid to take pain medications because of constipation, since although it is a common side effect of the opioid analgesics, it is easily prevented.

Be Sure to Get a Recommendation for a Laxative

As with most conditions, prevention is always the preferable means for dealing with chronic constipation. Since many of the drugs administered by the doctor, especially the opioids, can produce constipation, each time an opioid is prescribed, it should be accompanied by a recommendation for a laxative. Tolerance to these constipating effects occurs only slowly, if at all, and treatment with laxatives usually is required for as long as these medications are taken. Likewise, as the dose of opioid is increased, the dose or strength of the laxative should be increased as well. Just as more than one type of painkiller may be needed, it is not unusual for more than one type of laxative to be needed.

Fecal Impaction

If constipation persists despite treatment, the doctor will check for a condition called fecal impaction by performing a rectal examination. This is occasionally overlooked, because such an examination—even though brief and relatively painless—can be unpleasant. In fecal impaction, dried stool becomes hard and lodges itself in the rectum, usually near the anus, blocking the passage of other wastes. This is dangerous if unrecognized, because if increasingly strong laxatives are given, they may produce severe cramps and even a rupture or perforation of the bowel. Another reason that fecal obstruction is sometimes missed is that liquid stool (produced by laxatives) may leak around the impaction, causing confusion by creating the illusion of diarrhea.

One way to treat this condition once it has become established is for the doctor or caregiver to place a gloved finger through the anus into the rectum and remove the hardened stool manually. This is painful and may require anesthesia or a sedative. Sometimes fecal impactions occur higher in the colon and can be relieved with enemas. When combined with enemas (especially with mineral oil or milk and molasses) and laxatives, the impaction can usually be relieved, and with continued treatment with laxatives, repeated episodes can often be avoided.

Practical Strategies to Prevent Constipation

There are a number of strategies that can help to prevent constipation.

- Drink eight to ten glasses of water or other liquids daily. Fruit juice or warm tea upon awakening is often suggested. Prunes (preferably stewed) or warmed prune juice twice a day (morning and evening) can help produce more regular bowel movements.
- Try eating high-fiber foods, including bran, fresh raw fruits and vegetables, prunes, dates, whole-grain cereal products (whole wheat bread, brown rice, barley, whole-grain couscous, etc.), nuts, corn, raisins, and coconut.
- Avoid foods such as cheese and highly refined grain products, such as cookies, cakes, doughnuts, and crackers.
- Exercise as much as possible to stimulate intestinal activity. Even just regular walking will help.
- Keep a chart of bowel movements; they should occur around every two days. If the patient does not have a bowel movement within three days in spite of stool softeners and stimulant purgatives, a rectal suppository or stronger laxative is usually recommended to prevent severe episodes of constipation and fecal impaction.
- Encourage the patient to defecate as soon as he has the urge; a commode close by can often help. A squatting position is ideal for the patient, if possible. A toilet seat may be adapted with a plastic ring, which is often used on toilets for the handicapped, to make the seat higher, but patients will probably need a footstool to support their feet so they can bear down. Bedpans should be avoided as much as possible, since they are difficult to use for defecating; if necessary, however, try to help the patient maintain a crouched position on it, with the feet bearing down on the mattress or over the side of the bed onto a chair or table (avoid leaving the feet dangling).
- One home remedy is to freeze rolls of petroleum jelly (one-quarter teaspoon each) and then roll them in powdered sugar for eating. A few doses can often relieve mild to moderate constipation.

Medical Management of Constipation

STARTING WITH A LAXATIVE

As stated before, as soon as a person starts taking opioid medications regularly, he should also start taking action to prevent constipation. Although a stool softener (which keeps stools soft by retaining water) is useful, if constipation is already present a stool softener alone is probably not adequate, especially if fluid intake is low. That is why most doctors recommend starting treatment with a stool softener and a mild stimulant laxative (which enhances bowel activity) combined.

Common softeners include methylcellulose, psyllium (Metamucil), and natural fibers such as bran. If using Metamucil, drinking eight to ten glasses of liquid a day is very important. Common mild stimulant laxatives include Doxidan, cascara sagrada, senna (a natural product that is available alone [Senokot] or combined with a softener [Senokot-S]), bisacodyl (Dulcolax), and docusate (Colace). *Note*: Avoid laxatives with magnesium in patients with kidney disease and laxatives with sodium in patients with heart disease.

These medications are usually taken once in the morning and once in the evening, in increasing doses as needed, to produce a bowel movement of appropriate consistency at regular intervals. (For example, one tablet of laxative will usually counter the constipating effects of 60 mg of codeine or 30 mg of oral morphine. Higher doses of morphine will often require higher doses of laxatives; if on 60 mg oral morphine, for example, then two tablets may be needed.) Many patients prefer to use laxative medications that they have taken in the past because they have worked well; that's fine, as long as the doctor knows.

Treatment should proceed on what doctors often call a "sliding scale" basis. This means starting with regular treatment with a laxative that is strong enough to produce bowel movements regularly. If two to three days have passed without activity, patients should then take a stronger medication; if constipation still persists, their medication should be increased. Other laxatives such as lactulose, magnesium hydroxide (milk of magnesia), and especially magnesium citrate may be used as needed if several days without activity have elapsed. Mineral oil can be used occasionally, but not in patients who are very sick and thus prone to breathing and swallowing problems (aspiration). A variety of enemas are available, but regular use of enemas should be avoided.

An enema made at home from milk and molasses has gained considerable popularity at the M. D. Anderson Cancer Center and elsewhere because it's gentle but thorough. As opposed to many enemas, which are administered superficially or "low" by means of a short, stubby, hard plastic applicator, a milk and molasses enema is intended to be given higher, by using an applicator consisting of an enema bag connected to long soft, flexible tubing. After liberal lubrication, the catheter tip is gently inserted past the anus and, as long as no resistance is encountered, advanced an additional twelve inches or so. Eight ounces of warm water and 3 ounces of powdered milk are shaken in a jar; 4.5 ounces of molasses are added, and the solution is mixed again, after which it is administered every six hours until formed stool is no longer produced.

Interestingly, a novel opioid medication, methylnaltrexone (MNTX), has shown great promise in late-stage clinical development tests for reversing constipation associated with traditional opioid medications. Naltrexone is an opioid antagonist that reverses all effects of opioids (including pain relief). It was chemically altered to prevent passage across the blood-brain barrier; the resulting substance, methylnaltrexone, reverses the constipating effect of opioids but does not cross into the brain and thus does not affect the opioids' pain relief. Most test subjects experienced the immediate need for a bowel movement with no loss of pain relief. Similarly, naloxone (Narcan), an opioid antagonist that is used intravenously to reverse the effects of drug overdoses or severe respiratory depression, has been administered orally to treat constipation with good preliminary results. Used orally, the drug's chemical structure prevents passage to the bloodstream, where it would otherwise provoke a return of pain, but its action on opioid receptors in the gut helps reverse constipation.

By exploiting what would normally be regarded as its side effects, use of the weight loss drug orlistat (Xenical) also has some exciting applications for refractory constipation. This drug keeps weight down by blocking lipase, the body's usual mechanism for digesting fats, and produces an increased passage of stool after fatty foods are eaten, an effect that is welcome in most cancer patients. Orlistat, however, like naloxone, is expensive.

Diarrhea

Diarrhea is relatively uncommon in cancer patients and may actually result from the overzealous use of laxatives. The presence of diarrhea may require the physician to perform a brief manual rectal examination to be certain there is not a blockage around which liquid stool is leaking. Diarrhea may occur in conjunction with chemotherapy (especially 5-fluorouracil [5-FU]and rinotecan [CPT-11 or Camptosar]), or with radiation treatments to the abdomen or pelvis. It may persist for several weeks after such treatments, and in the case of radiation injury to the gut may be a permanent although treatable feature. Diarrhea also can be caused by anxiety and stress, lactose intolerance (when the body can't digest milk products), and the use of certain dietary supplements.

Recommended Diet

Eat low-fat and low-fiber foods, such as cottage cheese and other low-fat cheeses; eggs that aren't fried; natural yogurt; broth; baked, broiled, or roasted fish, poultry or ground beef; rice pudding, custard, or tapioca made with low-fat milk; gelatin; hot cooked cereals; bananas; applesauce or apples without skins; apple or grape juice; white bread or toast; white crackers; white pasta or rice; potatoes; and cooked vegetables such as green beans, carrots, peas, spinach, or squash, or soups made from these vegetables. Many nurses and the American Cancer Society suggest using nutmeg as much as possible because it is believed to help slow down the gastrointestinal tract.

Foods to avoid include all those mentioned above to help constipation; fried or greasy foods; raw fruits and vegetables; pastries; potato chips; strong spices (chili powder, licorice, pepper, curry, garlic, horseradish); olives; pickles; gas-producing foods such as beans, broccoli, onions, and cabbage; caffeine-containing drinks; alcoholic drinks; and tobacco products.

If the patient with diarrhea is fatigued as well, it may be a sign of low potassium. High-potassium foods such as potatoes, bananas, green beans, halibut, and asparagus tips should be eaten or potassium supplements taken. Those with kidney problems should be especially concerned with eating adequate high-potassium foods.

To prevent dehydration during episodes of diarrhea, at least eight to ten glasses of liquids should be taken daily, especially fruit juice, bouillon or broth, weak warm tea, gelatin, and flat caffeine-free sodas (those in which the carbonation has been allowed to escape).

If significant weight loss is associated with the diarrhea, or if adequate fluid intake cannot be maintained, contact the doctor at once.

Eat small but frequent meals, and stick to liquid foods if diarrhea is severe. Extremely hot or cold foods may aggravate the condition, so consume foods that are of moderate or room temperature.

Medications

For milder cases, over-the-counter medications such as Kaopectate, Pepto-Bismol, or Imodium can help. Some of these products contain loperamide, which can be also prescribed by a physician in capsule form as a preventive measure.

For more severe cases, when diarrhea lasts longer than two or three days, the doctor may prescribe Lomotil, paregoric, or tincture of opium. Although the latter two medications have withstood the test of time, they are controlled substances, and thus physicians try to avoid them even though they are safe and unlikely to promote addiction. Octreotide (Sandostatin), an analog of one of the body's own pancreatic hormones (somatostatin), is a newer alternative that is reserved for specific settings. Initially used just for diarrhea produced by certain hormonally related tumors (carcinoid tumor and VIPoma), because octreotide is so effective it is increasingly considered for persistent diarrhea due to other causes such as chemotherapy, AIDS, and radiation injury, among others. Its other main use in cancer is treatment of bowel obstruction that occurs in the course of some cancers. It is also used to treat acromegaly (a growth hormone disturbance).

In addition, this medication is helpful for certain types of nausea and vomiting; it dries gastrointestinal secretions and reduces obstructions. It is currently being tested by the spinal route for pain. The main limitation of octreotide, however, is that it is expensive and must be injected. As already mentioned, all of the opioid analgesics work to slow bowel function and should help reverse diarrhea. Discuss this with the doctor if relevant.

Making the Patient More Comfortable

Frequent diarrhea can irritate the bottom. To soothe it:

- Clean up after each bowel movement with warm water, rinse well, and pat the area dry with a soft towel. Don't rub.
- Creams for the anal area that can help soothe irritation include Desitin or Proctodon.
- If the area is very sensitive, a topical local anesthetic prescribed by the doctor or a corticosteroid spray or cream may be applied.
- Warm baths or salt baths may be soothing to the region.
- Allow the area to be exposed to air. If the patient has difficulty controlling the liquid stool, a disposable brief or pad (such as Depends, which is made for adults) can be helpful.
- Lay a disposable, plastic-lined bedsheet under the patient.

Nausea and Vomiting

Although many patients may never experience nausea or vomiting, those who do can be miserable. And unfortunately, nausea and vomiting are relatively common—either as occasional problems associated with chemotherapy sessions (usually during administration or within hours afterward) or as a chronic problem. Nausea and vomiting most commonly occur together but may occur separately. Since the causes and management of both symptoms are usually similar, most of the comments made here about nausea can also be applied to vomiting, and vice versa, unless specifically stated otherwise.

Causes of Nausea and Vomiting

Chronic nausea and vomiting may result from many factors. They may be triggered by tumors partially or even completely obstructing or blocking the gastrointestinal tract, in which case swelling of the abdomen (distension) may or may not be present. They may be caused by radiation injury to the bowel, scarring (adhesions) from surgery, and even by simple constipation.

Injury to the kidneys or liver can reduce the purifying functions of these organs, and nausea may result from a buildup of the body's toxic waste products. Nausea may be caused by a tumor in the brain, either one that starts there (primary tumor) or one that has spread from elsewhere (metastatic tumor). Metabolic imbalances—changes in the body's fluid and salt (electrolyte) content—are common causes of nausea as well, especially when there is an excess of calcium, which is particularly common in patients with bone cancer. Nausea can be caused or worsened by mouth problems—such as infection, sores, or tumor growth.

Nausea is also a potential side effect of many medications, including those used to treat pain. The NSAIDs can irritate the stomach lining and produce ulcerlike symptoms, including nausea and vomiting. All of the opioids, including morphine, have the potential to produce nausea and vomiting that are usually transient. In fact, up to one-third of patients will experience nausea after first starting to take an opioid medication, as well as after its dose has been increased. Such nausea can usually be effectively treated with a simple antiemetic (see later in this chapter), and since it rarely lasts for more than a few days, treatment with the antiemetic can, in most cases, be tapered and then discontinued with continued use of the opioid.

Tip: Whenever an opioid is prescribed, ask for a prescription to treat both constipation and nausea. Also, be sure to ask if the antinausea medication should be tapered off. Most people become tolerant to the nausea induced by painkillers and can begin tapering antinausea medications after just a few days.

Finally, nausea may be psychological in origin (which is not to say that it is less severe or significant or any less real). Doctors have recognized a specific nausea of this type, which they call anticipatory nausea and vomiting. It usually occurs in patients who have had nausea after chemotherapy, who then go on to become nauseated at the next session, even before treatment is started. This reflex may be so strong that simply driving by the hospital or seeing one's nurse at the supermarket can trigger an episode of nausea and vomiting.

Practical Strategies to Counter Nausea and Vomiting

Several simple techniques that don't involve medication can help with nausea and vomiting.

- Encourage the patient to eat plain crackers (saltines, for example) or to sip room-temperature flat cola or ginger ale when feeling nauseated.
- Switch, at least temporarily, to a clear liquid diet including foods such as apple juice, cranberry juice, broth, ginger ale, gelatin, tea, Gatorade, frozen fruit juice pops, cola or lemon-lime drinks, and so on.
- If the patient has no mouth sores, sometimes sour foods such as lemons, pickles, or sour hard candy can help ward off nausea. Rinsing with a dilute mixture of lemon juice and water may also help.
- Avoid sugary, high-fat, highly salted, greasy, or spicy foods, or those with strong odors, such as cheese or salami.
- Foods that usually are well tolerated include bland foods, such as toast, potatoes, applesauce, crackers, broth, and cottage cheese. Eat slowly.
- Avoid smells or sounds that could trigger nausea, such as cooking smells and perfumed body scents.
- When in chemotherapy, some relaxation exercises (see Chapter 12) before the treatment may help. During chemotherapy, sucking on hard or sour candies or mints may counter the distasteful metallic flavor that some patients taste during sessions. If nausea consistently occurs, try switching appointments to a different time of day.
- Experiment with different eating patterns. Some patients do better when they don't eat or drink for several hours before chemotherapy; others do best when they eat heavily three or four hours before a session and then continue throughout the day with light meals or snacks. Others prevent nausea by switching to a liquid diet for the day before and after the chemotherapy session. Still others prevent nausea by eating only light but frequent meals

throughout the day. Some doctors recommend avoiding favorite foods on days the patient may become nauseated so the patient does not come to associate the nausea with those foods.

- Get plenty of fresh, cool air, either through an open window or with a fan.
- Use the relaxation, distraction, imagery, and breathing techniques in Chapter 12. Acupressure or acupuncture may also help.
- Other distractions may help, too, such as watching a movie or television, doing a craft, or talking with a friend.
- Try to sleep after chemotherapy, when nausea may be expected.
- If the patient vomits, keep a log of the time, amount of vomit, and what it looked like (color, consistency) to report to the doctor or health care team. Avoid eating solids until vomiting spells pass; sometimes that might be up to twenty-four hours. Rinse the mouth after each episode with a dilute mixture of lemon juice and water. Afterward, try sucking ice chips or taking one of the liquids already mentioned as part of the clear liquid diet.

Medical Management of Nausea and Vomiting

Medications known as antiemetics can help prevent nausea and vomiting. When nausea and vomiting are the result of chemotherapy, the antiemetic should be taken six to twelve hours before the next chemotherapy session to avoid anticipatory nausea. The doctor will recommend that medication be continued every four or six hours for at least twelve to twenty-four hours, or longer if any nausea persists. Since many chemotherapy drugs have the potential to produce nausea, patients are often treated in advance of any problems with a combination of antiemetics, many of which are given intravenously. Even so, nausea and vomiting may still occur and may occasionally be severe enough to require hospital admission.

Choosing an antiemetic can be difficult. Nausea may be triggered by several different mechanisms, and since the antiemetic drugs work by different mechanisms, a trial-and-error approach using different drugs is usually taken. The first medication selected to treat mild nausea, including chemotherapy-induced nausea, most often comes from the group of drugs known as the major tranquilizers. These drugs are usually tried first because they are effective in most cases, can be given orally, are relatively inexpensive, and are unlikely to cause serious side effects. These medications include prochlorperazine (Compazine), trimethobenzamide (Tigan), promethazine (Phenergan), and haloperidol (Haldol). Interestingly, Haldol is commonly regarded in the United States as the treatment of choice for resolving severe psychotic reactions, but it is actually the least sedating of these agents. For this reason in the United Kingdom it is not stigmatized and is also usually the antiemetic of first choice. These agents are commonly prescribed in tablet form but are readily available as rectal suppositories (and even injections) if the nausea is accompanied by such severe vomiting that oral medications cannot be reliably kept down. Again, they are usually prescribed every four to six hours, and when nausea is persistent, they should be taken regularly for a period of time and then tapered off. The main side effect of these medications is drowsiness. Rarely they trigger a side effect that produces sudden involuntary movements (called extrapyramidal signs), which can be frightening but are not harmful. Extrapyramidal signs are more common in younger individuals and, fortunately, can usually be easily reversed with diphenhydramine (Benadryl).

The medications mentioned so far are the ones used most commonly. If they are not effective, however, new or overlapping strategies are then instituted. If one of the major tranquilizers has been only partially effective or produces undesirable sedation, a medication that works by an alternative mechanism can be added or substituted. Although treatment with the major tranquilizers is sufficient in most patients, sometimes several different medications must be tried, often together.

Metoclopramide (Reglan, Maxeran) is probably the most common second-line antiemetic drug. It has dual effects: its main action is to increase the speed at which the stomach and intestines empty food, while its secondary effect is on the brain's dopamine receptors. It is much less likely than the standard major tranquilizers (described above) to produce drowsiness and is especially effective when the stomach is slow to empty due to pressure from a nearby abdominal or chest tumor, which may produce bloating or appetite that is satisfied by just a few bites of food (early satiety). Metoclopramide may help stimulate appetite, and preliminary evidence suggests that it may also possess pain-relieving effects. Propulsid, another promising agent that works by a similar mechanism, has recently been restricted due to the recognition that it can interfere with normal cardiac rhythm.

Scopolamine (Transderm Scop) is another second-line drug that is usually administered in the form of a patch placed behind the ear. It is reapplied every seventy-two hours. Due to added actions at the inner ear, it is used primarily to treat vertigo and nausea from motion sickness and may be especially effective in cases where nausea is more prominent when patients are upright and moving around, and especially when the room seems to spin (vertigo). Treatment with scopolamine may also produce some degree of relaxation. Also useful at times is a similar drug, hyoscyamine, which is normally used to control spasms associated with irritable bowel, but can prevent nausea and vomiting and relieve stomach or intestinal cramps or spasms.

The corticosteroids, such as dexamethasone (Dexone, Decadron, Hexadrol), prednisone (Deltasone, Sterapred), and prednisolone (Prelone), are often used as second- or third-line drugs here, and even more commonly in the United Kingdom. Although their mechanism of action is not well understood, they relieve nausea very effectively and in the short term may have other beneficial effects, such as improving appetite, breathing, mood, and some types of pain. Although when used chronically (over months to years) they may produce serious side effects (see Chapter 8), they are generally beneficial and well tolerated for days, weeks, and even months.

Tetrahydrocannabinol (THC), the active ingredient of marijuana, can be an effective second- or third-line drug for both acute nausea due to chemotherapy and chronic nausea. Despite some states' efforts to the contrary, the medical use of marijuana is currently restricted to research, but THC can be prescribed in pill form (as dronabinol or Marinol). Doses that are usually sufficient to relieve nausea do not produce a high. And when grogginess or dysphoria (an unpleasant mental state) occasionally occur, they can usually be managed by reducing the dose. Of equal importance, the use of marijuana and treatment with its medical formulation, dronabinol, may also improve appetite, a medical correlate of the "munchies" depicted in popular culture. Effects on pain are more controversial, with research tending to be clouded by political considerations. Results are in part confounded because the smoke of marijuana actually contains hundreds of chemically distinct cannabinoids, but recent research suggests that the active ingredient in marijuana appears to be no more effective for chronic pain than codeine. Although clearly effective for nausea and appetite stimulation, effects on pain appear to be more closely linked to some subjects' ability to become more relaxed and easily distracted from unpleasant stimuli.

An entirely new class of agents, including ondansetron (Zofran) and granisetron (Kytril), that selectively block the action of certain subtypes of the neurotransmitter serotonin have come into vogue because they are extremely effective and very unlikely to produce side effects. Their actions are so potent that they may permit patients to tolerate new doses and combinations of chemotherapy that would otherwise be unheard of, but their costs (often exceeding $10 and even $20 per pill) are so excessive as to limit their use.

Another medication commonly employed as a component of an antiemetic "cocktail" is lorazepam (Ativan), an antianxiety medication that helps prevent nausea by inducing a more relaxed state. Given intravenously with chemotherapy, it may erase the memory of a vomiting episode, thus also reducing the risk of vomiting in the future. Occasionally, a defoaming agent such as simethicone (contained in Mylanta, Riopan Plus, and Maalox Plus), is useful to relieve gas pains.

Severe Vomiting Due to Obstruction or Pressure on the Digestive Tract

Disturbances in gastrointestinal function can range considerably in severity, character, and mechanism. Obstruction is a serious GI problem that should first be distinguished from simple irritation or an ulcer, conditions that are common with or without cancer. Irritation or erosion of the lining of the GI tract can be due to gastritis, reflux of stomach contents (GERD or gastroesophageal reflux disease), or ulcers. Symptoms are predominantly those of heartburn, indigestion, and pain, and unless a surgical emergency such as perforation or bleeding arises, treatment is with antacids and similar medications. In contrast, obstruction refers to a blockage to the passage of stomach contents somewhere between the mouth and anus.

After swallowing, food is transported along the digestive tract, where it is processed and eventually eliminated as waste. It goes from the mouth to the esophagus, stomach, small intestine (jejunum and ileum), large intestine (colon), rectum, and out through the anus. Should the digestive tract be blocked at any of these points, problems typically occur. These kinds of problems may arise with any tumor that grows within or near the abdomen, especially in esophageal and gastric (stomach) cancer, colon and liver cancer, as well as any primary tumor that has metastasized (spread) to the abdomen. Compression from outside of these organs (somewhat like the blockage that occurs when you step on a garden hose) can result from tumors, swollen lymph nodes, or adhesions (scars) from previous surgery or radiation treatment.

The symptoms of obstruction depend on whether the blockage is partial or complete and whether it is persistent or intermittent. Depending on these factors, there may be loss of appetite, bloating, swelling of the abdomen, pain, intermittent or persistent nausea, retching, vomiting, weakness, dehydration, constipation, and failure to pass gas. A complete bowel obstruction is associated with rapidly progressing deterioration that if untreated can progress to shock, infection, sepsis (a serious systemic response to infection), and ultimately death.

Ideally, an obstructing tumor would be surgically resected or bypassed with a colostomy, shrunk with chemotherapy or radiotherapy, or treated with combined therapy. However, the size, location, and type of tumor as well as the patient's overall condition may make this not feasible or advisable. Even so, symptomatic or palliative treatment that is aggressively instituted, is often surprisingly effective.

If the blockage is severe and persists, dehydration and malnutrition follow over time, and patients may become weak. These factors go hand in hand with the progressive weakness and failure ultimately associated with advanced untreatable cancer. It is obviously hard to sit by and watch while a friend or relative appears to be starving before one's eyes. When intestinal blockage cannot be relieved with surgery, several alternatives still exist. The traditional and most common method used by doctors in the United States is to hospitalize the patient and to insert a plastic tube through the nose and into the stomach (nasogastric tube) to drain its contents, while simultaneously administering fluids through an intravenous line. This method is costly, uncomfortable to the patient and, because it requires hospitalization, disruptive, inconvenient, and expensive. In addition, although the administration of routine IV fluids sounds reasonable because it can help counter dehydration, it neither helps reverse malnutrition nor extends life. The less invasive, home-based palliative care treatments (described below) have gained increasing support. Proponents argue that extended treatment with IV fluids in patients who don't eat much actually makes matters worse, since for a variety of reasons it usually leads to fluid imbalances, with swelling, strained breathing, wet cough, and frequent urination. In difficult situations, patient and care providers alike must sometimes make difficult decisions that may feel like "giving up" or "doing nothing" but are ultimately sensible and even courageous.

The alternate method of treating obstruction, practiced extensively in the United Kingdom and more and more in the United States, especially by hospice and palliative care teams, takes a very different approach and usually allows the patient to stay at home. Antiemetic medications, which have already been described, are administered very vigorously, often subcutaneously by a portable pump—a method that is much more convenient and comfortable than maintaining an intravenous line. In this manner, nausea can usually be controlled, often for a period of months (if needed), and sometimes the blockage opens a bit; even vomiting may cease. Patients are allowed to eat what they wish, although most prefer to restrict their intake mostly to liquids or soft foods. When a blockage is severe, nausea may be controlled so that patients can still eat; they may still vomit once or twice daily, but they feel good otherwise. While this sounds unpleasant, patients generally do not mind the occasional episode of vomiting, once the nausea is controlled, and they are spared the discomfort of hospitalization, IVs, and a suction tube in their nose. If covered by insurance, the new availability of ondansetron and subcutaneous octreotide (see above) can be used to help even more patients than in the past.

Occasionally, when nausea and vomiting still cannot be well controlled with these methods alone and patients are otherwise relatively well, a minor surgical procedure called a venting gastrostomy is recommended. It involves placing a short plastic tube from the stomach to a small bag that collects its contents; this relieves the pressure and eliminates the need to vomit. This is different from a feeding gastrostomy, which administers nutrition through a feeding tube. Decisions concerning whether a patient would benefit from a feeding tube depend on the nature and stage of the disease. (See Chapters 11 and 15 on nutrition in advanced stages of cancer.)

11

Dealing with Other Side Effects and Discomforts

Patients with cancer, even the same cancer, can have very different experiences, some of them more distressing than others. Many families will find over time that the status of their ill loved one will unexpectedly change. Families frequently feel unprepared and may be caught off guard about how to help when what feels like an emergency occurs (sudden nausea, difficulty breathing, coughing spells, increased pain, etc.). Caregivers should not be alarmed that there are so many different symptoms described here; it is unlikely that a given patient will experience many of them. Even when these symptoms do occur, their intensity, frequency, and duration vary greatly among patients.

Breathing Problems

Difficulty breathing is generally referred to as dyspnea and may include a variety of altered patterns of breathing. Hyperventilation, or rapid breathing (sometimes also called tachypnea or hyperpnea), is a normal response to illness and stress, but it is an inefficient form of breathing. When breathing excessively fast, there is no time to take a deep breath. Most of these shallow breaths go only in and out of the mouth and throat without enough air getting to the lungs, where the actual exchange of oxygen and carbon dioxide occurs. While rapid breathing usually starts with a lung problem, the air hunger excites fear and anxiety, making it all the more difficult to catch a breath or slow down breathing, a vicious cycle that only makes breathlessness worse.

Apnea refers to an absence of breathing. Minor episodes of apnea can occur in children and in healthy adults during sleep, but they can also be signs of progressive illness. In patients who are weak and very ill, episodes of apnea that last from a few seconds to half a minute are fairly common. Cheyne-Stokes respiration is a breathing pattern in which periods of apnea alternate with periods of deeper or more rapid breaths. While these changes can be a sign that the end of life is approaching, especially when severe or sudden in onset, these conditions can also persist, on and off, for days or weeks.

Causes of Breathing Problems

Difficulty breathing may arise from many factors and is a symptom that should be followed carefully by a doctor. The most common cause is a tumor growing in the lung, either one that has started there (primary tumor) or one that has spread from another site (metastatic tumor). If this is the case, breathing problems can often be reduced, at least temporarily, with radiotherapy and sometimes chemotherapy.

In some cases a tumor causes fluid to build up around the lung (pleural effusion) or heart (pericardial effusion). Breathing and fatigue will often improve dramatically when the fluid is removed from around the lung with a needle (thoracentesis) and a chest tube is used to prevent it from reoccurring.

A more common cause of breathing difficulties is pressure on the diaphragm, our main breathing muscle, from fluid or from a large incurable tumor in the abdomen. A drainage procedure (paracentesis), sometimes followed by the insertion of a catheter that can be cleared by staff or trained family members, can dramatically improve breathing and comfort.

Pneumonia is another treatable cause of breathing difficulties and is usually signaled by the presence of fever, weakness, and productive cough. Once the type of pneumonia has been identified, antibiotics are usually helpful.

Breathing difficulties that predate the cancer, such as from smoking, include diseases such as chronic obstructive pulmonary disease (COPD), emphysema, bronchitis, and asthma. Even when made worse by cancer, they can still be treated with some success using standard measures.

The functions of the heart and lungs are very closely related, and heart failure, from a variety of sources, may produce breathing difficulties. The most common is pulmonary edema, a condition involving fluid buildup in the lungs (rather than around them) because of the heart's lack of strength. It is usually treated with diuretics (pills that remove fluid by increasing the volume of urine) and various heart medications, including digitalis or digoxin.

Pulmonary embolus, a condition in which the lungs' blood supply is partially blocked by a blood clot, can cause sudden and severe breathing difficulties. Special support stockings, regular movement of the legs, and blood thinners can sometimes prevent this condition. Medical treatment involves prescribing blood thinners, either heparin or Coumadin, which need to be monitored with frequent blood tests.

Finally, psychological causes are an important part of most breathing difficulties. Feeling breathless can be terrifying, and frequently patients panic, causing them to breathe all the more rapidly and inefficiently. An important part of managing breathing problems is to offer reassurance and to try to eliminate the element of panic. Comforting the patient and instructing him in relaxation techniques can be very beneficial; in some cases, as we'll see, antianxiety medications can also help a great deal.

Practical Strategies

Specific techniques may not only help keep the lungs clear but also promote circulation, which is important since the blood carries oxygen to the lungs.

- Breathing properly and more efficiently can help ease shortness of breath. If possible, inhale through the nose from the stomach, not the chest. When this diaphragmatic breathing is performed correctly the abdomen should enlarge when you inhale. Exhale about twice as slowly as you inhale, and breathe out through pursed lips, as if blowing out a candle.
- When one is short of breath in bed, be sure the head and chest are elevated on pillows to take advantage of gravity. When possible, sit up and lean shoulders forward, either with arms spread out on either side or leaning forward on a support such as a table. If sitting up, foot support is more helpful than allowing feet to dangle. While in bed, patients should frequently change sides to keep lungs clear.
- When possible, improve circulation by standing or even walking. Take it slow and ask for help if breathing is strained.
- Patients should not stay in any one position too long because this will inhibit circulation. When sitting, they should try not to cross their legs for long periods. Special pressure stockings can be helpful to prevent blood clots, especially if the patient is on steroids.
- Keeping a patient moving, even when bedridden, can be helpful. Nurses or physical therapists often help patients with range-of-

motion exercises for the arms and legs, and families may, if they wish, ask the nurses how best to help with the exercises in their absence.

- If possible, the patient should drink as much as ten glasses of water a day to help mucous membranes clear lung secretions. This also helps relieve constipation.
- Ask a nurse, physical therapist, or respiratory therapist about proper coughing techniques to clear the lungs. One technique involves breathing deeply twice and on the third breath bracing the feet on the floor or other support to hold for three seconds. While braced, cough as deeply as possible three times.
- Keep air moist with a vaporizer (cold water), humidifier, teakettle, or even pans of water near a heat source. A fan to help circulate air can help relieve stuffiness.

Since breathlessness can be severely aggravated by anxiety, patients should be reassured and may be trained and coached in relaxation techniques, as described in Chapter 12. These exercises include progressive muscle relaxation, meditation, autogenic, cognitive, and imagery techniques.

Medications for Breathing Difficulties

Oxygen therapy involves keeping an oxygen tank handy or even in continual use if needed. Despite its relatively high cost, which is not always reimbursed by insurance, simply having oxygen available often has a reassuring, psychological value that can be quite important. Be certain that no one smokes, lights a match, or even has a pilot light engaged nearby because any of these could trigger an explosion. Be sure tubing is untwisted at all times and not kinked. Oxygen is usually delivered, at least initially, through nasal prongs. This is effective even if the patient is predominantly a mouth breather.

Opioids have a variety of complex effects on breathing, which are beneficial overall in the cancer patient. Because opioids slow breathing, doctors had in the past been cautious about prescribing morphine to patients with both breathing and pain problems. There is a growing positive experience with the use of opioids, in low doses, specifically to ease distress and breathing problems in cancer patients. They reduce the sensitivity of the brain's breathing center while also relieving the sensation, pain, and anxiety of having trouble breathing. The overall result is that the distress is lessened and patients are able to take slower, deeper breaths.

The anxiety related to dyspnea, which aggravates the condition, is also sometimes treated with tranquilizers such as diazepam (Valium); these medications can reduce anxiety and are muscle relaxants as well. Other medications that may help, depending on the cause of the problem, include steroids, bronchodilators, antibiotics, diuretics (which help expel extra fluid), heart medications, and blood thinners.

When a patient is very sick and near death, he may not be strong enough to cough up accumulated secretions in the back of the throat. Scopolamine or hyoscine (administered by injection or patch, marketed as Transderm Scop) may be used to dry up these secretions, and may have the effect of sedating the patient as well.

Coughing

Coughing occurs in about 30 percent of patients with advanced cancer and in about 80 percent of patients with cancers involving the lungs or bronchial tubes. It may also be caused by irritation to the lower throat or lungs or from factors unrelated to cancer, such as a postnasal drip, asthma, tobacco, or heart failure. Some simple measures can help alleviate coughing:

- Keep air moist with a vaporizer or humidifier.
- Avoid lying directly on the back, since this position makes coughing difficult.
- If cigarettes seem to be part of the cause, realize that if the decision is made to give up smoking, it will still take two to four weeks for coughing to gradually diminish. Families and patients need to consider how much gratification is obtained from the cigarettes, how difficult it would be to quit, and whether the attempt is worth it. A decision to eliminate smoking should be discussed with the doctor, who can usually recommend several treatments to make this transition easier.

Medications for Problems with Coughing

If the patient has difficulty coughing up secretions that make him nauseated or cause vomiting, medication can be given by mouth to help break up the secretion.

Although over-the-counter cough medicines are sometimes effective, if coughing persists or is disturbing, painful, or dry, the doctor may recommend a medication containing codeine or a related compound. When the patient has a tumor involving the lung area that is responsible for the coughing, an opioid such as hydrocodone or morphine may be needed. Corticosteroids may also be prescribed for persistent cough.

Mouth or Throat Sores

Chemotherapy, radiation, reduced intake of liquids or food, altered hygiene, and infection can all contribute to mouth sores or inflammation in the mouth. The sores may be like canker sores or they can be open ulcers, both of which may bleed or get infected. They may make eating painful and difficult but are often overlooked.

The need for mouth care may present an opportunity rather than be viewed as just a problem, according to some authorities. Sometimes, when patients are very sick, loving caregivers feel frustrated that they cannot do more to help. Learning the basics of mouth care and applying them regularly can be an excellent way for family members or other caregivers to spend time with the patient in a loving, meaningful, and helpful way.

The best strategy to manage these conditions, known as stomatitis and mucositis, is prevention. Simple daily routines should be undertaken twice a day, or even every four hours if the patient is undergoing chemotherapy treatments. Physicians more accustomed to managing acute medical problems may forget to advise how to prevent mouth problems, and an oncology nurse may be a valuable resource in providing instructions.

Mouth Hygiene to Prevent Problems

Brush the teeth with a soft nylon bristle toothbrush only. To soften the bristles even more, use hot water on the bristles before and after use. If toothpaste is irritating, try a paste composed of baking soda and water. If brushing hurts too much, clean teeth with cotton swabs or commercial sponge-tipped sticks called Toothettes. Floss with unwaxed dental floss; avoid flossing if there are bleeding problems or if platelet count is low. Using a Waterpik can help keep the mouth clean, too.

A mouthwash should be used as often as every two hours, such as one composed of half-strength hydrogen peroxide (one part 3 percent hydrogen peroxide to one part water) or baking soda in water. Avoid lemon, glycerin (which will make the mouth drier), or commercial mouthwashes containing alcohol (alcohol is a common ingredient in these and may irritate or dry the mouth). A very effective commercial preparation is a chlorhexidine mouth rinse.

Keep dentures clean and use them only if they fit properly; if they don't fit, they may injure the mouth during eating. If weight loss has occurred, dentures may need to be refitted.

Keep gums stimulated by encouraging the patient to chew foods or by gently rubbing a finger over the gums.

If the patient is on long-term chemotherapy, ask about using a fluoride preparation on the teeth to prevent cavity formation, which is common during chemotherapy. Also, radiation therapy in the region of the mouth greatly increases the risk of dental cavities. To prevent them, frequent fluoride applications are often recommended—consult with the doctor or a dentist. Avoid sugary foods. To avoid complications later, many physicians and dentists will recommend pulling high-risk teeth before radiation is administered.

When the Mouth Is Irritated

Keep lips moist with petroleum jelly, cocoa butter, or a water-based lubricant. Avoid hot, cold, acidic, rough, or salty foods. These may include spicy foods, vinegar, citrus foods, toast, pretzels, crackers, and other snacks. Also avoid alcoholic drinks and tobacco products.

Rinse frequently with mouthwash, as described above, as often as every two hours. Do not floss. If brushing is too painful, teeth and gums should be wiped regularly with moist paper towels or cotton.

Warm tea or a paste made from an antacid such as Maalox, diluted milk of magnesia, Mylanta, or Gelusic may encourage healing. Place the antacid into a warm liquid and let settle. Once settled, pour off excess liquid and apply the paste with a cotton-tipped stick or gauze. Rinse fifteen minutes later with water.

Offer a high-protein, high-calorie diet served at room temperature.

Medications for Mouth and Throat Sores

When irritated, mouth sores can be treated with a topical anesthetic, such as lidocaine (Xylocaine) or benzocaine (Hurricaine), to reduce the pain and promote healing; these are effective not only for mouth sores but for sores in the throat too (some sprays are available). To reduce pain, Benadryl liquid or lozenges may help.

When mouth infections (usually yeast infections such as candidiasis or thrush) occur, mouth rinses with hydrogen peroxide and a saline or sterile water solution with the addition of flavored nystatin (an antifungal medication) or an antifungal pill may be prescribed by the doctor. The nystatin should be applied four times a day to each side of the mouth, kept there three minutes, and then swallowed. The doctor may prescribe another antifungal medication (such as ketoconazole) for certain infections.

Expect medications to take several days to become initially beneficial and about two weeks to be fully effective.

Dry Mouth

Radiation to the head and neck area can cause dry mouth, known as xerostomia. The reduction of saliva production may last from six months to a year and in some cases may be a permanent side effect of radiation therapy. But the most common cause of dry mouth in cancer patients is from the side effects of certain medications, especially tricyclic antidepressants, antihistamines, opioids (narcotics), some chemotherapeutic agents, and major tranquilizers (phenothiazines). Reviewing the medication list with the doctor may make it possible to delete problematic medications and substitute others. Dry mouth can also be caused by a tumor near the salivary glands, mouth infections, and tobacco and alcohol use. Sometimes a patient's general dehydration, lack of eating, or breathing through the mouth can contribute to dry mouth as well.

Dry mouth causes food to taste different and may contribute to poor appetite. This condition can cause the patient a number of problems: it may make it more difficult to digest starches, promote mouth irritation and sores, inhibit taste, make it difficult to chew solid foods, promote cavities and mouth infections, and even make it difficult to form words.

Practical Strategies

Some attention to diet and oral hygiene can often relieve the problem of dry mouth. Try some of the following suggestions:

- Avoid spicy, very hot, or very cold foods, citrus products, and carbonated beverages, as well as foods that are hard to chew. Serve foods well moistened with gravies, sauces, or mayonnaise.
- Consume as much water or other nonirritating liquids as possible— at least several times an hour. Frequent small sips of water and rinsing the mouth with cold water also help. Keep a thermos or pitcher near the patient with a straw or spout, if necessary.
- Keep lips lightly lubricated with lip balm, cocoa butter, Vaseline, or similar product.
- Sucking on peppermints, sour hard candies, lozenges, Popsicles, and pineapple chunks as well as chewing gum may also help promote saliva production.
- Keep something in the mouth, such as a pipe or lollipop.
- Keep air humid with a vaporizer (cold water), humidifier, teakettle, or pans of water near a heat source.
- Maintain mouth hygiene as described above (see under "Mouth or Throat Sores"). That means brushing the mouth with a soft toothbrush after eating anything. Every two hours use a mouthwash,

such as one that produces an effervescent wash (a mixture of one part Cepacol, one part saline solution, and one part 3 percent hydrogen peroxide) or glycerin and citric acid washes, which may help stimulate salivation. Ask the doctor or oncology nurse for a recommendation.

Medication for Dry Mouth

Dry mouth occurs despite being well hydrated because it's such a common symptom of medication. When dry mouth is severe, artificial saliva products such as MoiStir or MouthKote are available by prescription. A medication called pilocarpine (Salagen) may also be prescribed to treat dryness of the mouth and throat. It can help the patient talk without having to sip liquids and can help with chewing, tasting, and swallowing. Pilocarpine can interfere with many other medical conditions such as glaucoma, asthma, and heart disease and may interact with other medications, so the physician should be fully informed when prescribing. Products such as Salivart and similar products also can provide relief, as can water-soluble gels such as K-Y for dry tongue in mouth-breathing patients.

Drooling

Tumors in the mouth can cause excessive drooling (sialorrhea), which may be upsetting to the patient and family. There are few practical treatment measures other than wiping the mouth as necessary and reassuring the patient.

Medication the Doctor May Recommend

Atropine drops can provide temporary relief; for longer-term relief, atropine tablets can be used, although they can cause dry mouth and, occasionally, irritability.

The antidepressant amitriptyline (Elavil) can work for some patients. The antiemetic Transderm Scop can also help dry up secretions.

When very troublesome, in selected circumstances, radiotherapy can be used to modify salivary gland function.

Difficulty Swallowing

Chemotherapy and radiation may interfere with the function of the esophagus, which can make it difficult to swallow (dysphagia). Tumor growth into muscles or nerves involving the pharynx (the area around and including the esophagus) may also be a cause of this condition.

Practical Strategies

Try these suggestions to ease swallowing problems:

- Avoid tobacco and alcoholic drinks, as well as spicy, acidic, hot or cold, hard, crunchy, or coarse foods.
- Serve a high-protein but well-balanced diet.
- Use milk and dairy products, such as yogurt, sour cream, or cottage cheese, to coat the throat.
- Keep foods well moistened with liquids, gravies, sauces, and so on.
- Keep bites small; when swallowing problems are severe, foods may be liquefied in a blender or food processor.

Medications for Difficulties in Swallowing

If swallowing is painful, liquid aspirin or acetaminophen may be helpful, as well as anesthetics applied directly in the mouth. For more severe pain, other nonsteroidal anti-inflammatory medications in liquid form or morphine can be used.

If tumors are involved, corticosteroids (such as dexamethasone) can temporarily shrink a tumor and improve swallowing. In some cases, radiation may also be able to shrink the tumor.

If cancer in the esophagus is involved and radiotherapy doesn't help, a feeding tube may be considered.

Stomach Pain

Chronic use of some medications, particularly some of the NSAIDs, can irritate the stomach and other areas of the gastrointestinal tract or may actually damage the mucous lining of the gastrointestinal system. In this case, medications to treat and prevent ulcers may be used, such as sucralfate, which helps form a coating that helps protect the ulcer from acids of the stomach. Other medications, classically used to treat ulcers or GERD (gastroesophageal reflux disease), a severe form of heartburn, that reduce or eliminate acid production—such as Tagamet, Zantac, Aciphex, Prilosec, Prevacid, and Protonix—are often considered as well.

Problems with Taste

Cancer can alter taste perceptions in a variety of ways, a problem that affects about half of all cancer patients, regardless of the type of cancer they have. Doctors believe several factors may contribute to the problem.

The taste buds themselves may lose their sensitivity because chemicals produced by the cancer or poor dental hygiene may lead to loss of taste. Usually food tastes bland or slightly "off," having a metallic or medicinal flavor. Some people find they either want no sweets or want more sweets; many lose their desire for meat and bitter foods. When taste problems occur, an extra effort should be made to prevent or treat sores and dry mouth (see preceding sections on mouth and throat sores and dry mouth).

Practical Strategies

When tastes seem to be altered, try one or more of the following strategies:

- Brush teeth often, and use a mouth rinse such as a mixture of water and baking soda.
- Assuming the patient doesn't experience nausea, the aroma of foods cooking may stimulate the desire for food.
- Flavoring food with mild spices such as salt, vanilla, cinnamon, or lemon may enhance flavors.
- When all foods taste bitter, good selections may include white meat, eggs, and dairy products. Some suggest adding honey, NutraSweet, or sweet fruits to foods that taste bitter. Adding beer or wine to soups, marinades, sauces, and seasonings may also help. Marinate meats and fish, use strong seasonings, and avoid hot foods—wait until they are room temperature or even cold.
- Unpleasant aftertastes can be masked with mints, chewing gum, or mildly sweet or pleasant desserts.

Loss of Appetite

Cancer patients may lose their desire to eat (anorexia) either temporarily or chronically at various stages of the disease; it may, in fact, be one of the first symptoms of cancer, and is also common in advanced cancer. Foods may taste different, have metallic or medicinal "off" flavors, or be downright unappealing. It is often disorienting to patients when they find that foods they have enjoyed for a lifetime no longer hold much pleasure and that they can suddenly tolerate foods they never cared for. They should be reassured that this is a common side effect of cancer and its treatment, and patients should be encouraged to experiment with different foods.

Failure to eat is one of the most distressing aspects of cancer for patients and their families. The degree of concern that this symptom should raise depends very much on the specific case, the prognosis, and stage of the disease.

Practical Strategies

When a patient has a chance for a cure or is in the early or middle stages of cancer, aggressive methods to counter malnutrition should be undertaken. These may include:

- Providing small but frequent meals.
- Selecting the patient's favorite foods.
- Offering a milkshake-like dietary supplement if solid food can't be taken. Ask the physician to recommend one of the highly nutritious food supplements available on the market. They range from common products such as Carnation Instant Breakfast to more specialized ones such as Ensure or Boost. Patients frequently find these most palatable when served chilled or over ice; the manufacturer may also be able to provide information on how to prepare these foods in interesting ways.

Medication for Loss of Appetite

Preliminary research suggests that treatment with medications may stimulate appetite, with a relatively low risk of serious side effects.

Corticosteroids (dexamethasone, prednisone) administered in moderate doses may be successful for a short time. The administration of high doses of megestrol (Megace), a hormone, may be effective for longer periods with fewer side effects. Taken at night, the antidepressant amitriptyline or the tranquilizer chlorpromazine may boost appetite and general attitude as well.

The active ingredient in marijuana, THC, currently only legally available in pill form as dronabinol (Marinol), may also be effective in some patients.

Reglan (metoclopramide), a medication commonly used for nausea, works in part to minimize sensations of bloating and early satiety (feeling full after just a few bites) by its prokinetic activity, meaning that it helps energize or jump-start the GI tract by encouraging it to empty more rapidly.

In some cases, aggressive treatment that includes tube feeding (gastrostomy) or intravenous feeding (total parenteral hyperalimentation) will be recommended. These methods, however, are appropriate in only a small proportion of cases.

Lack of Appetite in Advanced Stages of Cancer

When patients do not have a good chance of long-term survival and are in the advanced stages of cancer, lack of appetite is relatively common. Yet patients and families are often unable to admit that the patient's prognosis is poor. Doctors often find it difficult to discuss a poor prognosis, either because they do not have specific training in discussing such difficult topics with patients, because they are not comfortable admitting that some cancers are beyond cure, or because they simply do not want to upset their patients. Since even experts in palliative and hospice care cannot always predict life expectancy with certainty, many experts will be hesitant about conveying that death is imminent. Finally, patients and their families are often naturally reluctant to receive unpleasant news and may discourage doctors from engaging in such conversation.

Nevertheless, patients with progressive cancer commonly lose their appetite, and families often feel helpless when this occurs. Many families equate preparing and offering food with providing love. Some view their central role or job as providing food and feeding the patient; when the patient won't eat, they feel like failures. Families in this situation should not be discouraged: they are witnessing an unavoidable but natural part of the disease process. Patients with advanced cancer usually don't want to eat and may try to do so simply to make their families feel better. Most experts concur, however, that dehydration and missed meals are not particularly uncomfortable for a very ill person with cancer. Forcing the person to eat or drink may not help him and can make a very ill patient feel guilty and even more uncomfortable. Although it may be difficult to witness the progressive loss of appetite in a loved one, it is unkind to pressure someone to eat when he is unable to do so. Families must try to find more direct, verbal ways to show that they care. This is one of many challenges that face all caregivers of gravely ill loved ones.

Loss of Weight

Many cancer patients will lose weight and, over time, may appear emaciated. Weight loss can be caused by a variety of factors, such as loss of appetite, diarrhea, vomiting, hemorrhaging, ulcers, poor absorption in the gastrointestinal tract, a failing metabolic or digestive system, and even the chemical by-products of a tumor.

Patients who lose a great deal of weight (a condition known as cachexia) may look ill, feel weak, look pale, and feel full when they have eaten only a little. Their changed appearance can cause distress, fear, and feelings of being isolated as friends and family members note the marked change in appearance. Clothes will no longer fit well; dentures may become loose and may not only cause problems with eating but also be painful.

Unfortunately, cachexia is common and can't be avoided or treated in many cases. Although the medications mentioned under the section "Loss of Appetite" can be tried, attention should really be focused on relieving the social implications associated with the changed appearance, dealing with more practical matters such as obtaining clothing that fits better, and using coping strategies to ward off depression and other potential psychological problems. Dentures may be refitted (even at bedside) and can help the patient chew and look better. Caring for the skin and mouth is important during this time, as described in this chapter (under "Skin Problems").

Do not force foods aggressively. The person will have a fickle appetite and will feel full with a small amount of food.

Fatigue and Weakness

For a variety of reasons, cancer patients often suffer from fatigue. Fatigue is said to be multifactorial, meaning that it is usually caused by many combined factors. As a result, it is often difficult to determine which is the main culprit. Reasons for fatigue include side effects of chemotherapy or radiotherapy, poor nutrition, infection, the effects of chemicals made by the tumors, the effects of other medications used by the patient, liver or kidney failure, imbalance of the body's salts and electrolytes (calcium, potassium, and sodium), depression, fever, and anemia. Even so, the doctor may recommend some simple tests to find correctable causes. Although medications prescribed to treat pain may contribute to fatigue, reducing them to heighten alertness does not usually make sense, because patients will suffer more from untreated pain, and they will become tired out from fighting the pain.

Practical Strategies

Sometimes fatigue or weakness will be a temporary side effect of treatment. To help relieve it during treatments:

- Be sure the patient rests often. The patient should stay relaxed, go to bed earlier, and sleep later. Several short rest periods may help more than one long rest. However, some studies show that too much rest may affect your body's production of energy. When fatigued, spend less time lying down and more time sitting or doing gentle activities.
- Try to maintain a normal but somewhat slowed routine that can be stepped up gradually as tolerated.
- Encourage the patient to keep drinking plenty of liquid—ideally, eight to ten glasses of water daily.

- Offer the patient foods that are complex carbohydrates (rice, beans, grains, vegetables), which provide more energy than highly processed foods or sweets.
- Encourage the patient to accept help with simple chores he can't easily do, such as cooking and cleaning. However, keep the patient's mind busy with car rides, movies, visiting, listening to music, and so on.
- A careful regimen of fresh air, exercise, and physical therapy may be helpful. However, these remedies are situation-specific ones: rest instead of exercise may be the best thing for many patients who are weak.
- When fatigue is a sign of depression (see Chapter 14), it will sometimes get better when the depression lifts. Simple measures are often sufficient, such as conversation, companionship, reassurance, hugs, and encouragement with small activities. When depression persists, professional counseling or treatment with one of the antidepressants should be considered. Patients need to be reassured that depression is common in patients with cancer. If the fatigue is attributed to a major depression, then antidepressants may help.
- If pain or anxiety is preventing normal sleep, it should be treated aggressively (see Chapter 12).
- Ensuring that sleep and rest are maintained is a key factor in minimizing fatigue. Pay attention to the sleep-wake cycle, which often gets reversed in ill patients. It is very common that, for one reason or another, patients are unable to sleep well at night. As a result, they are drowsy during the day, nap at odd times, and then are even less likely to sleep well at night, perpetuating a vicious cycle that is hard to reverse. If this seems to be occurring, minimize or eliminate daytime sleeping so that patients are more tired at night, and talk to the doctor about adding either a nighttime sleeping pill or a daytime stimulant.
- Be attentive to what has come to be regarded as "sleep hygiene." In other words, create a setting that promotes sleep. Make sure that at bedtime the patient is reclined and in comfortable garments, with relaxing music, a candle, incense, a cup of tea, or other environmental cues that promote restfulness. Avoid having the television on incessantly, frequent interruptions, uncomfortable postures, and restrictive clothing.
- Consider renting a hospital bed, bedside commode, wheelchair, ramps, raised toilet seat, walker, and stool for the bath or shower. These simple measures will help conserve the patient's strength and are typically covered by most insurers' home health programs as well as by hospice, should it be necessary.

- In more advanced stages of the disease, when weakness and fatigue can be expected, distractions such as conversation, music, television, and so on will continue to bring pleasure to the patient who is weak.

Medications and Other Treatments for Fatigue

Review the patient's medication list with the doctor periodically. Sometimes patients continue to take medications that are no longer essential and which, if eliminated, may give them more strength.

Blood tests may indicate an abnormality, such as anemia, potassium that is too low, or calcium that is too high. A transfusion or other treatment may be recommended. Keep in mind that not all abnormalities require treatment; for example, a blood transfusion does not make sense if it will only correct the problem for a few days or is unlikely to promote well-being. Remember, the important thing is to treat the whole patient. Often abnormal test values are well tolerated when they are the result of gradual changes. Not every abnormality can be fixed or needs to be. Working with the doctor will help determine when comfort versus strict attention to the numbers is the best guide to choosing therapies, especially when the treatments themselves may be uncomfortable or disruptive.

Simple multivitamins, especially those that include iron, may be sufficient to help combat anemia and fatigue. If fatigue has been determined to be a likely consequence of anemia (reflected by a low hematocrit or hemoglobin on blood work), weekly (or more frequent) injections of a medication that stimulates the bones to produce more red cells may be extremely helpful, and avoids transfusion. Medications such as Procrit or Epogen (epoetin alfa) help increase the body's supply of erythropoietin, a hormone produced by the kidney that stimulates the production of new red blood cells, which carry the oxygen needed to rekindle lost energy. These injections are very costly but are covered by most insurers when given under recommended circumstances.

Fatigue may also result from excessive blood levels of calcium (hypercalcemia, see Chapter 8). The input of your physician is critical to determine whether hypercalcemia is a minor problem that does not require aggressive treatment or may be life-threatening if allowed to persist. Depending on the situation, hypercalcemia may be treated with the regular use of oral or nasal medications intended to combat osteoporosis, or may require periodic injections of a bisphosphonate, which sometimes dramatically reverses fatigue and mental confusion.

To boost a sense of well-being, steroids (including dexamethasone, prednisone, and prednisolone) are very commonly used for patients with advanced cancer, usually helping them feel stronger and hungrier.

The stimulants methylphenidate (Ritalin) and dextroamphetamine may be useful to reduce sleepiness and fatigue, especially when these problems are caused in part by the treatment of pain with the opioids and other medications that can contribute to drowsiness. Although less highly regulated, Cylert (pemoline) is less frequently prescribed as a stimulant today since it has been shown to be occasionally associated with liver failure. Provigil (modafinil), currently approved just for the treatment of the sleep disorder narcolepsy, is being used more frequently to promote daytime arousal in fatigued cancer patients. Many physicians may be reluctant to prescribe stimulants, in part because, like the opioids, their use is regulated to minimize potential for abuse. Nevertheless, some patients respond favorably to stimulants and can be intensely grateful for the return of energy and alertness. The stimulants are prescribed for use mostly in the early morning and at noon, just as some use coffee to start the day without interfering with needed nighttime sleep. There is a limit to these medications' effectiveness, since sometimes fatigue needs to be respected as the body's signal that additional rest is needed. These medications are usually avoided in patients with rapid or irregular heartbeats, seizure disorders, or brain tumors, and when anxiety or paranoia are present.

Finally, remember that fatigue and lack of motivation are common symptoms of depression. If it is present, depression can be addressed by counseling, antidepressants, or a combination of these.

Hair Loss

Hair loss, known as alopecia, is a fairly common side effect of chemotherapy or radiation to the scalp. Severity may range from hair thinning to complete loss of hair. Strangely, when hair grows back, it may be softer, thicker, or of a different texture than before. Sometimes gray hair that falls out is replaced with hair of the patient's original color. Occasionally, patients may also lose hair in other area of the body, such as from the eyebrows, arms, groin, and so on.

Although much less disturbing to the body's functioning than nausea or other side effects, patients are often devastated psychologically by hair loss because hair is frequently an integral part of the patient's body image.

To minimize hair loss and protect new hair that's growing in:

- Though unproven, some patients wear an "ice turban" or keep cold compresses on the head during chemotherapy treatments to inhibit the drugs from reaching the hair follicles.
- Before treatments, cut hair into a manageable style that won't require a lot of brushing or combing.

- Use mild products on the head, and keep shampooing to a minimum. Pat hair to dry.
- Avoid hair dryers, curling irons, clips, elastic bands, hair spray, and all other hair products, including brushes and combs.
- Satin pillowcases may help prevent hair tangles.
- If hair loss is expected, choose a wig before treatment. Synthetic wigs are more comfortable and less expensive than wigs made from real hair. Consider obtaining a wig through the American Cancer Society, the hospital, or support groups. Check with insurance about reimbursement.
- Use a hat, scarf, or turban if hair loss has occurred. A hairnet at home can help contain hair and minimize shedding.
- In summer, keep head covered to avoid sunburn; in winter, keep head covered to prevent heat loss.

Bleeding Episodes

While it is relatively rare, bleeding can be a side effect of chemotherapy or radiation, a result of the cancer itself, the result of an allergic reaction to some medications (especially quinidine, quinine, digitalis, sulfonamides, or thiazides), or caused by stress and anxiety. Bleeding may occur directly from the skin or may arise from the mouth, nose, groin, or elsewhere.

Practical Strategies

To prevent bleeding, be sure the patient:

- Avoids activities that might be too physically strenuous and that may cause even minor trauma
- Avoids hand razors, cuticle scissors, tight-fitting clothes that could irritate the skin, tourniquets, and aspirin
- Avoids strenuous activities, such as lifting, bending over from the waist, or straining during a bowel movement
- Drinks plenty of liquids to keep the mucous membranes moist
- Follows hygienic precautions listed under "Mouth or Throat Sores," earlier in this chapter, to avoid mouth bleeding
- Keeps stools soft and avoids using anything in the rectum (thermometers, enemas) to prevent bleeding from the anus
- Takes an antacid or milk with oral steroids to prevent irritating the stomach
- Uses a lubricant before sexual intercourse (for women) to prevent friction and bleeding; avoids douches and vaginal suppositories

- Blows nose very gently through both nostrils and keeps air humid with a vaporizer or humidifier to avoid bleeding from the lungs or nose

If bleeding occurs, apply pressure to the area for five to ten minutes, and if a limb is involved, elevate it. Apply ice to cause the local blood vessels to constrict. If the nose bleeds, squeeze the nostrils gently shut below the bridge of the nose; tilt the head forward to prevent blood from backing up. If it persists, place an ice pack on the bridge of the nose. Contact the doctor if bleeding of any kind doesn't stop after five minutes.

Sexual Problems

Cancer can interfere with sexuality in many ways—the patient may be tired, nauseated, anxious, or fearful; he may lose sexual desire or may be unable to function normally. Cancer reminds us of our mortality and vulnerability. Just the psychological impact of being diagnosed with cancer, let alone the body changes that might occur, can affect our body image and make us feel less sexy, attractive, and lovable. Couples need to communicate during this stressful time about their needs, fears, and anxieties. When intercourse is not possible, physical intimacy (hugging, holding, caressing) can go a long way in maintaining needed closeness. Sexual partners may be fearful to initiate intimacy out of concern that they will hurt their mate. This concern can easily be overcome with communication.

During chemotherapy, women are more prone to bleed heavily during their periods, and many doctors advise that women of childbearing age take birth control pills to stop menstruation during this time. During radiation to the genital area, women may be advised to have regular intercourse or even to use a dildo-like device to retain the vagina's natural shape. If these matters have not already been brought up by the health care team, patients and their families should make a special effort to discuss them with a nurse or doctor.

Skin Problems

Itching and Dry Skin

Chemicals produced by the tumor, side effects of treatment, dehydration, and even anxiety or boredom may cause or aggravate dry, itchy skin, a condition known as pruritus. To relieve it, patients should:

- Use water-based moisturizers and avoid oil-based ones. Use these moisturizers after bathing and every night.
- Drink plenty of fluids (eight to ten glasses a day).
- Protect skin from wind, heat, hot sun, and cold.
- Avoid hot baths and soap. Use soothing bath solutions that include cornstarch, baking soda, Aveeno, or soybean powder. Pat the skin dry rather than rubbing it.
- Keep cool, wet packs on the itchy area for twenty minutes at a time.
- Don't exercise excessively.
- Keep clothes loose and light; avoid heavy fabrics such as wool and corduroy.
- Avoid scratching by using ice packs, by practicing distraction or another relaxation technique (see Chapter 12), or by applying a vibrator or extra pressure to the area. Cut nails if necessary and encourage rubbing instead of scratching.
- For dry patchy areas, try placing a wet cloth over the area for fifteen minutes and then apply cream before allowing it to dry.
- Lidoderm, a new medication in patch form that delivers numbing medication directly to the irritated area, may be useful. Approved for treating the pain associated with shingles and postherpetic neuralgia, it may be effective for localized itching.

MEDICATIONS FOR DRY, ITCHY SKIN

Physicians may prescribe an antihistamine if the patient feels itchy all over; for local patches of itching, a corticosteroid cream or local anesthetic may be used. Small doses of naloxone can relieve itching when it is severe and is due to treatment with a narcotic.

Bedsores

With prolonged bed rest, weight-bearing surfaces such as the hips, tailbone (sacrum and coccyx), ankles, and heels may develop pressure sores, also known as bedsores or decubitus ulcers. Factors that increase the risk of developing pressure sores include weight loss, poor nutrition, numbness and loss of sensation (feeling uncomfortable ordinarily prompts the patient to shift position), anemia, infection, paralysis, incontinence, spasticity, heart failure, poor circulation, friction, irritation, dry skin, excessive moisture, and wrinkled or unclean bedding or clothing.

While pressure sores are largely preventable with good nursing care, once they are established they can be difficult to treat as long as the underlying conditions that caused them persist. They can range in severity from very mildly irritated skin with a little redness that disappears promptly when pressure is relieved (stage I) to blisters (stage II; similar to a first-degree burn) and even open, deep, and very serious wounds that are prone to infection and can burrow down to the bone or into internal organs (stage III or IV).

PRACTICAL STRATEGIES

Bedsores can usually be prevented by following these guidelines:

- Make sure the patient moves or is moved at least every two hours so pressure does not persist on the same areas.
- If the patient doesn't move much, avoid skin contacting skin: put a pillow between the legs, a folded towel between the arm and body, and spread out the fingers.
- Keep the patient clean, dry, well hydrated, and well fed.
- For patients who are bedridden, consult with a home care nursing expert (through your doctor's office or insurer) to consider the use of special equipment such as foam or sheepskin padding, an air mattress, silicon gel pads, sponge rubber mattresses (egg crates), or in selected circumstances even highly specialized flotation beds, such as a Ken-Air bed, which, though costly, are covered by some types of medical insurance.

If blisters or ulcers do start to form, dead tissue should be removed, pressure should be minimized, and efforts to improve nutrition should be increased.

MEDICAL MANAGEMENT OF DECUBITUS ULCERS

To promote healing, the health care provider will dress the wound with a moist dressing and may use any number of products, such as synthetic dressings, saline dressings, acetic acid compresses, and various antibiotic dressings (since bedsores are vulnerable to infection). For severe wounds, surgery is sometimes considered to remove large areas of dead tissue so that healing may commence.

Tumors That Break Through the Skin

Tumors that ulcerate, or break through the skin, are distressing for the patient and the family. Although not very common, such sores can be unpleasant, may devastate a patient's body image, and can escalate feelings of helplessness. Such tumors may also leak or drain fluid and may produce embarrassing odors.

Caring for these problems requires plenty of support from health care professionals, such as a visiting nurse and, when available, a wound care team. Wounds should be kept dry and, when appropriate, cleaned twice a day. Certain creams may be recommended to clean and dress the wound. To control any odor, special charcoal dressings may used; an effective home remedy is yogurt gently spread over the wound. Certain antibiotics, especially metronidazole (Flagyl, Protostat), reduce odor when administered directly onto the wound or by mouth. When such a tumor constantly oozes blood, the wound can be dressed in gauze that has been lined with a gelatin sponge material, the most specialized of which contain chemicals that inhibit fresh bleeding. Protect the surrounding area with petroleum jelly or zinc oxide. An air freshener may also help minimize the odor. When a large wound is involved and massive bleeding is feared, an entire blood vessel can sometimes be closed preventively with minor surgery.

Medications for Problem Tumors

When a tumor has an odor, an infection is probably involved and should be treated. Antibiotic treatment often helps reduce pain.

The antibiotic clindamycin or the antibacterial medication metronidazole can be effective. Metronidazole can cause nausea and nerve damage and is dangerous if taken with alcohol; clindamycin can severely irritate the gastrointestinal tract. Powdered and cream preparations of metronidazole, however, hold promise for topical treatment and are now available.

Urination Problems

The urinary tract is particularly sensitive in the cancer patient; problems such as burning during urination or a constant urge to urinate are fairly common. Symptoms of an infection include local discomfort, dark or strong-smelling urine, fever or chills, and low back pain.

When a Bladder Infection Is Diagnosed

If a bladder infection is present, encourage the patient to drink up to three quarts of fluid a day (especially water), avoiding coffee, tea, and other caffeine-containing products, as well as alcoholic beverages. Avoid foods that could be irritating to the bladder lining, such as alcohol, coffee, tea, and spicy foods. Vitamin C or large quantities of cranberry juice (up to three quarts) may help reduce infection by acidifying the urine.

Emergencies

Dehydration and kidney failure can result from hyperuricemia (excessive blood levels of uric acid), which is most common in cancer patients as a result of tumor lysis syndrome (TLS), an emergency that may follow some chemotherapies, especially for leukemia or lymphoma.

When chemotherapy results in especially rapid destruction of massive numbers of tumor cells, tumor lysis syndrome may occur due to the accumulation of toxic waste products. This is a potentially life-threatening medical emergency that must first be identified by the treatment team. In addition to medical management, the following dietary recommendations should be considered:

- Drink at least three quarts of fluid a day (especially water), but avoid tea and wine, as they are high in purines. These substances contribute to the formation of uric acid, which can overwhelm kidney function.
- Avoid lentils, dried beans, liver, sardines, or anchovies, which also contain higher amounts of purines and so can make the condition worse.

Other Guidelines

When incontinence (leakage) is a problem, sometimes a medication to increase the sensation of having to urinate (an anticholinergic drug) or a catheter may be used.

Urinary retention, an uncommon side effect of opioids and a few other drugs, is most common in elderly men. Tolerance to the drug often eventually develops. If it is not particularly uncomfortable or severe, it may be left untreated.

Occasionally the outflow of urine becomes completely blocked due to medications, swelling, or pressure from a tumor. This is usually accompanied by swelling of the lower abdomen, feelings of pressure, and discomfort. If simple measures to help the urine flow do not work, the doctor should be informed; if he is unavailable, the patient may need to go to an emergency room to have a catheter passed to empty the bladder. Usually bladder catheterization is not uncomfortable, especially for women.

A catheter is often left in place when patients chronically leak urine or are bedridden and do not have the strength to get to the bathroom. The use of a catheter may increase the risk of a bladder infection, but it can make life much easier for patients who are easily fatigued by frequent trips to the bathroom.

Sleeping Problems

If the patient can't sleep, try to determine whether it's because of pain, anxiety, night sweats, fear of urinating, or other reasons. To help monitor a sleep problem, try to keep track of how long it takes to fall asleep, how long sleep lasts, how many times premature awakening occurs and why, whether returning to sleep is problematic, and how rested the patient feels in the morning. Counseling, applying practical tips, and using medication may help manage insomnia, especially when anxiety or fear are its cause (see Chapter 14). If night sweats persist, underlying causes should be sought, such as fever, hormonal abnormalities, seizures, strokes, and the use of certain medications. If they cannot be reversed, a nonsteroidal anti-inflammatory drug, such as indomethacin, often helps, as does attention to the simple elements that constitute good sleep hygiene, such as regular changes of bedclothing and using a gentle fan.

Practical Strategies

Some simple techniques may ease sleep-related problems:

- If anxiety is the root of the problem, any of the relaxation and distraction exercises in Chapter 12 (breathing, progressive muscle relaxation, music therapy, guided imagery) can be used to soothe patients, allowing them to more easily drift off to sleep.

- Opioids used for pain will help induce sleep, especially when pain stimulates wakefulness; families should not be overly concerned if the patient seems oversedated at the beginning of an opioid regimen, since this may represent catch-up sleep. Most patients build up a tolerance to the sedative effects of opioids within a week or two (see Chapter 7 on morphine and the other strong opioids). A soothing back rub or massage can often reduce anxiety and relax the person, helping sleep come.

- Pay attention to whether the sleep-wake cycle has undergone reversal. It is very common that, for one reason or another, a patient is unable to sleep well at night. When this occurs, he becomes drowsy during the day and eagerly grabs a nap at odd times, and then is even less likely to sleep well at night, perpetuating a vicious cycle that is hard to interrupt. If this seems to be occurring, minimize or eliminate daytime sleeping so that the patient is more tired at night, and talk to the doctor about adding either a nighttime sleeping pill or a daytime stimulant. Maximizing exposure to daytime sunlight is believed to stimulate natural circadian rhythms.

- Avoid stimulating substances before bed. Avoid caffeine after noon, limit coffee to two cups per day, and avoid nicotine and chocolate at night. When possible avoid medications known to interfere with sleep (caffeine-containing painkillers such as Excedrin, Darvon,

Esgic-Plus, Fioricet, Fiorinal, Hycomine, Norgesic, and Wigraine; sinus and cold medications containing pseudoephedrine or phenylpropanolamine; supplements containing phenylpropanolamine, ephedra, ma huang, or ginseng; corticosteroids such as cortisone, prednisone, and dexamethasone; bronchodilators and asthma inhalers like theophylline and albuterol; some sinus medications, such as Entex and Profen; cimetidine; Demerol; certain antidepressants, especially the SSRIs, or selective serotonin reuptake inhibitors; hyperactivity remedies such as Ritalin; beta-blockers such as propanolol, atenolol, timolol, or metoprolol, which are associated with nightmares; and some glaucoma medications).

- Avoid excessive laxatives and the evening use of diuretics to minimize nocturnal voiding.
- Avoid alcohol. Although sometimes helpful to initiate sleep, it has a rebound effect that disrupts routine sleep and causes frequent early awakenings.
- Avoid food within two hours of bedtime, especially large meals. If you must eat, stick with an easily digestible light snack (nothing greasy or spicy) that will not produce heartburn; avoid protein and stick with carbohydrates.
- Include activities likely to lead to sleep, such as listening to soothing music or recordings of nature sounds, reading, taking a warm bath, or getting a massage.
- Keep the bedroom conducive to sleep and relaxation; keep it quiet, cool (about 65 degrees), dark, comfortable, and well ventilated.
- Eliminate disruptive lights, sounds, temperatures, or touch sensations and adopt corrective measures (eyeshades, earplugs, monotonous low-volume background noise, new bedlinens).
- Behavioral approaches, such as progressive relaxation training, meditation, autogenic training, yoga, self-hypnosis and biofeedback, cognitive therapy, and mindful living, can encourage relaxation and promote sleep (see Chapter 12). These tools help empower the individual to control a sleep problem by relying on internal coping mechanisms, thus boosting self-esteem, rather than relying on external factors such as medications, which tend to reinforce the patient's role as a victim.

Medical Conditions

Work with your doctor to identify the presence of conditions that may interfere with normal sleep. These can include depression, arthritis, kidney disease, heart failure, asthma, sleep apnea, restless legs syndrome, chronic pain, Parkinson's disease, and hyperthyroidism. Illicit and prescribed medications can contribute to insomnia (see above).

Of Possible Use

While their relaxing effects have not been confirmed, some people claim success with folk remedies: warm milk; a cut-up onion in a jar at the bedside inhaled before bedtime; herbal supplements or teas containing valerian, chamomile, lavender, passionflower, lemon verbena, lemon balm, peppermint, red clover, calendula flowers, California poppy, hops, linden flower, skullcap, St. John's wort, or vervain; other supplements, such as GABA or tryptophan (amino acids), melatonin, and certain vitamins and minerals, such as calcium, B vitamins, zinc, magnesium, iron, and copper. No matter how unscientific, such remedies certainly have a chance of working if the user believes in them.

Prescribed Sleeping Aids

While well accepted for short-term use, tremendous controversy surrounds the regular, chronic use of sleeping pills. Despite physicians' reluctance to provide such medications on an ongoing basis, they are among the most widely prescribed. Over-the-counter sleep remedies, usually containing antihistamines such as dopodramamine or diphenhydramine (Benadryl), are generally safe but may cause dry mouth, constipation, rapid heartbeat, and urinary retention. Using a prescribed sleep medication on a daily basis is usually best avoided. Older sedatives or hypnotics, including the barbiturates (Nembutal, Seconal), chloral hydrate, and glutethimide, are no longer be recommended due to risks of oversedation, addiction, seizures, and even death. The most widely used agents, the benzodiazepines, include clonazepam (Klonopin), flurazepam (Dalmane), quazepam (Doral), estazolam (ProSom), temazepam (Restoril), triazolam (Halcion), alprazolam (Xanax), lorazepam (Ativan), and diazepam (Valium). Although effective, they may cause daytime fatigue (hangover), and prolonged use is discouraged due to concerns about the need for increasing doses (tolerance), habituation, and abuse. The newer medications zolpidem (Ambien) and zaleplon (Sonata) are preferred today because hangover and abuse seem much less prevalent. Tricyclic antidepressants may be used to treat insomnia in cancer patients because they help induce sleep and enhance the pain-relieving effects of opioids. However, they should not be taken as needed; instead, they are usually prescribed to be taken regularly so that they can help relieve pain as well.

Confusion and Delirium

Many conditions can trigger confusion in patients with cancer. Unlike delirium, which is a more established condition, a confused patient will be mixed up from time to time, but overall behavior remains normal. The patient is not agitated, and even if he occasionally hallucinates or seems to be "losing his mind," he becomes aware of these episodes. If this condition becomes more profound or the patient becomes agitated, then the patient may be described as delirious. Delirium, by definition, is marked by passing episodes of disorganized thinking or incoherence, in which the patient is disoriented as to the time of day and displays impaired attention. Patients with delirium can hurt themselves, especially without supervision. Delirium tends to be worse at night.

The terms *confusion* and *delirium* represent a continuum that is not sharply defined, and they need to be distinguished from dementia, a gradual intellectual decline that occurs over months or years, usually in association with aging. Patients with dementia may be unaware of commonly known facts but are usually more alert and aware of their surroundings than those with delirium.

Delirium and confusion can stem from many causes, including infection, stopping a medication suddenly, or the side effects of certain drugs, such as diuretics. Confusion may also occur from too much insulin, especially if a patient has suffered great weight loss and persistently shows a lack of appetite. Many medications, including benzodiazepines, narcotics, steroids, and anticholinergic drugs, and even nonprescription drugs such as aspirin or antihistamine, if taken often, can trigger confusion. Other causes include poor pain control, lack of sleep, fecal impaction, urinary retention, and brain tumors. In most cases, the cause is a result of the disease and not a form of any kind of mental illness. Families should be prepared, however, for episodes of confusion or delirium, because they occur is some 85 percent of terminally ill cancer patients. Almost all patients will experience some degree of confusion or delirium at least intermittently in the last few days of life.

It is important not to panic if patients experience confusion. Most spells pass quickly, although they may return. If persistent or severe, the doctor should certainly be consulted. Keep in mind that patients may be very embarrassed by such episodes and often will try to keep them from others. They should be reassured that these events are expected for patients in their condition.

When possible, drug substitutions can be tried. If a patient is taking cimetidine (Tagamet), which carries some risk of delirium as a side effect, sucralfate (Carafate) can be substituted. Similarly, nortriptyline (Pamelor), which has less chance of causing this side effect, can be substituted for amitriptyline (Elavil).

Symptoms and Management of Delirium

Delirium, usually associated with agitation, is a confusional state in which the autonomic nervous system is overactive. Symptoms include flushed face, dilated pupils, sweating, and rapid heartbeat. It may be caused by a physical problem, such as by a tumor affecting the central nervous system, organ failure, infection, or other complication. It may also be caused by the indirect effects on the central nervous system of certain medications (including chemotherapy agents). In contrast to agitated delirium (described above), some patients experience hypoactive delirium, where the confusion is associated with sleepiness and reduced activity and response.

Some 15 to 50 percent of hospitalized cancer patients have episodes of delirium. Often just the change of scenery, frequent interruptions, and absence of familiar surroundings are disorienting. When sudden episodes of agitation, cognitive impairment, change in attention span, or levels of consciousness occur, chances are these changes are from the cancer or side effects rather than a new psychological problem. If there is severe agitation or hallucinations, an antipsychotic medication that helps calm the patient may be called for. Haloperidol (Haldol) is commonly used because it is sedating and has fewer side effects than other antipsychotic medications. It can be given orally, intravenously, or intramuscularly. Some sedatives, especially the benzodiazepines—diazepam (Valium), alprazolam (Xanax), lorazepam (Ativan), and others—although usually calming, sometimes will paradoxically make things worse by reducing inhibitions, like the effects observed in someone who has consumed too much alcohol.

Caring for a confused or delirious patient can be difficult because patients may become unintentionally violent and disruptive. The following strategies may be appropriate for either confusion or delirium.

Practical Strategies

If the patient seems to be confused or suffering from delirium:

- Repeatedly reassure the patient, keep familiar objects near him, and speak simply and clearly. Don't be frightened. Acknowledge the abnormal behavior, stressing that it will probably be temporary, is likely to be the result of needed medications, and is harmless. Sometimes it is even appropriate to joke about it together.
- Keep the patient's room quiet and well lit at night with a nightlight. Try not to awaken the patient during the night.

Medications for Delirium

Families and physicians usually prefer to make the patient less restless and aggressive with an antidepressant, haloperidol (Haldol), or the antipsychotic medication chlorpromazine (Thorazine, Promapar) if needed. For more on sedation in patients who are very ill, see Chapter 15.

Hiccoughs

In cancers affecting the stomach, diaphragm, and brain, hiccoughs are not uncommon. They may also be triggered by kidney failure (uremia) or infection. Many of us don't realize how exhausting and demoralizing hiccoughs can be when they last a long time.

Practical Strategies

Hiccoughs can sometimes be managed with simple physical maneuvers such as holding the breath or breathing in and out of a paper bag (to boost inhaled carbon dioxide).

There are a number of folk remedies, mostly scientifically unproven, but which cannot hurt. They include:

- Sipping water from the "wrong" side of a glass (lean forward, as if trying to touch the toes, and tilt the glass until you can drink from the far edge).
- Drinking water with two heaping teaspoons of sugar to stimulate the esophagus.
- Running a cold key down the back of the person hiccoughing.
- Drinking peppermint water, which can relax the sphincter of the esophagus—which may be useful when the hiccoughs are due to pressure on the stomach.

Medications for Hiccoughing

When the hiccoughs are due to pressure on the stomach and peppermint water doesn't work, an antiflatulent such as Maalox might, as might metoclopramide. When the hiccough reflex is stimulated by a tumor or fluid pressing on the diaphragm, chlorpromazine often helps; possible side effects include drowsiness, light-headedness, and heart palpitations. When hiccoughs are caused by a brain tumor, phenytoin or carbamazepine may help. Other medications that are occasionally used to suppress hiccoughs include quinidine, benzonatate, atropine, and methylphenidate.

If hiccoughs persist despite all these efforts and are troubling to the patient, a phrenic nerve block (see Chapter 9) or surgery to the phrenic nerve may even be considered.

Muscle Jerking

No one knows what causes muscle jerking (myoclonus), which can be much like twitching, or why high doses of opioids can have this effect. The movement is not sustained, but sudden and uncontrollable, and usually involves single jerks of the entire body, much like many of us normally experience as we fall asleep. Muscle jerks may awaken patients and can make drinking a cup of water unpredictably difficult but otherwise are not particularly bothersome to the patient. Although they may disturb family members, reassure them that these involuntary movements are an expected side effect of medications and would stop if the medication was stopped. Sometimes jerking causes pain. If so, the doctor may consider clonazepam for this side effect, or the pain medication may need to be changed.

Muscle Cramps

Muscle cramping may be totally unrelated to cancer, or it can be a symptom of a systemwide problem such as uremia (a buildup of toxic substances in the blood due to poor kidney function), cirrhosis, or other metabolic condition. In cancer patients, muscle cramps may also be caused by the tumor exerting pressure on certain nerves or by dehydration (from sweating or diarrhea), or it may be a side effect of medication (such as diuretics), radiation, chemotherapy (when vinca alkaloids or cisplatin are used), hormone therapy (such as those used for breast cancer), or surgery, which may cause nerve damage.

Practical and Medication Strategies

Muscle cramps can often be treated by one or more of the following strategies:

- In cases where the cramping is caused by dehydration or medications that aren't vital, withdrawing suspect drugs, if possible, might help.
- When the culprit medication can't be withdrawn, other medications may help so the patient can more comfortably continue with chemotherapy or hormone therapy. Quinine taken at bedtime can

prevent cramps that typically occur during the night. Doses are kept low.

- For bothersome cramping during the day, the anticonvulsants phenytoin (Dilantin) and carbamazepine (Tegretol) are considered most useful and have been well studied. Other substances that have been reported to help cramping but for which studies are scant include baclofen (Lioresal), tizanidine (Zanaflex), diazepam (Valium), dantrolene (Dantrium), procainamide (Pronestyl), diphenhydramine (Benadryl), fluoride, riboflavin (vitamin B_2), vitamin E, verapamil (Calan), and nifedipine (Procardia).

12

Mind-Body Approaches to Easing Pain

Mind and body are inextricably linked, and their second-by-second interaction exerts a profound influence upon health and illness, life and death. Attitudes, beliefs, and emotional states ranging from love and compassion to fear and anger can trigger chain reactions that affect blood chemistry, heart rate, and the activity of every cell and organ system in the body-from the stomach and gastrointestinal tract to the immune system.
All of that is now indisputable fact.

—Kenneth R. Pelletier, Ph.D., M.D.

So far we've discussed how doctors ease the pain and discomfort of cancer by drawing from an arsenal of drug therapies and medical treatments. But limiting our focus to treatment of the body neglects the very powerful influence of the mind on the body. In recent years, more and more Western physicians in almost all fields of medicine are recognizing that the mind and body are not two separate entities but integral parts of the whole body system. Physical illness, the immune system, and the mind are all, in fact, intimately connected, and as we'll see, many studies are showing how feelings, thoughts, attitudes, and behavior can all have powerful and pivotal influences on well-being, health, illness, and pain.

In 2001, a report in the *Journal of the National Cancer Institute* that reviewed fifty-four published studies on various mind-body techniques found that many of the techniques have great promise for relieving cancer pain and suffering.[1] Behavioral therapy (discussed below), for example, was particularly effective in controlling anticipatory nausea and vomiting in both children and adults undergoing chemotherapy and in reducing anxiety and distress associated with invasive medical procedures. Hypnosis, relaxation, and distracting imagery, on the other hand, seemed particularly effective for alleviating pain.

We know now how chronic pain can increase muscle tension. As the tension causes escalating pain, a patient may get anxious and depressed, which in turn may magnify pain sensations. To break this vicious cycle, pain clinics typically include recommendations for a range of mind-body techniques, such as:

- Relaxation techniques to interrupt the pain-tension-spasm cycle
- Physical therapy to stretch and strengthen muscles in order to help correct muscle tension
- Psychotherapy and antidepressant medication to help relieve depression and feelings of despair
- Occupational therapy to learn how to do everyday tasks with a reduced risk of reinjury

Though not miracle cures, mind-body approaches can help harness the power of the mind to better control thoughts and emotions such as worries, pessimism, negativity, hostility, and depression and to promote relaxation, hope, control, and optimism. Some evidence even suggests that such techniques may help arrest or perhaps even reverse the disease process and promote longevity. Whether or not these benefits will be substantiated by further research, most doctors nevertheless acknowledge that these techniques can greatly improve the quality of life for cancer patients and others by helping them better cope with the fear and anxiety of having cancer and with the treatments for cancer, which may have very unpleasant side effects. By helping patients improve their spirits, mind-body techniques can go a long way in reducing the severity and frequency of medical problems, including pain. As we'll see, a growing body of evidence is showing that these mind-body approaches can relieve nausea, for example (a common side effect of chemotherapy), reduce the amount of pain medication that cancer and surgical patients need, and even speed up recovery.

These mind-body techniques range from meditation and yoga to biofeedback and music therapy, among others. Most of these alternative therapies were considered totally unconventional and on the fringe just twenty years ago. Today they are becoming more widespread and accepted in hospitals and clinics throughout the country as effective, no-risk strategies that can ease distress, muscle tension, anxiety, and depression—all of which can improve quality of life and enhance the medical treatment of pain and other discomforts associated with cancer.

Although none of these techniques is meant as a substitute for medical treatment and none has been shown to actually cure pain or cancer, they can usually help enhance relief to allow patients to regain some control and mastery over their lives.

How Distress Aggravates Pain and Illness

First, let's look at how the stress of cancer can make pain and illness worse. Obviously, having cancer is enormously stressful. The disease turns a person's and the family's lives upside down, and in many ways the individual feels out of control. Stress bombards the cancer patient on all fronts: worry and anxiety about the disease, its progression, its treatments, potential disabilities, and perhaps disfigurements; concerns about its negative impact on the family's emotional, financial, and even physical well-being; anxiety over losing control of one's life and independence. At one time or another, the typical cancer patient is plagued by despair, depression, hopelessness, and helplessness. And a cancer patient will naturally be fearful about pain and dying. (See Chapter 14 for more about psychological aspects of cancer and cancer pain.)

There is little doubt that emotional distress can lower a person's pain threshold and increase pain. Stress also takes a serious physical toll: many studies show that stress causes muscles to tighten, disturbs appetite and sleep habits, and triggers the production of stress hormones. These hormones, such as adrenaline and cortisol, increase heart rate, blood pressure, muscle tension, and blood sugar and, over time, can lower one's pain threshold and weaken the immune response.

Another way that stress may influence health is through the chemistry of our emotions. Researchers have discovered that emotions can influence the production or activity of chemical messengers called neuropeptides, which travel through the body and influence the nervous, immune, and endocrine systems. Thoughts and feelings may also influence levels of brain chemicals such as endorphins, the body's natural painkillers, which are chemically similar to morphine.

Whatever the exact mechanisms between interactions among the brain, nervous system, and immune system, growing evidence demonstrates their intimate and dynamic connections. Studies at Ohio State University have shown, for example, that people under stress—those taking important exams, family members caring for loved ones with Alzheimer's disease, and women who have recently endured a difficult divorce—had lower levels of immune cell activity. Other studies have shown that people who had experienced significant levels of stress were much more likely to become ill. Similarly, studies at Duke University have shown that people with "angry" personalities or those who are easily upset by life's stressors are more prone to heart disease.

If psychological states such as stress and anger can wear down or inhibit the immune system, making one more vulnerable to illness and infection, can the mind work to promote health? The answer appears to be a resounding yes. The evidence that reducing stress, loneliness, and depression and boosting control, relaxation, hope, and optimism may bolster the immune system has been gaining such momentum in recent years that a new medical subspecialty called psychoneuroimmunology has been born. Psychoneuroimmunology is the study of the relationships among the mind, the brain, and the immune and endocrine (hormonal) systems. Although the evidence is far from conclusive, current findings have been so provocative that the National Institutes of Health now includes the National Center for Complementary and Alternative Medicine. It will take many more studies to validate the effectiveness of many of these treatments, yet increasing numbers of researchers now agree that mind-body techniques have merit and can play a definite role in pain management and cancer treatment.

These positive results, however, should not be interpreted to mean that negative emotions can cause an illness or that positive emotions can

Strategies for Cancer Pain That Do Not Involve Drugs or Surgery

To relieve muscle spasm	Massage Ice or heat packs Walking, stretching, and other exercises Repositioning chair, bed, and pillow
To disrupt nerve pathways to interfere with the transmission of pain to the brain (counterirritants)	Menthol cream rubs Heat or ice packs Vibration, pressure, rubbing, or massage Transcutaneous electrical nerve stimulation (TENS) Acupuncture
To relieve tension and stress, which aggravate pain	Relaxation techniques, deep breathing, distraction and imagery exercises, progressive muscle relaxation Autogenic exercises Music therapy Mindfulness and yoga Meditation and prayer Hypnosis and self-hypnosis Biofeedback
To cope more effectively	Group support Cognitive coping strategies Desensitization techniques
To relieve movement-related pain	Splints and other orthopedic supports (collars, corsets, slings)
To promote movement	Strengthening and stretching exercises Compression cuffs for swelling Walking aids (cane, crutches, walkers)

cure it. What researchers are growing more convinced of is the positive effect emotions have on overall well-being. Even if these mind-body approaches prove to be ineffective in actually influencing the course of disease or indirectly relieving pain, patients can benefit from these strategies by reducing stress, improving outlook and coping strategies, and regaining some control over their thoughts and feelings, all of which can enhance quality of life and help reduce the intensity of perceived pain.

Cognitive Skills: Find Out What to Expect

Having accurate and detailed information on the illness, treatment, and prognosis is a fundamental key to helping patients and their families cope, because such knowledge helps restore autonomy and a sense of some control over one's life. Knowledge is key, and avoiding surprises can make a big difference. Before any procedure, for example, be sure that the physician or technician reviews details about what will happen before, during, and after the procedure, such as possible sensations that might be felt— pulling, bloating, stinging, and so on. Some studies, though not all, have even found that such information can raise pain tolerance, can reduce the need for painkillers, and is linked to faster recovery rates and shorter hospital stays. However, some patients prefer to cultivate trust in their care providers and receive minimal details of risks that they may find disturbing. In patients who tend to repress their anxiety and avoid seeking information, training in coping skills may be helpful (explained later in this chapter).

How Counseling or Supportive Therapy Can Help

Once patients and family members have clear and straightforward information about the disease, simple supportive therapy may be very useful in allaying fears, anxieties, and emotional conflicts. Many doctors do this automatically; in other cases, patients and families may benefit from talking instead to a nurse on the staff, a social worker, or other type of medical or mental health professional who specializes in working with cancer patients and families. The professional listens carefully to the patient's and family's concerns and responds with understanding and empathy, providing knowledgeable reassurance, support, and advice about any concerns. Supportive counseling should also focus on helping the patient and family communicate openly and on enhancing their coping skills.

GROUP SUPPORT AND SUPPORT GROUPS

Participating in groups with other cancer patients can also help; a professional or even a specially trained patient may lead the group. You can benefit from talking with others who have similar problems, helping you feel less isolated, different, alienated, and alone. The support provided in settings such as this may help promote communication among the family as well.

Studies find, for example, that people with few social supports have higher death rates from a variety of diseases (including cancer) than people who are the same age but have more social support. Evidently, support groups seem to reduce stress and isolation and improve one's outlook on life; these factors help the patient regain control and mastery over life. Unfortunately, many patients are initially reluctant to join such groups and share their feelings with strangers. Many people are more inclined to suffer in silence, especially if they are depressed or scared. Many are not used to asking for help or admitting fear, particularly to people they don't know. Caregivers may seek the help of a professional mental health worker to initiate discussions or to encourage the patient to just try attending a group, initially without having to say anything.

How Coping and Relaxation Skills Can Reduce Pain

To help cancer patients cope and improve their psychological well-being, families and loved ones can help by providing information and support. It can be helpful to show the patient certain techniques that can break the vicious cycle of anxiety, which intensifies pain and, in turn, causes more anxiety. Coping and relaxation skills are among the most studied and recognized of these techniques.

How Coping Techniques Work

A study at the University of Southern California School of Medicine compared how fifty-six children coped with bone marrow procedures, a traumatic and often painful treatment. At different procedures several weeks apart, the children received either (1) Valium, a tranquilizer, (2) training in breathing exercises, imagery lessons (imagining they were at Disneyland or on the beach), and distraction techniques (imagining scenarios in which the children help Superman or Wonder Woman), with a small reward at the end; or (3) distraction by viewing cartoons during their procedures.

When the children used the cognitive-behavioral techniques in the second alternative (breathing, imagery, and distraction), they had significantly lower distress, pain ratings, and pulse rates than when they took a tranquilizer or were distracted by cartoons alone.

Source: Jay SM, Elliot CH, Katz E, Siegel SE.
Cognitive-behavioral and pharmacologic interventions
for children's distress during painful medical procedures.
J Consult Clin Psych 1987; 55(6): 860–5

Although studies showing the effectiveness of psychological approaches abound, some patients are still skeptical about trying them. Some resent being asked to try these kinds of techniques, believing they are mere "mental tricks." Others feel that being asked to use them minimizes the legitimacy of their pain and suffering, implying that their problems are all in their head. Others feel silly doing them or lack faith that they can help. One way to help convince these skeptics might be to get them to acknowledge how their pain escalates when they're upset. Then ask them to consider how the opposite could be true—how their pain could be soothed if they were relaxed. Also, they can be reassured that these techniques are safe and noninvasive and have no risk of side effects. In other words, trying them can't hurt in any way.

A few cautionary notes: These exercises are skills and, as such, must be learned, practiced, and mastered. Don't be easily discouraged—it may take up to two weeks to feel comfortable with these skills and to experience any noticeable benefits. While these methods will not *cure* pain, they do have the ability to help change the perception and experience of the pain and responses to it.

If a pain is sharp and stabbing, a patient may try to think about it as dull and spreading. If the pain is burning, the sensation can be countered with thoughts of a colder pain.

By changing the perception of pain, cancer patients can regain some control over their thoughts and feelings, over their pain and discomfort, and even over life in general. They may also benefit physically when physiological factors aggravated by stress are improved: they may experience reduced muscle tension, increased blood flow, and reduced heart rate, among other benefits.

These techniques are most appropriate for patients in mild or moderate pain. Those with minimal pain may not be very motivated to practice new skills if simple analgesics can relieve discomfort. Patients in severe pain, on the other hand, may have a hard time concentrating and may not find these techniques particularly beneficial. Patients with lung cancer may wish to check with their doctor before initiating deep breathing exercises.

Enhancing Coping Skills

An important skill for any patient (and any person, for that matter) is to learn how to notice and change negative attitudes, pessimism, and automatic, self-defeating thoughts. By monitoring thoughts, feelings, and behaviors, you can identify and modify ones that are self-defeating, negative, or unproductive. These would include thoughts that may exaggerate or take things out of proportion, such as always imagining the worst. For example, a patient experiencing an unfamiliar stomach pain may immediately jump to the unwarranted conclusion that it means that the cancer has invaded the stomach. When a patient finds himself automatically interpreting a flare-up as a sign of worse things to come, it not only escalates feelings of anxiety, depression, and helplessness, but also makes it difficult to concentrate on productive ways of dealing with the problem.

When a person is ill, it is common to have good days and bad days, as well as to experience new feelings and symptoms that sometimes include pain. When pain can't be wished away, it might as well be acknowledged. This is a good first step in dealing effectively with a tough situation. Know, too, that it is natural for negative feelings and fears to arise; they need to be dealt with head on, which can sometimes be a harder job than managing the pain. Although anyone with cancer has good cause to be concerned, fretting and worrying will not make things better. Worrying can only make it worse. In fact, numerous studies have shown that people who chronically think about the negative aspects of life—in other words, pessimists—fare worse than optimists in warding off illness and depression and gaining control over their life (see "Sustaining Hope" in Chapter 14).

Whenever possible, the patient should take a positive and action-oriented approach—one that confirms that he is in charge and is not a helpless, passive victim. Review and use the techniques and medications available. If the pain persists, the doctor and the rest of the health care team should be informed so they can reevaluate the case and prescribe new doses or new medications. If negative feelings persist and seem overwhelming, it is important to communicate them. Identifying and sharing the problem is the first step to resolving what is troubling the patient. A good heart-to-heart conversation with a close family member, friend, member of the clergy, or professional counselor may help, as might a new medication. These strategies are action-oriented: when a problem arises (for example, a new side effect or symptom), the individual communicates it to a doctor, discusses it, and works through the problem without imagining the worst every step of the way.

It may sound like a questionable exercise, but focusing on the positive rather than the negative is a powerful means of bringing life's circumstances into perspective. More and more long-term studies have found a link between pessimism and earlier death, showing that optimists—people who look on the bright side and who explain adversity to themselves as temporary or as specific problems—are healthier and live longer.[2]

In sickness, many people naturally dwell on negative thoughts, so we have to make a conscious effort to look for the life-affirming, meaningful, and positive aspects of life, even in the face of serious illness.

THE GLASS CAN BE HALF FULL, NOT HALF EMPTY

Instead of a negative thought such as "This pain must mean that the tumor has grown—the pain will probably get worse and worse until I can't take it," try this type of positive, conscious thinking: "This new pain is unpleasant, but I can deal with it. I will practice deep breathing and consider taking more pain relievers. I will write down what I'm feeling as best as I can, so my family and doctors can know what I am experiencing. It will help them take care of me."

Instead of the negative thought "This pain only gets worse—it's never going to go away," try this type of positive thinking: "This is a bad pain. I know my doctor is committed to my well-being. I must let him and the nurse know that the pain treatment needs to be stepped up. In the meantime, I will take my medication and practice relaxation techniques."

Instead of thinking negatively, "I'm all alone—everyone's given up on me. The doctor and my family haven't come to visit," try "Just because I've been alone all afternoon, I can't jump to the conclusion that everyone's giving up on me. The doctor has always shown up before, and so has my family. I should take this time to focus on what's good in my life. Perhaps I will listen to that new tape I received, or write my niece a letter."

Instead of the negative thought "This pain is killing me. I can't take it," try this type of positive thinking: "It is a bad pain, but I must not panic. Relaxing will make it better. Remember to breathe deeply, in and out. Relax. The more I relax, the faster the pain will subside."

Instead of thinking "I can't go shopping anymore, I can't drive anymore, and I can't even clean the house anymore. I am useless and helpless," think positively: "I've started to read novels again after all these years, and to listen to all the works of Mozart, something I've always wanted to do. Also, spending so much time with my daughter has really strengthened our relationship."

Such statements not only highlight the personal goals a patient has attained but empower him, allowing him to feel a greater sense of control over his life and to acknowledge that some good changes have come out of misfortune and illness. This kind of approach can shift a patient's point of view from pessimism, helplessness, and hopelessness to resourcefulness, control, and optimism. Learning to replace automatic, self-defeating assumptions and interpretations with more positive ones is an important coping strategy for everyone. By acknowledging, communicating, and dealing honestly with fears, feelings, and thoughts, the patient can ultimately gain a greater sense of mastery over life as he copes with the many losses that cancer can entail.

GAINING CONTROL AND RELIEF BY CHANGING THE MEANING OF PAIN

How a person thinks about pain can have a direct impact on the perception of pain and the ability to cope. Consider the different meanings people associate with their pain: one person might believe the pain is a punishment for something done in the past, while someone else sees it as an enemy, another views it as weakness, and yet another considers it an overwhelming loss. All of these perspectives will make it harder to maintain a sense of control and power over one's life, since they all generate stress from self-defeating thoughts. The muscle tension and anxiety from these thoughts can exacerbate pain and keep the mind focused on the pain and its negative meanings.

On the other hand, considering that the pain is perhaps a relief from other demands, or is a challenge or a vehicle for growth, can help maintain a sense of mastery and control over life. A study by researchers from Ohio University and the University of West Florida, for example, found that tension headache patients who learned to think about their pain differently experienced at least a 43 percent improvement in pain relief, with some experiencing as much as 100 percent improvement; the control group who received no counseling in these skills showed no improvement.[3]

Cancer patients who can view their pain as a challenge may be more apt to feel they can exert some control and try to master the situation. Those who view pain as punishment, on the other hand, have a more resigned, helpless, and hopeless outlook. By using cognitive techniques to reframe reactions and thoughts about pain, it may be possible to transform the experience from a threat to a challenge, which in itself is linked to lower pain levels.

Another way to help develop this skill is by using a pain diary (see Chapter 3). The patient can chart when pain is at its worst and what was going on at that time: What was the patient thinking or feeling? What was the situation? How did the patient try to reduce the pain? What worked? In looking for patterns, try to understand what might have aggravated the pain—perhaps certain emotions, particular problems, or thoughts about the meaning behind the pain.

DESENSITIZING THE FEARFUL PATIENT

When patients have uncontrollable fears about a treatment or avoid doing things because of unjustified concerns, which will in the long run make things worse, an approach that relies on using very small steps to overcome fears can help. This method is called desensitization. First, the patient should be taught one of the relaxation techniques described in this chapter (see next section). While deeply relaxed, the patient can be guided to imagine a pared-down, less stressful version of the fearful stimulus (such as a very thin needle in the case of fear of injections) and then may actually be shown a thin needle. With success at this level, progressively larger needles can be substituted. Likewise, if a patient is afraid of moving or performing some activity, he can be encouraged to master it in a series of smaller steps, in which the process or procedure is broken down into more manageable chunks. By systematically exposing the patient to feared thoughts or realities in a gradual way, the feared object or idea is rendered significantly more approachable and less threatening. Personal control and mastery are thus gained. This process of desensitization is usually best carried out under the supervision of a mental health professional, like a psychologist, psychiatrist, or psychiatric social worker.

Methods to Promote Relaxation

Because stress, muscular tension, spasm, distress, and the body's responses to these phenomena (sweating, increased blood pressure, changes in brain chemicals and blood flow, or heart rate) can increase pain and make it harder to deal with, techniques to reduce these negative feelings may help alleviate pain. Some conditions—such as irritable bowel, headache, and muscle spasm—may be direct results of tension states. Even when pain is unrelated to tension, relaxing muscles can prevent or alleviate increased pain due to tension. Although relaxation and self-hypnosis techniques have been used in Eastern cultures for centuries to produce physiological changes, Western science has only recently acknowledged the powerful effects of these techniques. A robust body of studies has shown relaxation to be very effective in producing physiological reductions in heart rate, blood pressure, respiratory rate, and oxygen consumption. In addition, these changes, along with increases in brain waves associated with peace and tranquility (low-frequency alpha, theta, and delta waves), reduce anxiety and ease muscle tension, thereby inducing a calm mental condition.

Studies have also shown that relaxation can be directly responsible for reducing pain. Studies at Duke University have shown that relaxation techniques are effective for various kinds of persistent pain, such low back pain,[4] while studies at the State University of New York at Albany demonstrate success with relaxation and chronic headache.[5] Relaxation techniques have also been shown to be effective for reducing the nausea and vomiting that commonly occur before chemotherapy treatments. As a result, more and more cancer clinics are employing these techniques.

Intriguing studies also suggest that the beneficial effects of relaxation meditation are specifically linked to reduced secretions of the stress hormone cortisol. Cortisol helps the body muster more energy needed to cope with stress—often, however, at the expense of immune system function and the effectiveness of tissue repair. When neurochemists at the Maharishi International University in Fairfield, Iowa, measured cortisol levels in people before and after they practiced meditation for four months, they found a 15 percent drop in cortisol. Another study indicated that meditators experienced up to a 25 percent drop in cortisol levels.[6]

A number of techniques are used to achieve deep relaxation, a state that has also been called the relaxation response, or self-hypnosis—including relaxation exercises, meditation, hypnosis, and biofeedback. Whatever works for a particular patient, to enable him to quickly and easily restore an inner sense of calm and peace, should be used. Patients who are most willing to use their imagination and have the confidence to do so tend to benefit the most. Patients in severe pain or those who are on higher doses of opioids and other mood-altering medications may find it harder to concentrate on these exercises.

All of these techniques should be practiced in a quiet place and in a comfortable position, usually with the eyes closed. Soothing music in the background may help produce a calming environment. Paradoxically, a setting that is too comfortable may interfere with the patient achieving these goals by too easily inducing sleep.

Progressive Muscle Relaxation

Progressive muscle relaxation, or progressive relaxation training (PRT), involves tensing a body part for ten seconds and then releasing the tension. Each body part is "squeezed" separately, moving from the forehead, eyes, and mouth down to the arms and fingers, the trunk, and the feet and toes. At the end of the session (which may last from five to twenty minutes), the entire body is tensed at once, after which all of the increased pressure and tension are allowed to flow from the body, leaving the patient in a more relaxed state and perhaps ready for a mental (cognitive) relaxation exercise.

The reason why PRT is important is that so many of us don't recognize when we are tense. Signs of tension in the body include hunched shoulders, a tight lower back, and tense facial and jaw muscles. By actually forcing us to tense a body part and then relax it, this procedure helps us recognize the state of relaxation and its desirability. Several studies have shown that PRT can significantly reduce nausea before chemotherapy in patients who have learned to associate nausea with cancer treatment (anticipatory nausea and vomiting). PRT can also markedly reduce how long such nausea lasts and its intensity, which is why experts at Memorial Sloan-Kettering Cancer Center in New York City and elsewhere are using it more and more.[7]

CONTROLLED BREATHING

As part of PRT, a patient can learn controlled breathing. The patient progressively relaxes his muscles and then focuses all his attention on breathing slowly and rhythmically, in and out. Inhalation is preferably through the nose, deep into the back of the throat where breaths become more audible, and is held for several seconds. Exhalation is through the mouth, slow, complete, and even. Progressive relaxation and controlled breathing can be combined by tensing different muscles when inhaling and relaxing others when exhaling. Upon exhaling, some trainers suggest that a calming word be repeated in the mind (such as *peace, beauty,* or *love*).

AUTOGENIC TRAINING

Patients using PRT may also want to add autogenic training to their relaxation sessions. Autogenic training is a relatively simple technique in which the patient repeats self-affirming statements involving warmth, heaviness, and calmness. The repetitions are aimed at lulling and calming the patient into a state of tranquility, eliciting the relaxation response.

Although it sounds so simple, this technique can have dramatic effects on the body, much like the other techniques that prompt the relaxation response—including increased blood flow to various body parts, which can relieve pain and promote a sense of well-being. In fact, electronic skin temperature monitors can be used to provide physiological feedback to the patient, showing what works to achieve the desired effect and what doesn't. This process of monitoring a person's ability to change a physiological response is called biofeedback. An electronic monitor indicates how effectively a patient's body is responding to a technique or procedure he is trying to learn and sharpen. Biofeedback is discussed in more detail later in the chapter.

Exercise for Autogenic Training

In a darkened, private space, lie on the floor or a sofa with eyes closed and body comfortably relaxed. Repeat the same thought in four or five different ways. For example: "My arms are heavy and warm, very heavy, leaden, and warm. My arms are getting even heavier and warmer. My arms are sinking, sinking down into the floor." While repeating these statements, the patient should try to visualize a warm bath, bright sunshine, a warm fireplace, or other things that suggest warmth and pleasure. Repeat with every body part in turn (substituting legs, neck, feet, back, and so on in place of arms in the example) for as long as possible, breathing deeply and slowly. The object is to put the mind and body into a relaxed, trancelike state.

VISUALIZATION, IMAGERY, AND DISTRACTION

Adding visualization, imagery, and distraction exercises to any of these relaxation techniques not only can distract the mind from focusing on the pain but can promote relaxation, which may indirectly promote pain relief. The distraction may be as simple as singing, watching television, counting the ceiling tiles, or making conversation. Other kinds of visualization techniques involve conjuring up pleasant images in the imagination—being on a sailboat, on a beach, or on a mountaintop. Any relaxing or peaceful scene the patient imagines or remembers will do. As in a daydream, patients can follow any train of relaxing thoughts, perhaps capturing the image of a loved one or reliving a special experience from the past, like walking through a childhood home, imagining a magical holiday moment, fantasizing about a romantic interlude, or spinning a fictional tale of themselves from a favorite novel—all with a body that is free of pain. The key is to concentrate on the scene as much as possible and imagine as vividly as possible all possible details, using all the senses, including smell, taste, touch, sound, and so on. Scientists have in fact found that the parts of the brain that are stimulated during the visualization are the same as those that would be stimulated when actually experiencing the tranquil scene.

The patient can also use imagery to soothe the painful area in a more direct way—imagining, for example, that a sparkling wand of healing energy, a flow of vitality, or a series of colors are coursing through the body and bathing the problem area and the pain. By coordinating breathing with the imagery, the patient can picture the tension and poisons exiting the body with each exhalation. Try holding the incoming breath, and

---

Sample Imagery Relaxation Exercise

Find a comfortable position, and close your eyes.

Imagine you are floating on a raft at a tropical beach. A warm gentle breeze is blowing over you. The sun is beating down on your lightly clad body. Your raft is gently bobbing up and down.

Feel the warmth in your fingertips, your arms, your toes, up your legs.

Enjoy the gentle rocking motion, lulling you into a gentle, weightless state.

Breathe slowly, deeply. Each breath brings in warmth; each exhalation pushes out poisons.

Imagine that you begin to float. Soon you're on a large, billowy cloud, floating through the sky.

Let yourself be calmed by the rhythms, the warmth, the peace.

during that time, imagine painful joints easing into their sockets, tense muscles softening, and even tumors shrinking.

Another technique is to imagine transforming the pain into another sensation or image. The patient imagines that, instead of pain, the sensation is an ice cube, a trickle of sand, the tickle of a feather, or a piercing light. The patient can then try to modify the sensation by imagining the ice melting, the sand blowing away, and so on.

Many people benefit from using professionally prepared audiotapes that are readily available through bookstores and health magazines. Bernie Siegel, author of *Love, Medicine and Miracles*, for example, has produced audiotapes intended specifically for the cancer patient. In them he leads the listener through meditations and thoughts that can induce relaxation, accompanied by soothing background music or sounds (a seashore or sounds from a night forest, for example). Although not for everyone, such tapes may help the patient drift into a trancelike state far from the unpleasantness of the cancer bed. Some report emerging from the experience feeling relaxed, refreshed, calm, and peaceful. Others prefer to use tapes they have produced themselves, with or without the help of a professional, using music and imagery that uniquely suit and soothe them.

The reason such techniques work is that they help the patient elicit the relaxation response, which, as we've discussed, can create beneficial physiological, psychological and behavioral changes. Later in the chapter we'll discuss the use of imagery for purposes other than relaxation. (See Appendix 3 for detailed instructions on using a relaxation technique.)

Imagery can also be used in an effort to fight the cancer rather than to just induce relaxation or control pain. During chemotherapy sessions, some patients find it helpful to visualize the drugs being injected as little angels or white knights, coursing through the bloodstream and annihilating each and every cancer cell. Others picture their tumors being bombarded by an army of white cells. Although some researchers believe that such imagery can actually bolster the immune system, studies have not yet confirmed this. Nevertheless, using this kind of imagery may help the patient feel more in control and regain a sense of mastery and power.

One way to determine whether this (or other techniques) is working is to keep a log of when such techniques are used, and how the pain or use of pain medication changes. Over a week or two, if positive changes are noticed, then the technique may be helping.

MEDITATION AND REPETITIVE PRAYER

According to Herbert Benson, M.D., of the Mind/Body Medical Institute and associate professor of medicine at Harvard Medical School, who coined the phrase "the relaxation response," meditation and prayer may also elicit a relaxation response. By emptying the mind of all intruding thoughts and therefore tensions, and by repetitively repeating a mantra, or simple word or sound, in one's mind to minimize distractions, Benson found that the same physiological changes occur as they do with other methods of relaxation already described in this chapter. This form of meditation is called transcendental meditation (or TM). Benson's group also tested the responses of persons of different religions while praying—he included a davening (a type of prayer) from Judaism, a rosary-type prayer from Catholicism, and a centering prayer from Protestantism—and again observed the same physiological responses. Like the deep breathing exercise and TM, repetitive prayer helps draw attention away from distress and pain and induces relaxation by emptying the mind of distracting thoughts.

Using Yoga and Mindfulness Meditation

Another type of meditation, known as mindfulness meditation, also induces relaxation and well-being, but instead of tuning out all thoughts, mindfulness focuses on them. As with other techniques, it is not used instead of medical treatment, and it has not been shown to slow or reverse disease, but it can help people cope more effectively with their illness. The process involves facing and even welcoming stress, pain, fear, and other negative feelings, because acknowledging these negative states or emotions is the first step in transforming them. First the practitioner begins with a deep breathing or standard meditation exercise. Yoga, particularly hatha yoga, is often used, because it promotes physical strength and flexibility while focusing on breathing and calmness.

Once the patient is relaxed, if the mind wanders, instead of bringing it back to the breathing or the mantra right away, mindfulness involves observing where the mind goes—watching as if from outside what the feelings or thoughts are, without making any judgments or analysis. The premise of mindfulness is that by observing the thoughts and feelings, a person becomes more aware of what is really bothering him, or what his true fears or dislikes or preferences are. The object is to be aware of what one is feeling by simply observing. As a result, the practitioner is said to be more in touch with himself and his life, and more accepting of it.

According to Jon Kabat-Zinn, Ph.D., director of the Stress Reduction Clinic at the University of Massachusetts Medical Center in Worcester, where he is an associate professor of medicine, patients who have participated in mindfulness training for eight weeks experience a sharp drop in their medical problems, as well as significantly less anxiety, depression, and hostility. They also feel more in control, are more self-confident, and can better view life's stressors as challenges rather than threats. He says the practice works because it reduces the suffering associated with problems such as chronic pain. Patients can learn to separate their physical discomforts from negative emotions and thoughts, and thereby feel more in control.

Biofeedback Techniques

Biofeedback is a training method that uses painless sensors or electrodes (which are like stickers placed on the skin) to monitor various functions electronically, such as breathing rate, temperature, muscle tension, blood pressure, brain activity, and pulse. In this way, physiological changes during training become observable and quantifiable. Through monitoring their bodily responses, patients can learn self-regulation techniques and relaxation, imagery, meditation, or any of the other techniques already mentioned. Patients can thus tangibly monitor their progress with this electronic feedback and hone their skills. Once patients learn how to master the relaxation skills effectively to reliably produce desirable physiological changes, the equipment is usually no longer needed, although portable biofeedback equipment is now available for home use.

Most pain clinics and hospitals have some biofeedback equipment; however, hospital-based sessions may be costly. For more information and referrals, see Appendix 1.

Hypnosis

In 1995 the National Institutes of Health endorsed hypnosis as an effective adjunct to help relieve the chronic pain associated with cancer after several studies have supported its effectiveness. By helping patients achieve a state of deep relaxation in a state of altered consciousness, the subconscious mind can override the conscious mind. While being hypnotized, patients can learn from the hypnotherapist how to retrain the brain to achieve more control over the body and mind to manipulate the perception of pain and reduce fear and anxiety. The panel pointed out that although medications to relieve the pain and suffering of irritable bowel syndrome, for example, help only about half of patients, hypnosis can help some 85 percent of those who try it.

In various studies, hypnosis also has been shown to be useful for some pain patients and can play a supplemental role in cancer patients. When researchers at Stanford University reviewed the studies on hypnotherapy, they reported that in some cases it could significantly reduce the pain of cancer.[8] Other studies have found that it could significantly reduce anticipatory nausea and vomiting[9] and help children, for example, cope with painful procedures associated with cancer treatment.[10]

When hynotherapy doesn't relieve pain directly, it can still benefit the cancer patient by reducing distress and tension and inducing relaxation, all of which may help relieve pain and boost one's sense of control. Similar to relaxation, deep breathing, and imagery techniques, hypnosis usually involves deep breathing to harness one's attention, closing the eyes or fixing the gaze, deep relaxation, and imagery to transform the pain sensations. A person in a hypnotic state, which is somewhat like the floating, drifting feeling we get just before we fall asleep, becomes very receptive to the directions of the therapist, which might be something along these lines: "You are feeling totally relaxed. You are more and more comfortable with each breath you take."

Any unpleasant experience—say, a boring meeting or a particularly painful episode—can often seem interminable. Hypnosis can help by changing our perceptions, especially of time. With hypnosis, the sense of the passage of time can be altered, much like the feeling of losing all sense of time when completely absorbed in an activity.

Of course, not everyone is responsive to hypnosis. Only about one-third of the general population can be induced into a deep hypnotic state; about 10 percent seem completely resistant, and the remainder fall somewhere in between. Nevertheless, that means that up to 90 percent of people may derive some benefit from it. Those who respond the most strongly may find relief in concentrating on changing the temperature associated with their pain, or even its sensation, or by using their harnessed concentration to focus on an area of the body that feels no pain.

SELF-HYPNOSIS

Some patients also respond well to self-hypnosis, or autosuggestion, a state that can be reached by the patient without the aid of a practitioner through meditation, breathing, imagery-based relaxation exercises, visualization exercises, or progressive muscle relaxation techniques. The physiological and psychological effect is very similar to the relaxation response, the main difference being that the patient deliberately incorporates a suggestion such as "When you complete this exercise you will feel rested and energetic." Like many of the approaches described here, self-hypnosis requires that the patient actively participate by learning new skills, but its practice can go a long way to increasing independence and restoring a sense of control and mastery.

Although very much like a relaxation or autogenic session, experts say that if deep relaxation can truly be attained through hypnosis, then trained patients may be able to achieve the same state at different times merely by counting backward from twenty, feeling themselves going deeper and deeper into a relaxed and restful state.

As with any alternative therapy, consumers need to beware of quacks and price tags. (For more information and referrals, ask your doctor or medical center; see Appendix 1 for specific information.)

Exercise for Self-Hypnosis

Get in a comfortable position, and close your eyes.

Let all the muscles in the body relax, one at a time if necessary. Each part of the body should feel limp, loose.

Start at your feet. They should feel heavy. Release all the tension in them.

Feel your legs; they should feel heavier and heavier. Let go of all the tension in them. Let go of everything; let yourself relax . . . completely.

Continue to move through the body, repeating these phrases for each part. Constantly repeating to yourself that you need to let go completely, to relax, to feel limp and loose. Every muscle is relaxed.

You feel sleepy and more relaxed. Go deeper, sleepier, more and more relaxed.

At the end of any session, open your eyes and sit up slowly.

Music Therapy

Music therapists, employed at some clinics, know how music can capture the patient's mind and mood like nothing else, and, when properly employed, may distract the patient from pain and distress. Music therapy involves using music of the patient's own choosing with the aim of improving psychological, mental, and physical health, and promoting improved well-being.

Over the past two decades, studies have revealed a link between music therapy and diminished pain reactions in patients after surgery, in patients attending cancer centers, and in those with chronic pain. Research demonstrates the effects of music on mood, which may in turn indirectly influence pain levels. A 1999 study funded by the National Institute of Nursing Research, for example, found that simple relaxation exercises or listening to soothing music can significantly reduce patients' pain after major surgery, supporting these techniques' roles as adjuvants to opioid therapy.[11] Other researchers have found a host of other benefits from soothing music, such as its influence on reducing blood pressure, heart rate, pain, and the amount of anesthesia needed for surgery and dental work.[12] Although studies on music's effect on cancer pain are very limited, music therapists are part of the pain teams in some of the leading cancer pain clinics in the country, including Memorial Sloan-Kettering Cancer Institute in Manhattan.

In choosing selections of music that will appeal to a patient, music therapists take into account a patient's mood—a depressed patient, for example, may respond well to music in minor keys, a lonely patient to a solo instrument or a song expressing the need for contact, an emotionally fragile patient to a soft and comforting piece. The music therapist next attempts to progress from a piece that matches the patient's mood to one that may transform it. Thus, a solo instrument for the lonely patient would change to a full orchestral piece. The music for the emotionally fragile patient might progress to something more upbeat and dramatic.

At Memorial Sloan-Kettering, patients report that after a music therapy session they generally feel less pain, experience better mood (with less anxiety, depression, or anger), and are more communicative—that is, they talk more freely and feel less lonely and isolated, while feeling more peaceful.[13]

Professional music therapists are not necessarily needed; family members can choose music, provide the patient with headphones, and may even arrange for live presentations. Shared music sessions may be helpful to family members, who can reminisce with the patient and communicate closeness, support, or whatever else is on their minds.

Acupuncture

Practiced for some five thousand years, this ancient Chinese treatment came to the attention of the West just decades ago. Today acupuncture is used around the world, with an estimated twelve million visits yearly to acupuncturists in the United States alone. In 1995, some ten thousand certified acupuncturists were practicing in the United States, one-third to one-half of whom are medical doctors. Supported by the World Health Organization, the U.S. Food and Drug Administration, the National Institutes of Health, and the American and British Medical Associations, acupuncture can help many function better and with less pain.[14] Acupuncture is now routinely used in many medical centers before, after, and in between chemotherapy sessions. A study at the University of California, Los Angeles, School of Medicine, for example, found acupuncture could significantly reduce the nausea and vomiting associated with chemotherapy.[15] Similarly, a recent study at Duke University Medical Center found acupuncture just as effective and sometimes even more effective than the leading medication used to reduce nausea and vomiting after major breast surgery; the same researchers also reported patients with acupuncture treatments experience much less pain after surgery.[16] And a study at the University of San Diego in California found that in cancer patients receiving acupuncture treatments, about 60 percent experienced at least a 30 percent improvement in their symptoms.[17]

Acupuncture bases its success on reestablishing a balance between the body's yin and yang, which, according to Eastern thought, are two opposing forces at work in the human body and the cosmos. They are like opposite sides of a coin, and together they make up the body's primal energy. Although scientists don't know exactly how acupuncture works, they think that acupuncture points, of which there are about five hundred, are related to nerve receptors that, when stimulated, somehow muffle pain, perhaps by triggering nerve cells to produce endorphins, the body's natural painkillers.

The acupuncturist inserts any number of hair-thin stainless-steel needles into selected groups of points on the body's meridians or energy pathways, the function and integrity of which are believed to be the key to good health. Some acupuncturists twirl the needles, stimulate them with mild electricity, or heat them to enhance the effectiveness of treatment.

While many studies have found acupuncture useful for nausea and pain, more studies are needed to determine its effectiveness for chronic cancer pain. When improvement does occur, it tends to be short-term, up to several days or weeks, with repeated treatments often needed.

In 1996 the NIH estimated that between 70 to 80 percent of U.S. insurers now cover some acupuncture treatments. To find an acupuncturist, first ask your doctor for a referral (see Appendix 1 for more details). The American Academy of Medical Acupuncture can recommend licensed medical doctors who have had acupuncture training As with any nontraditional form of health care, it is important to inform the primary physician of all treatments being pursued.

Using Therapies Involving the Skin

Families should not forget some of the simplest of pleasures—the bliss of a warm bath or the soothing relief of a firm but gentle massage on the back, arms, face, legs, or feet.

A bath can be revitalizing and may promote a sense of well-being. If getting out of bed is not too much effort, a warm (not hot) bath can be relaxing. It may be helpful to line the tub with towels so the patient can lean back and rest comfortably; others find a bath chair helpful. If the patient is particularly weak, a caregiver may want to wear a bathing suit and sit in the tub with the patient. Another helper might be needed to get the patient in and out of the tub safely.

Stimulating the skin directly can reduce pain by exciting nerve endings in the skin. Vibration, friction, or even applying a menthol cream is sometimes used to stimulate the skin and modulate the same nerve pathways that transmit pain. By rubbing a cream on the arm, for example, the barrage of stimuli transmitted along nerves that transmit nonpainful sensations may flood the spinal cord, thus blocking out some of the pain signals. The theory that explains why this works—the gate control theory of pain—speculates that the activation of one nerve pathway may close off others, thereby reducing pain. It is used to explain the pain relief associated with our usual first responses to smacking our thumb with a hammer—to suck on it or run it under water. Many forms of bodywork and massage, including Feldenkrais, therapeutic touch, Pilates, Rolfing, and deep tissue mobilization, reduce pain not only by relieving tension and increasing blood circulation but also perhaps by closing these "gates" at the spinal cord and other levels of the nervous system.

Menthol preparations include such creams as BenGay, Heet, Icy Hot, or Mineral Ice. Rubbing them on the skin can feel warm and soothing. But be sure to avoid sensitive areas, such as the mouth, eyes, and genitals, and avoid any areas of broken skin or rashes.

Similarly, using a vibrator or electrical stimulation (see the discussion of TENS in Chapter 9) near a painful area may ease the pain temporarily. For headache, for example, the scalp or neck may be vibrated gently. Other areas may also be particularly responsive and stimulation there can be very soothing, especially the lower back, the bottom of the feet, and the buttocks.

When considering a massage, avoid alcohol-based lotions that may dry the skin and, unless requested, deep muscle massage. Choose the scent of the lotion, cream, or oil with the patient or use an unscented variety, since patients can be hypersensitive to scent when they are ill. Sometimes slow circular motions feel best, while other people prefer light stroking or brushing. For the patient who can't be massaged or who doesn't want to be touched, try bathing just the feet. With a warm bowl of water near or under the foot, lift the leg and drip water from a saturated washcloth over the foot. Massage with cream afterward, if desired. Avoid massaging any areas that are being exposed to radiation unless authorized.

Similar to massage, acupressure involves applying variable pressure for a short time, from ten seconds up to a minute, to areas such as the heel of the hand, the ball or heel of the foot, fingers or fingertips, or around an arm or leg. Try pressing near and around a painful area, looking for particularly sensitive "trigger points" under the skin. Experiment, asking the patient what feels good and what doesn't.

Hot or cold compresses can be used to alter the pain threshold, relieve muscle spasms, and reduce congestion in a painful area. Cold can minimize the response of the tissues when injured, while heat may help flush out toxins and fluids that have accumulated. Patients are sometimes not sure which to use. Try both to see which is more successful. For warm compresses, use either warm, moist heating pads (only those that are specifically made to be wet), hot-water bottles, or even a washcloth dipped in hot water. For cold compresses, cold gel packs wrapped in a towel, ice bags wrapped in a towel, or wet washcloths from the freezer or refrigerator can be used. Be sure to always cover the skin with a towel or sheet to protect it from the source of heat or cold.

Experimenting with these simple activities can bring soothing relief and may enhance the patient's sense of well-being, as well as affirm a loved one's importance and compassion. Moreover, these activities can serve to help communicate love and acceptance between patient and caregiver.

A few precautions: Avoid areas that are being treated by radiation therapy or that are irritated already; check with a doctor or nurse if unsure. Do not use heat or cold on areas that have poor circulation or poor sensation. Keep treatments to five or ten minutes. Do not use heat on any new injuries, and if a cold compress causes pain or shivering, stop. Avoid sleeping with a heating pad on high settings to prevent burns, and do not apply heat or cold to transdermal drug delivery patches such as Duragesic or Transderm Scop.

Occupational Therapy

Although not a routine part of the cancer or pain team, consultation with an occupational therapist may be warranted to assess function status and to help the patient and family achieve practical goals. Occupational therapists can help patients assess what tasks they may need help with to enhance quality of life. They can use creative means to modify the environment, thus helping patients adapt to their illness. They may be knowledgeable about the cognitive-behavioral techniques described earlier in this chapter and about support groups that may be available to patients, which include meeting with people who are coping with similar disabilities.

Making the Patient Comfortable: Splints, Pillows, Cushions, Commodes, and Beds

If the patient is at home and having trouble getting around, simple measures may go a long way to conserving energy. These may be useful in the rehabilitation of someone recovering from cancer or surgery, as well as for patients whose reserves of energy and strength are reduced. Even though it may be difficult, the family should try to be attentive and accepting of changes in the patient's condition and needs, and realistic goals should be established. Although a large electric hospital-type bed may seem intrusive, it can be extremely helpful. Alternatively, it may be sufficient to add an extra pillow or a foam roll under the knees, one at the lower back, one under the head, or an extra "hug" pillow for the patient to manipulate.

Frequent trips to the bathroom may elicit pain and fatigue, in which case a bedside commode, rented, purchased, or provided by an insurer or home health service, can be surprisingly helpful. These simple portable toilet chairs allow the patient to relieve himself right next to the bed with very little fuss and are surprisingly well accepted. The idea that using a hospital bed or portable commode is symbolic of "giving in to the cancer" may need to be overcome, especially if the patient's best interests are served by its use. Remember, these items can always be returned when they are no longer needed. Often, especially in two-level homes, the patient is best served by converting a large downstairs room. By cutting down on isolation, this can be a positive move for the whole family.

Many types of splints or supports for joints and the spine are available that can help prevent movement-related pain. When walking is painful or difficult, the safety of a walker can increase self-confidence, and many find that leaning forward on them eases back pain. Pain from swelling (lymphedema) can be reduced by using wraps. Pressure stockings or sleeves can also improve function in this setting and after limb pain from a deep venous thrombosis (DVT or blood clot). Simply wrapping a painful joint in an empty plastic bag sealed to the skin with tape can elevate the temperature around the joint by trapping the body's own heat. If moving an arm, a leg, or even the back is very painful, talk to the doctor about whether splinting would reduce the pain. When joints or muscles are weak or paralyzed, a variety of splints are used to provide support and reduce pain. Pain in the spine is common in patients with prostate cancer, breast cancer, or a tumor that has spread to the spine and weakened the vertebrae. Doctors who specialize in bones and joints (orthopedists) may be consulted. If a commercial splint isn't available, you may be directed to the hospital's orthotics lab, which will fashion a custom device and provide adjustments and instructions.

If a patient's condition dictates that he spend most of his time in bed and he can't easily turn himself, bedsores may be prevented with an inflatable mattress pad or a pad made of convoluted foam (called an egg crate pad). These items are usually covered by insurance. During a hospitalization they are often charged to the bill and later disposed of, so ask if they can be taken home. Be sure that the patient turns frequently or is turned and that skin is not dragged across the mattress or rubbed against other skin surfaces; it can be helpful to lift the patient when he turns and to position a pillow between the patient's thighs, use towels between the trunk and arms, and spread the fingers apart. Keeping bedsheets and skin dry is another important step. Families can recognize red areas on the skin that indicate where bedsores may soon appear. These areas can be rubbed gently or massaged, and cushioned to reduce pressure on them. Special bandages (such as OpSite) are now available to protect vulnerable areas; they allow air in but still provide protection. Inquire about these and other products from a home health care nurse or a drugstore that specializes in home care products. (Treating bedsores is discussed more fully in Chapter 11.)

Prostheses (artificial body parts) can sometimes be used to ease the pain due to cancer, such as a well-fitted leg prosthesis to help control amputation pain.

Movement, Exercise, and Physical Therapy

If a patient is bedridden, ask a nurse about gentle exercises to prevent the development of stiffness in the joints. If it's not too painful, gently moving the arms and legs several times a day to the extreme in each direction helps maintain range of motion. It is often helpful to dispense an extra (bolus) dose of analgesic before such exercise, as well as before other strenuous activities such as going to the bathroom or bathing, to prevent pain that is triggered by movement.

If a physical therapist is available through the pain or home care team, consultation may be useful after surgery, or when a patient's activity and strength are compromised. Physical therapists can be helpful in suggesting a range of exercises to maintain flexibility, strength, and stamina. They are knowledgeable about whether to elevate an extremity; how to gently "milk" a swollen limb or apply a special type of pump called a compression pump for swollen limbs; how to massage; how to use breathing exercises, coughing, and posture techniques; and whether applying a splint, garment, or brace may help relieve pain.

Nutritional and Other Alternative Treatments

Herbs

Because the use of herbal and nutritional supplements is not formally supervised by the Food and Drug Administration (unless medicinal claims are stated), few studies have carefully evaluated their effectiveness and safety. Nevertheless, numerous anecdotal reports recommend various herbs, and scientific studies are on the rise. Despite confusing claims, herbal products can have not only favorable but also unfavorable effects (like thinning the blood) and can interact with standard medications, so be sure to tell your physician what the patient is taking and consult a competent, well-trained expert before use.

Among the most popular recommendations are:

- Yerba maté tea, available in tea bags, for nerve pain associated with chemotherapy.
- Valerian (*Valeriana officinalis*) to reduce pain and promote rest and sleep.
- Feverfew (*Tanacetum parthenium;* also called featherfew, bachelor's button, featherfoil, febrifuge plant, or midsummer daisy) to reduce inflammation and the pain of migraine headaches. Usual dose in capsule form is 100–200 mg a day, or use ½ to 1 teaspoon of the dried herb per cup of boiling water and steep for five to ten minutes; drink up to two cups a day.
- Turmeric (also called curcuma or Indian saffron) as an anti-inflammatory. May be taken either as a tablet (available from 400 to 1,200 mg daily) or as a tea, 1 teaspoon of turmeric powder per cup of warm milk; drink up to three cups a day.
- Ginger (also called Jamaican ginger, African ginger, or Cochin ginger) as an anti-inflammatory and to reduce nausea and vomiting. Use 1,500 mg daily in supplement form, or drink as a tea, using 2 teaspoons of powdered or grated ginger root per cup of boiling water and steeping for ten minutes. Sip all day. Beware that excessive amounts can cause heartburn.
- Emu oil, often combined with other substances for various aches and pains involving the body's soft tissues.
- Aloe vera for irritation of the skin (many skin creams have aloe vera).
- Boswellia (*Boswellia serrata*) for its anti-inflammatory properties.
- Calendula for skin inflammation.
- Cat's claw for joint pain.
- Eucalyptus for sore joints and muscles.
- Glucosamine sulfate and chondroitin sulfate for arthritic pain.

Aromatherapy

Aromatherapy, which uses scent as therapy, has been used for hundreds of years. Irritating or irrelevant to some patients, aromatherapy may be soothing to others. You can either add a few drops of scented oil to water and spray the mixture in the patient's room or dab a few drops of the scented oil on a cotton ball and place it in the patient's shirt pocket or next to his bed. The scents of lavender, juniper, and sandalwood may help to sedate an agitated patient; grapefruit, rose, or neroli may help depression; orange, jasmine, or frankincense may help to reduce anxiety; peppermint, rosemary, and lemon may stimulate a sedated patient.

In general, when interested in pursuing an alternative treatment, patients should gather all relevant viewpoints, pro and con, including costs and any potential risks. If after such investigations a patient is still interested, consult the primary physician to determine if there is any potential harm or if such a treatment could interfere with current medications and therapies.

As mentioned earlier, the therapies, techniques, and exercises discussed in this chapter don't cure pain. With relaxation and other mind-body techniques, however, we do know that the beneficial states achieved may have favorable effects that endure longer than the few moments it takes a trained patient to perform these exercises. They not only help reduce the patient's pain threshold and break the vicious cycle of anxiety and pain but, because the patient has taken an active role in the treatment that has helped him to cope, may promote an overall and enhanced sense of well-being by boosting self-esteem, a sense of control, and confidence.

13

Special Cases: Children, the Elderly,
and Patients with Special Needs

So far we've discussed techniques that are generally effective for controlling cancer pain. Yet certain groups of individuals have special needs—namely, the very young and very old, as well as those with a history of substance abuse.

Cancer in Children

When confronted with a diagnosis of cancer, most people grapple with the injustice of the situation. Childhood cancer is perhaps the most vivid proof that cancer strikes with neither rhyme nor reason—and that while it follows certain known rules, fairness is not one of them. It is sad whenever cancer is diagnosed, but it is especially tragic when this occurs in an innocent child.

Unfortunately, the younger the child, the more often his pain and suffering are overlooked or undermedicated. Only recently have doctors become convinced that youngsters experience pain as acutely as adults and need to be treated just as aggressively.

Most Common Types of Cancer Pain in Children

In general, adults tend to get solid tumors, and pain from solid tumors is usually due directly to the tumor growing into pain-sensitive tissues. Cancers in children, on the other hand, are more likely to be a leukemia (cancer of the blood cells) or lymphoma (cancer of the lymph cells). These types of tumors spread through the bloodstream first; if not stopped, they usually eventually invade the bone marrow, where blood cells are produced and stored. Only later, if at all, would the leukemic cancer cells spread to distant organs.

As a result, children experience pain from the extension of a tumor much less often. Most of their pain problems come from treatment, not from the tumor. Thus, children's most common problems with cancer are with infection, bleeding, and blood clots rather than pain. Pain, whether from the tumor or from treatment, should be treated aggressively.

PAIN FROM TREATMENTS

Children receive similar pain treatments as adults for problems such as mouth sores, bone pain, and nerve pain stemming from radiotherapy and chemotherapy. But unique to children—and by far the most common and challenging problem with children—is procedural pain.

It is easy to forget, even for doctors, that the small tribulations that arise during a hospital stay and which are usually relatively insignificant to an adult can be both painful and terrifying to a child inexperienced with hospitals, their routines, and an ever-changing staff. Depending on the type of cancer, various diagnostic tests may be required. Tests such as X-rays may be frightening but are rarely painful. However, children must often also undergo more painful tests, sometimes daily, because of the kinds of cancers that afflict them.

BLOOD TESTS, SPINAL TAPS, AND BONE MARROW BIOPSIES

Blood tests, spinal taps (also called lumbar punctures, which involve inserting a needle between two bones of the spine to remove spinal fluid), and bone marrow biopsies (obtaining material from within a bone through a needle) are common tests that children with cancer undergo in order to monitor the effectiveness of treatment, especially when the child has leukemia.

Blood tests, or venipuncture, may be simple procedures for an adult but not necessarily for a child. That's because youngsters have much smaller and more fragile veins than adults. They also tend to be fearful, may be less cooperative, and may require more attempts to obtain satisfactory test samples. Usually, as treatment continues, more and more venipunctures are needed, and the easily accessible veins can collapse. This may result in both more needle sticks as well as efforts to obtain blood from less conventional areas, such as the ankle, thigh, wrist, chest, or neck—sites that can generate both more pain and more fear. This is one of the most common reasons to surgically insert a more durable IV line or port, as well as a less invasive PIC line that can be inserted by specially trained nurses. These same problems may occur with lumbar punctures and bone marrow biopsies.

Communication Problems

Because pain is a personal experience that can't be measured or detected with a machine or test, doctors rely heavily on a patient's report of pain. While most adults can easily describe the nature of their pain, children generally communicate in very different ways.

NEWBORNS, INFANTS, AND TODDLERS

Newborns are completely unable to communicate feelings other than by crying, just as they do to convey hunger or a wet diaper. Up until a few decades ago, scientists assumed that newborns did not even feel pain, thinking that their nervous systems were insufficiently developed. As a result, many procedures, even surgery, were performed with little or no anesthesia. Now there is good evidence that newborns are sensitive to pain, and most doctors work to prevent and minimize pain in infants, though this has been slow to universally catch on. For any procedure in a baby—even a circumcision—it is reasonable to ask the doctor what will be done to prevent pain.

Although an infant may experience distress when separated from a parent, most infants can be comforted simply by being held, even by a stranger. Toddlers, on the other hand, are attached more specifically to their parents, making separation much more difficult. They also easily interpret an unfamiliar setting as threatening. As a result, unless special care is taken to reassure the toddler and even, when indicated, to treat him with a sedative or analgesic medication, he is likely to react intensely to events that, even if painless, are strange to him.

SCHOOL-AGE CHILDREN AND ADOLESCENTS

Obviously, as children mature they can better understand what's going on, can communicate, and can begin to learn coping skills. Yet even without pain, children may suffer intensely from the experience of being sick, from having their lives disrupted, and on encountering each new hospital routine, all of which are typically interpreted as shocking and terrifying invasions of their self. This is all the more difficult because it is at this stage of development that children begin to establish a sense of themselves that is independent of their parents but still fragile. Children need

---

Pain Behavior in Young Children

Infants
- Move less than normal
- Cry more
- Appear pale and sweaty
- Have loss of appetite
- Cry upon being touched, moved, or stimulated

Toddlers
- Cry more frequently
- Are cranky, less active
- Can point to the "boo-boo" or "owie" or "ouchie"

Young children
- Can point to the "owie"
- Can color on a body outline to show where the pain is
- Can use the McGrath face scale described in Chapter 3

---

constant understanding and support, and parents "rooming in" with their hospitalized child, which is increasingly accepted, can be extremely comforting, as can bringing in familiar toys and video games.

As children mature into adolescents, they can often communicate important information effectively, such as where and how much it hurts. When stressed by illness and separated from their families, however, adolescents may revert to their childhood ways and become harder to communicate with; as a result, their problems may become harder to manage.

Usually, though, when given love and support, adolescents can deal effectively with the stress of illness. Such support should come not only from family and friends but also from doctors and nurses. Newly independent, adolescents may pride themselves on their ability to handle things and at times may even discourage attention from their family, a phenomenon that may be hard for parents to understand.

Pain Strategies in Children

PAIN VERSUS DISTRESS

Children commonly react to many different kinds of unpleasant events similarly, making it hard to distinguish whether the resulting distress is due to actual pain or just fear. A child who has stepped on a nail looks very much like a child who has been told he is going to get a needle. Both need attention, but distinguishing between distress rooted in pain versus that rooted in anxiety will help determine the correct response.

Preventing Pain

In the last few years experts have begun to realize that even when children can't tell us, they may be hurting. More and more, the prevailing attitude is that it looks as if a child may be in pain, and even when parents and doctors aren't sure, the suspected pain should be treated as if it is present.

Because doctors can't easily differentiate between a young child's response of fear or anticipation and a response to physical trauma or pain, doctors increasingly favor treating children's distress preventively, rather than using a wait-and-see-if-it-hurts attitude. Once a child learns that something the doctor does hurts, chances are the procedure will continue to hurt. Once this pattern of memory and anticipation of pain is established, it is hard to break, in children as well as in adults. On the other hand, if a child can get through a procedure without too much discomfort, he or she will gain confidence, and repeat procedures are likely to go more smoothly.

Pain Assessment Tools for Children

The three basic methods to assess or measure pain are relying on the patient's report, observing the patient's behavior, and assessing pain based on physiological changes, such as changes in heart rate or blood pressure. Ongoing research is focusing on how these methods can be best used in young people.

Most doctors agree that when children are old enough to report on their pain, this is by far the preferable way to assess discomfort. The sophisticated questionnaires to assess pain in adults (discussed in Chapter 3) are obviously not very useful in young children. Instead, special pain assessment tools for children use colors, poker chips, a thermometer, or faces.

As mentioned in Chapter 3, "face scales" are often used with children as young as three. They point to a face that best corresponds to how they feel. With the poker chip method, youngsters are given chips that represent a "piece of hurt," and they are asked to show how many pieces of hurt they have at a given time. They may also point to where their hurt is on a pain thermometer, or show which colors best describe their hurt.

When children are too young to report pain, doctors must rely on the observations of parents and health care providers and physical changes. The physical changes are not always that useful—even though blood pressure and pulse usually change when pain is present, these changes are not very specific. Although the child's pulse rate may go up during pain, it may go up for many other reasons too. A pale complexion, perspiration, and dilated pupils also suggest pain, but they don't indicate pain severity. Also, although the observation method is useful, it depends a great deal on who's watching (parent, doctor, other person). Researchers interested in perfecting the science of observation are at work analyzing how the quality of an infant's cry, specific facial expressions, and movement change with pain.

TREATING CHRONIC AND ACUTE PAIN IN CHILDREN

Chronic pain can usually be controlled with oral pain medication, usually avoiding the need for additional sticks of the needle. The adult pain medications used are primarily the nonsteroidal anti-inflammatory drugs (NSAIDs) and oral morphine (or similar opioids), but in child-size doses calibrated to the child's weight. Aspirin is usually not given to children because of its risk of triggering Reye syndrome, a serious condition that occurs in children and may cause sudden and severe changes in mental status, such as agitation, seizures, and coma. Acetaminophen and other NSAIDs, such as ibuprofen, are therefore used instead. Of the NSAIDs, tolmetin and naproxen are the other ones that have been approved for children, and they are particularly useful for mild to moderate pain caused by inflammation or bone tumors.

As with adults, since children tend not to ask for pain medication until their pain is severe, pain medications should be given on a scheduled basis around the clock, not only as needed. Around-the-clock dosing prevents bad bouts of pain and provides better overall relief.

Whereas doctors used to think children metabolized opioids more slowly than adults—and therefore were given fewer doses—today doctors believe that children as young as one month of age process morphine and related drugs the same way that adults do. Newborns, on the other hand, are more sensitive to the respiratory depressant effects of opioids and should be monitored closely for apnea (cessation of breathing) if younger than three months, just to be on the safe side. For special kinds of pain, such as nerve pain, the adjuvant analgesics (antidepressants, anticonvulsants, and others—see Chapter 8) may also be useful, but again, in lower doses than those prescribed for adults.

When oral medications are ineffective or cannot be taken because of nausea, doctors have other options, and parents can help by making procedures as pleasant as possible, to minimize a child's fear and apprehension. Since children hate needles, injections should be avoided whenever possible. If older children seem embarrassed by using suppositories, other forms of medication can be prescribed. Subcutaneous infusions (by pump), for example, require a needle, but it needs to be changed only about once a week. If it appears that the child will need medication by injection over a long time, or if many blood tests are planned, it may be best to have an indwelling catheter or port placed surgically. This is a durable plastic IV line that is placed (under anesthesia) in a large vein, usually in the chest, but sometimes in the neck or thigh. While not specifically approved for children, a skin patch, which is changed every three days, is another good option when pain is ongoing and chronic. A lollipop form of the same strong painkiller (fentanyl), available as Actiq, is the best option for intermittent or breakthrough pain. Only rarely are nerve blocks or spinal morphine required in youngsters, but when they are, they have been used successfully even in babies.

Although the risk of addiction in children treated with opioids is *extremely* rare, many doctors continue to maintain erroneous concerns about prescribing them to young children. In most cases, such concerns should not inhibit the use of these very effective painkillers for moderate to severe pain.

Short-term pain from procedures can be controlled by a combination of reassurance, medications, and psychological approaches. As opposed to chronic pain, the problem here is more often fear and apprehension. A good treatment, therefore, is using a sedative (such as midazolam, a benzodiazepine), either with or without a painkiller, by mouth whenever possible. Youngsters will often then sleep lightly through the procedure and not even remember it later. If the child should get even more distressed after such premedication, it is probably an indication that the child prefers to know what is going on and feels as though he is losing too much control when sedated. If this is the case, the relaxation or cognitive techniques described in the next section, and in more detail in Chapter 12, can help relax and soothe the child.

PARENTS AS COACHES

As with adults, the many cognitive and behavioral strategies discussed in Chapter 12—such as hypnosis, visual imagery, and distraction, among others—can help reduce anxiety and pain in children. Some pediatric oncology centers focus on using parents as coaches to help youngsters master these techniques. The parent must be calm and relaxed, speak quietly and calmly, and know how to coach the child through a relaxation technique. According to pediatric psychologist Dan Armstrong at the University of Miami Medical School, parents should not necessarily try to reassure the child directly, since such behavior is actually linked to more distress in the child. Rather than telling the child what to do (such as "Hold out your arm") or trying to reassure him (such as telling the child "It's going to be okay" or "It'll be over in a minute"), parents are most helpful when they stick to providing facts (such as "The little sting you are going to feel will make your arm numb so you can't feel anything else") or use statements of reinforcement in a calm voice (such as "That was a very good job").

Parents need to be as fully involved in treatments as possible, so that the anxieties and fears they communicate to the child are minimized. Parents can be particularly helpful by using the behavioral and relaxation strategies described in Chapter 12, which can ease their own stress as well as their child's. Breathing techniques, for example, may be modified for children by encouraging them to think about their bodies as balloons or bike tires. The goal is to fill the balloon up with air and to gently empty it. Taking the image further, the parent may ask the child to pretend he is a hot-air balloon or is on a magic carpet. Once relaxed with the breathing exercise, the child can imagine he is floating high above the bed in the balloon or on the magic carpet visiting distant lands. Imagery or distraction techniques may be particularly useful during a painful procedure. Parents can use their imaginations and bring with them party blowers, bubbles, video games, or pop-up books to help a youngster imagine pleasanter thoughts than those that overwhelm him in his hospital bed. Helping the child pretend he is visiting Disneyland, is Superman or Wonder Woman soaring into space, or is a character the child knows from the movies or a favorite book can ease the pain and pass the time. Parents can help prompt the child to imagine he is somewhere else, doing other things, or can help the child spin a story in which a hero or heroine has the same fears as the child but triumphs over them.

Children are particularly responsive to hypnosis and self-hypnotic techniques because they are used to harness their imagination in pretend play. With a few practice sessions, children can quickly learn effective self-hypnotic techniques to induce a tranquil and distracted state.

As with adult patients, the more control a child can exert—such as influencing the timing of procedures, the order of procedures, and the placement of an injection—the greater to extent to which feelings of helplessness associated with a chronic disease can be relieved. Another tactic that some hospitals use to prevent anxiety in children when a nurse comes close is to require that nurses who take blood wear a red apron, so that the child need not become distressed when other nurses approach.

If anesthesia is required, talk to the anesthesiologist ahead of time about staying with the child until he is anesthetized. Talk with the child about all the interesting things going on around him; calmly explain to him what's going on, allowing him to play with devices as permissible, such as a face mask. By remaining calm, the child will feel secure and follow the parents' lead in viewing the experience as a challenge or adventure rather than a worrisome and fretful experience.

Cancer Pain in the Elderly

The management of cancer pain in the elderly follows the same basic principles that have been described for mature adults:

- The mainstay of treatment for moderate to severe pain is still potent opioids, such as morphine, administered around the clock, supplemented with rescue doses of short-acting opioids for breakthrough pain.
- Pain that is slight or moderate may be treated primarily with the weak opioids, such as hydrocodone.
- Depending on the type of pain, treatment may be supplemented with other drugs, such as the NSAIDs and adjuvant analgesics (antidepressants, steroids, etc.).
- Occasionally treatment with the adjuvant drugs alone is sufficient.
- Individualizing and readjusting therapy to take into account the unique needs of each patient are essential.

Elderly persons do, however, differ in several important ways from younger patients, and knowing these differences can help guide treatment. First of all, older people tend to minimize their pain and tend to fear "bothering" or "annoying" family members or doctors and nurses with their "complaints." They may not mention or show their pain and may have to be asked actively about it. Some older people may not be able to communicate their pain concerns because of speech, hearing, or cognitive deficits, and many older people have been taught to be stoic about their pain. Also, as people age, various organs and systems (kidneys, liver, brain, etc.) tend to function less efficiently, becoming impaired or more vulnerable to change. As a result, the elderly patient may have a lower tolerance to analgesic drugs, so lower doses of medication can often be prescribed. Some doctors also recommend the use of short-acting painkillers rather than the use of long-acting ones, such as methadone (Dolophine) or levorphanol (Levo-Dromoran). Moreover, starting doses may not need to be increased as rapidly as in younger patients. To avoid serious side effects, the doctor usually starts medications at lower doses, being prepared to quickly raise or lower the dose depending on the patient's response.

Just as elderly patients may be more susceptible to the analgesic effects of painkillers, they may also be more susceptible to their side effects, especially constipation and sedation. The principles for managing side effects in elderly patients are the same as those for mature adults, and can be summarized as follows:

- Begin treatment with low doses to prevent side effects; if pain persists and there are no serious side effects, raise the dose quickly.

- As soon as an opioid is used, a laxative should be administered regularly to prevent constipation.
- Be prepared for mild grogginess, sedation, or catch-up sleep soon after treatment with an opioid is started, but don't be too concerned—these effects usually disappear after a few days. At the first sign of nausea or vomiting, ask the doctor to prescribe an antiemetic (an antinausea drug). Nausea tends to resolves itself quickly, so treatment can usually be withdrawn after a few days.
- If grogginess persists, the doctor may want to consider treatment with a psychostimulant, such as modafinil (Provigil), methylphenidate (Ritalin), or dextroamphetamine (Dexedrine).
- Keep records of the schedule and intensity of pain and the presence and severity of any side effects. Maintain regular contact with the physician so that medications can be adjusted upward or downward as needed.

Cancer Pain in Those with Histories of Substance Abuse

Patients who are either active or recovered substance abusers (alcohol or drugs) need special attention. It is essential that the doctor be informed, honestly and thoroughly, of any history with drugs or alcohol. If he is not, it could mean potential agony for a patient who is an active abuser of alcohol, narcotics, benzodiazepines (such as Valium), or other street drugs. That's because these patients often have higher levels of tolerance—that is, they may need higher doses of painkillers at the outset to quell their discomfort. If a doctor is unaware of a substance abuse problem, he is likely to unknowingly underprescribe appropriate medications. These patients also may have more problems getting their pain under control than other patients because they or their physicians may be concerned about worsening an addiction or rekindling an old one. On the other hand, these patients will be at higher risk for being undertreated because doctors may be reluctant to prescribe potentially addictive medications such as opioids. As we have emphasized throughout this book, the risk of addiction from cancer pain treatment in the general population (those without any history of abuse) is extremely low. When a patient has a history of abuse, however, that risk is substantially higher. This is not to say that the pain shouldn't be treated or that strong medications should not be prescribed; it just means that these risks need to be considered in making a treatment plan, which will usually include more rigorous education, monitoring, and involvement of family members.

Discuss with the physician any fears about whether the pain will be treated effectively and whether readdiction might occur. The risk of readdiction should be discussed frankly and balanced against the risks of undertreated pain. With certain precautions, the risks of rekindling a drug habit can be minimized. The physician may try to treat the pain with non-habit-forming medications (such as nonsteroidal anti-inflammatories, antidepressants, and anticonvulsants) for as long as possible. Many of the pain syndromes associated with HIV, for example, are due to nerve injury and will not require treatment with opioids. Maintain open and regular communication with the doctor, informing him if medications are not effective enough and stronger pain medications are needed.

Expect that the doctor may want to establish some ground rules—to protect both himself and the patient. Most doctors will insist that pain medications be taken exactly as ordered. Some may suggest that a pain medication diary be maintained to reflect the patient's responsible use of the drugs. The doctor will become uncomfortable and may lose some trust in the patient if given excuses that appear concocted, such as that the prescription was lost or that the medication was accidentally damaged or flushed down the toilet. If the medication is used as directed, there should be no need to ask for early refills or to call the doctor on nights or weekends for medication. Maintaining a trusting relationship with the doctor is essential, and the patient needs to continue being honest with himself and the doctor.

If stronger medications are needed, the doctor will probably want to prescribe long-acting ones (such as MS Contin or Oramorph), transdermal fentanyl (the skin patch Duragesic), or methadone, administered around the clock) rather than as needed (see Chapter 7), since these medications relieve pain most consistently and are less likely to produce a euphoric feeling or high. If the pain is treated with an inappropriately weak analgesic (such as codeine or propoxyphene [Darvon]) or with a stronger painkiller prescribed in too low a dose or on an inappropriately infrequent schedule, the patient may develop what is called pseudoaddiction. That is, the patient may ask for more medication in a manner that appears to resemble the drug-seeking behavior of an addict, because the pain is inadequately relieved due to undertreatment, not necessarily because of a drug craving per se. Around-the-clock dosing is important for pain control and avoids alternating peaks and troughs in the concentration of medication in the blood; such peaks are much more likely to be associated with a sensation of being high and may promote more erratic use of the medication. *It is important, therefore, that medications be prescribed as they are for cancer patients in general—with adequate doses, around the clock.* If the doctor is concerned about whether the medications are being used properly, you may mutually decide to obtain prescriptions for opioids in small quantities—say, on a weekly basis.

Another problem that may occur with patients who are recovered addicts is a reluctance to take the medications as prescribed. Patients may also be pressured by families or peers, especially if in a twelve-step program such as Alcoholics Anonymous or Narcotics Anonymous, to back off the needed painkillers. The patient or family may need to reassure the group that it is appropriate to take such medication for medical reasons.

Patients and families need be aware that physical dependence and tolerance will probably occur, as they would with patients with no history of substance abuse. As discussed earlier in the book, these reactions to opioids are not the same as addiction. (See Chapters 1 and 7 for fuller discussions of these topics.)

Should an active or recovered substance abuser use one of the increasingly popular patient-controlled pumps (see Chapter 7), in which the patient pushes a button for an extra dose of painkiller as needed (within certain limits set by the doctor on the computerized pump)? In fact, the risk of a recovered addict abusing such a medication pump is lower than doctors had previously thought. Again, the risk of addiction needs to be balanced against the need to treat the cancer pain. If the patient is expected to have a temporary pain problem, as opposed to a patient with advanced cancer, the risks and balances will obviously shift.

If a substance abuser is involved with Alcoholics Anonymous or another support group or with counseling, it is important to maintain these supports and to share freely with peers any problems or experiences the patient is encountering with his use of habit-forming medications. Sharing freely with others who can empathize and provide support may go a long way in helping the patient resist abusive behavior.

14

Dealing with Feelings

Finding out you or a loved one has cancer is a shock and usually signals a major crisis. For most people, the biggest terror is that the diagnosis is a death sentence, which of course it is not. But it is a vivid reminder of our mortality and is a very real threat to our security and all we take for granted.

Understandably, a diagnosis of cancer will throw most people into a psychological tailspin as they begin the process of coping with the news. Most of us regard ourselves as fit, healthy, and whole persons with a past and a future. Even if we have had some chronic illness, once we adjust to it we still tend to maintain a healthy self-image. Unexpected news of cancer causes doubt and uncertainty and suddenly threatens all of the things we relied on as being dependable and certain.

This aspect of threat is all-pervasive—the reliable and predictable things of everyday life are suddenly subject to change. The potential threats are many:

- To the image of ourselves as being healthy
- To our professional life and goals
- To our role in the family and household
- To our financial security
- To our dreams, hopes, and aspirations

In short, every aspect of our well-being is suddenly called into question. Concerns can arise almost automatically and cloud everything we think and do. We become victims of a roller coaster of reactions, including disbelief, shock, fear, anxiety, panic, sadness, depression, feelings of helplessness, despondence, and anger. And even once we feel we've gotten a handle on our current feelings, new ones flood in.

However painful, these reactions are common and normal. In fact, there's more cause for alarm when a person diagnosed with cancer doesn't express such feelings. Keeping strong negative emotions bottled up or denying the illness to oneself and to others can be psychologically and physically harmful. Mates need to catch themselves when they feel the need to overprotect their loved ones and are fearful of bringing up the cancer. Talking about feelings and fears is healthy and to some extent necessary, and family members may need to encourage each other to keep talking.

About half of people diagnosed with cancer adjust normally to the news, although obviously, no two persons' adjustment will be the same. Many experience sudden changes in eating or sleeping patterns or in how they relate to other people, including their loved ones. This is called an adjustment disorder and is viewed as a reasonable, normal reaction to a crisis, especially to a potentially life-threatening one like cancer. Adjustment disorders can have features of depression or anxiety but are usually short-lived. By and large, with time and support, most people manage to mobilize their psychological resources and support networks and adapt relatively well.

But when these changes persist for more than several weeks, they may be a warning sign that major problems are brewing. If ignored, they could seriously impair a person's functioning and well-being and could even interfere with medical treatment. Counseling, specifically short-term supportive psychotherapy, often works quickly—in as little as four to ten sessions. By helping the patient express his bottled-up feelings and fears, sort out the rational fears from the irrational, and learn how to cope with the rational ones, many of the psychological symptoms mentioned above will often subside.

Almost all people diagnosed with cancer will be fearful and anxious as they cope with the news of their diagnosis, tests, treatments, and symptoms of cancer. How distressing those emotions are for a particular person depends a great deal on specific personality traits and the coping strategies that have been learned over a lifetime, as well as the support that is available from family, friends, and the medical team.

A new science called psycho-oncology, the study of the psychological and psychiatric aspects of cancer, identifies what kinds of psychological issues are associated with cancer and the means to help by enhancing the person's supports and coping skills. This chapter will discuss how family members can be supportive and help the patient (and each other) distinguish between realistic and irrational fears, and how to cope with crisis while minimizing distress. These issues are discussed in a book about cancer pain because emotional distress can lead to anxiety and depression, which often increases physical tension and therefore the intensity of pain. Likewise, pain is much more difficult to manage when people are depressed or anxious, conditions that also affect pain threshold. Moreover, pain itself can cause psychological changes that may seriously impair physical, psychological, and spiritual well-being, or may make problems seem worse.

Psychological Responses to Cancer

As we've said, about half of cancer patients adjust normally to being ill with cancer, leaving about half whose psychological problems may become debilitating. Of those, about two-thirds suffer from reactive anxiety and depression—that is, new anxiety and depression that are a direct response to the illness. However, when in pain, patients are about twice as likely to develop anxiety and depression than those whose pain is well controlled.[1]

Undergoing chemotherapy may be a particularly emotional time—often more so than during radiation treatments or surgery, because of concerns about unpleasant side effects that may or may not occur. Often the first chemotherapy treatments and those with very high chances of success are first associated with upbeat and hopeful feelings. If the cancer advances, the frequency of psychiatric problems among cancer patients increases, as might be expected.

Symptoms of Depression	Symptoms of Anxiety	Symptoms of Panic
Insomnia	Restlessness	Chest pains
Loss of appetite	Jitteriness	Feelings of choking
Irritability	Aggitation	Feelings of dizziness
Isolation	Sweating	Feelings of unreality
Fatigue	Upset stomach	Hot or cold flashes
Loss of interest or pleasure in	Palpitations	Trembling
everyday things	Worry	Faintness
Sadness	Fear	Fear of "losing it"
Much less energy than usual	Irritability	
No interest in eating	Difficulty concentrating	
Difficulty concentrating,	Being easily startled	
remembering, or making decisions	Clammy hands	
Constant feelings of guilt,	Insomnia	
worthlessness, or helplessness		
Crying a lot		
Thoughts about death or suicide		

It is, of course, always difficult to know whether some of these symptoms (poor appetite and sleep, etc.) are due to depression, medication, cancer treatment, or direct effects of the tumor. Regardless of the cause, the effort to clear up these symptoms is well worth it, to enable the patient to be as strong as possible during tough times. You may be surprised at how much a consultation with the doctor, psychiatric or oncology nurse, or social worker can help.

The Typical Distress of Cancer Patients

As patients try to cope with their illness and its repercussions, they may experience a merry-go-round of changes. We will first discuss the most common ones, and later suggest how family members and other primary caregivers can help.

Anxiety

From the moment a lump is spotted, a mysterious and insistent pain nags, or sudden weight loss is noticed, almost everyone experiences some anxiety. First, an unspoken fear nags that it could be cancer. If a doctor confirms it, new fears arise—concerns about treatment, pain, disfigurement, and even death. The anxiety can mushroom into panic or chronic anxiety that can threaten the patient's ability to cope and comply with treatment recommendations.

Denial

Some people choose to ignore distressing signs, denying to themselves and those around them that something might be wrong. Although denial can sometimes be a useful coping mechanism, if it is severe or persists, problems can fester until a crisis develops later on.

Fear

Fear is pervasive in these circumstances: fear of the unknown, of pain, of mental and physical loss, of rejection by the family, of lingering illness, and of death. Every time a new pain or symptom surfaces, a fresh wave of fear may surge. This is to be expected and is best expressed so that it does not get out of control. Being afraid is bad enough—but handling it alone (perhaps to avoid "burdening" loved ones) makes it especially hard.

Isolation and Detachment

Some people react to cancer by detaching themselves from decisions about their medical treatment, discussions about their illness, and, in the advanced stages of cancer, thoughts of death and dying. This detachment is another form of denial and serves as a buffer for the patient and to protect family members. Like the other negative emotions discussed here, this is normal up to a point. This form of denial may be just another step in coming to terms with a very unpleasant situation, but if it persists, professional counseling can help.

Guilt

Sometimes patients blame themselves for having caused the cancer in the first place or believe that they are sick or in pain as punishment for something they've done. Smokers, for example, may feel shame and guilt for smoking despite warnings of increased cancer risks. Whether justified or not, this self-punishment does no one any good. Commonly, such guilt can lead to a major depressive disorder.

Worry

In addition to pain and other physical problems linked to cancer (such as nausea or vomiting, difficulty in breathing, or weakness), patients worry about losing control over their daily lives, losing their independence and personal freedom, and having to become more dependent on others. They also worry about whether they can continue working or not, finances, and being a burden to their family. All these factors contribute to the patient's overall suffering. These are legitimate concerns that need to be dealt with in a productive way, but worry doesn't help. Instead, constant fretting needs to be talked about with a loved one or mental health professional.

Loss

Cancer patients suffer many losses on different levels, and each one needs to be dealt with directly and, when appropriate, grieved for separately.

Use the Timeless Wisdom

Focus on taking one day at a time . . .
May you have the serenity to accept the things you cannot change
the courage to change the things you can,
and the wisdom to know the difference.

Esteem by others, self-control, future dreams, body image, sexuality, and reproductive abilities are just a few of the highly important attributes upon which we base our well-being, self-esteem, and quality of life, and cancer threatens many of these. Again, such concerns are best faced up front and discussed with a supportive person.

Withdrawal

Disfiguring surgery or side effects from treatment (such as hair loss) may trigger despair and depression, causing the patient to withdraw from seeing or even speaking to friends and acquaintances. Those who lose a breast or have had a colostomy, for example, may feel physically mutilated or unattractive and may withdraw from partners and friends.

Self-Pity

Patients who are terminally ill and debilitated may pity themselves, and although a certain amount of grumbling and anger may be therapeutic, it can be destructive if sustained. The patient may feel justified in being demanding, in complaining, and in being short-tempered. These behaviors, however, can end up being manipulative and exploitive, turning the patient's powerlessness into a negative form of power. As a result, caregivers and family members may start resenting the patient (and feel guilty as a result). Then the patient can accuse them of not caring or of abandoning him. This negative cycle breeds emotional distance.

Defiance

An opposite tack to self-pity is the decision to fight the disease and its pain at all costs. By fighting the pain without seeking medical help in controlling it, patients only end up hurting themselves more. By waiting and holding out, they usually end up requiring more medication to relieve the intensified pain when much smaller amounts could have been used to prevent the pain from turning severe. The defiant, fighting spirit, however, if channeled properly, can be a very positive and powerful response. Remember, every good fighter needs a coach.

Information-Seeking and Bargaining Behaviors

Some patients act exactly the opposite of those who deny or avoid; they try to read everything they can about their condition and may panic when the slightest little thing goes wrong or doesn't fit their mental pictures. These patients need to be active members of the medical team so that they can feel they have some input and control in the decision-making process.

Irritability and Anger

Patients fighting cancer may become surprisingly irritable when things don't go as predicted. They may easily come to believe that if something can go wrong, it will happen to them. They may feel they don't deserve their plight, believe that life isn't fair, and feel angry with God, who seems to have deserted them; this often occurs just at a time when faith can be a powerful ally. Many patients seek a sense of meaning for their suffering where none exists, and any expectation of equity and fairness in life is easily shattered. Cancer has no favorites. Typically, cancer patients may lash out at family members and loved ones, the most convenient and forgiving targets and the ones with whom they feel the safest. Though stressful for everyone, fits of anger, even screaming, crying, throwing dishes, or whatever it takes (without becoming a threat or danger) to get the anger out can be therapeutic. After acknowledging anger, patients can more easily harness that energy to fight the cancer.

Resignation

Some patients reject offers of help, choosing instead to suffer in silence and to be just left alone. It is sometimes hard to distinguish between a defeatist attitude and an approach that is realistic, especially since feelings change from day to day. Although it is hard to listen to expressions of negative or pessimistic thoughts—especially when trying to keep one's own attitude positive—they must be talked out and dealt with. Maintaining a positive attitude can help immeasurably during a crisis. With these and other changes, loved ones must be attentive to whether pessimism is a passing phase or a serious problem that needs professional attention. No matter how bleak the situation may appear, there are always things to be hopeful about.

Hopelessness and Helplessness

Since many patients feel that they have little or no control over the outcome of their illness, they feel helpless. When medical help seems inadequate, feelings of helplessness can evolve into feelings of hopelessness. Both of these feelings can contribute to depression and may make other mental and physical illnesses seem worse.

Hopefulness, as long as it is realistic, can be a very positive response that needs to be encouraged. To counteract feelings of hopelessness, patients need to set realistic goals and feel that their lives have meaning and value. Families can reassure their loved ones that time together is valuable. If cancer has rendered the future uncertain, the patient needs to be encouraged to take one day at a time and to work toward having a good morning, a good night's sleep, or a pain-free day. The more control the patient can have over his life—such as the timing of treatments, baths, or other activities, or being asked about everyday decisions (what to eat, whom to call, where to go, etc.), the less negative and hopeless he may feel. Priorities and goals need to be continually reframed and addressed, especially if the disease is advancing.

Cancer as a Post-Traumatic Stress Disorder

When people believe the diagnosis of cancer is a life-threatening event, they may be thrown into a series of psychological changes that are similar to those triggered by combat, rape, physical, sexual abuse, or other traumatic events that are outside the range of everyday experience. These psychological changes are collectively called post-traumatic stress disorder (PTSD), and in the cancer patient may include attempts to avoid all thoughts or feelings associated with the illness; forgetfulness about what the doctor has said; a sudden loss of interest in things that used to be meaningful, such as young children or a job one loved; feeling and acting estranged from others; inability to have or express loving feelings; and a sense of a suddenly foreshortened future.

The person also may have trouble falling asleep or staying asleep, find it difficult to concentrate, be irritable or quick to burst out in anger, have an exaggerated startle response, or suddenly break out in a sweat or hyperventilate if exposed to something that reminds him of his own trauma (in this case discovering and being told about the illness). These changes don't indicate that a person has suddenly "gone crazy." Instead, he is responding to a deeply disturbing and frightening event in his life.

How to Help

As a rule, cancer patients are at their most vulnerable. Some of their important needs are relatively simple; having such needs fulfilled can make them feel immeasurably safer and therefore more physically comfortable. Most can benefit by being well informed about the nature of the cancer and its treatment and by being reassured that physical complaints will always be aggressively treated. Family members can help by reassuring them about what the doctor really said and helping the patient see when he may be worrying about something excessively or focusing on something that is beyond his control.

In most cases, though, family members themselves are also under enormous stress, often feel physically and emotionally drained, and need help and support themselves. Naturally, loved ones try to always put the needs of the patient first. A son or daughter, for example, may see the illness as an opportunity to return the love and support experienced as a child. There are always limits, though, and relatives sometimes need to be reminded to take care of their own needs.

If the family members' basic needs are ignored, they may get too burned out to really be there when they're needed. Families should be sure that they have at least one member of the doctor's team or the home health care program (a nurse, pharmacist, social worker, or other mental health professional) in whom they feel comfortable confiding. They may want to take advantage of this person's availability, experience, support, and empathy to talk over their own concerns and emotions.

Psychological Needs of Cancer Patients

Family members and caregivers can significantly help satisfy the basic psychological needs of patients. Typically, cancer patients need to feel safe, needed, loved, understood, and accepted. Their self-esteem needs to be maintained, and they must feel as though they can trust others.

Feeling Safe

Feeling secure where they are and confident in the hands of caregivers is important and must be established as a foundation for working out other problems associated with the disease.

Feeling Needed

Many patients, as they become weaker, may feel like they are a burden. They will need reassurance that they are still needed and loved. In fact, the unexpected need to provide a patient's care usually is burdensome, in which case the patient needs to be reassured that it is a responsibility that the family is privileged to take on. The needs associated with the illness can be framed as an opportunity for family members to "give something back," which, given how helpless family members typically feel, is usually regarded as an honor that is satisfying to undertake.

Feeling Loved

All people benefit from expressions of love and affection; touching the patient, holding his hand, and massaging him are all important. Behaving warmly and touching are common ways for love to be communicated.

Feeling Understood

Family members and other loving caregivers can't make the illness go away, but they can express empathy for the patient's distress. Patients need their family to acknowledge the severity of their illness, but at the same time they may need to be reminded not to worry too much and that they should take one day at a time.

The patients may benefit from having his symptoms explained—why they're occurring, what can be done about them—as well as from information about the process and nature of the disease. Caregivers should try not to deny or minimize the patient's feelings, especially if the patient is gravely ill. Rather than saying something like "Don't be ridiculous, you're going to beat this and be fine" if it's obvious the patient is terminal, it would be more helpful to say something like "I know you're very sick, and you might die. Are you feeling scared? How can I help?" Acknowledge the patient's feelings and try to get him to talk about them. Don't push—keep communication lines open and be available to listen and offer input when asked.

Feeling Accepted

Patients must feel secure and accepted, regardless of their condition, appearance, mood, and demands. They need to be reminded that just because they may look dramatically different, they are no less the person whom family members have spent a lifetime loving. Their essence and self are just as unique, vital, and important to others as ever.

Maintaining Self-Esteem

Many cancer patients not only are devastated by their disease but, due to the various reasons described above, internalize their distress. They may be haunted by thoughts that they are somehow responsible for their illness, viewing it as a punishment for something they've done or not done—if only they had been a better person, hadn't been unfaithful, hadn't had that abortion, or whatever, they might not have gotten sick. They may need to be reminded and reassured that cancer can strike anyone . . . and does.

To maintain self-esteem, involve patients as much as possible in the decisions that must be made. Allow them to give advice or instructions and make decisions; by doing so, they are more likely to be accepting of what follows.

Trusting Others

Patients need to know that they are receiving the best care possible—that their doctors and family will aggressively pursue treatment and pain management to ensure the best possible outcome.

Helping the Patient Cope

Coping involves efforts to reduce stress in the face of adversity. Some coping mechanisms, such as prayer or seeking knowledge, are healthy. Alternatively, patients may erect psychological walls, or defense mechanisms, to avoid or deny the seriousness of their situation. Although less healthy, these responses can still help patients get through the difficult process of gradually accepting their illness; as a result, such responses are mainly a concern if they persist.

Patients with a tendency toward hypervigilance and who characteristically accumulate as much information as possible usually feel more in control if assured that they will be involved in all decision making. Finding or even starting a support group with other cancer patients, especially those close in age and of the same sex, can serve to alleviate many fears, help patients share their fears and problems, and reduce isolation (see the next section). Teens with any kind of cancer and women with breast cancer, for example, need to talk with others in their circumstance.

Families should try to be as open as possible about the cancer and the threat it implies. Try not to keep secrets from either the patient or close family and friends, and be as honest as possible with young children about relatives with cancer. Although we tend to avoid negative emotions such as anger, anxiety, and sorrow, expressing them openly helps the family feel closer and more bonded during this difficult time. Children need not be excluded from this emotional upheaval—they can understand more than many people give them credit for.

Children who receive a diagnosis of cancer can understand that they have a sickness, and they can also acknowledge that if they listen to the doctor, he can help. While we all need to vent our anger in such trying times, adolescents in particular need opportunities to express their feelings. In addition to cancer being a threat to health and welfare, cancer in teenagers may also be viewed as a threat to their emerging independence and desire to emotionally separate from authority figures. Cancer makes them dependent again. If possible, they need to feel independent and in control. Middle-aged patients, on the other hand, characteristically need support and help in coping with the needs of other family members. Middle-aged patients often feel sandwiched—responsible for caring not only for their children but for their elderly parents as well. They worry about how those dependent on them will cope while they are ill. Friends and family members can help out by providing practical assistance with the children or elderly parents. Friends and family can also help by offering emotional support, reminding patients of their strengths, and encouraging and guiding them to use coping strategies that have worked in the past. They can encourage patients to use relaxation techniques, help them observe thought processes and change them if they are self-defeating, offer help in practicing self-hypnotic pain control strategies, set realistic goals, work on asserting themselves, and improve communication skills. These skills are described in more detail in Chapter 12.

Again, while we tend to focus on the patient in these discussions, it is important for caregivers to care for themselves and their own needs. Relatives and friends will certainly want to know details and will offer help. Don't feel compelled to go into the details with everyone. Find ways of avoiding the need to tell everyone everything; it may be a good idea to appoint a friend or relative to tell a circle of common friends about the status of the patient. Be specific in communicating with others about how they can help. It is acceptable to tell acquaintances or even close friends who want to visit that the patient is not feeling up to having visitors that day. Thank them, and remember that this is a time when the needs of the patient and caregivers must come first. In general, consider a balanced approach that involves allowing loved ones access to the patient, but for short visits only.

Although caring for an ill member of the family takes a lot of time and effort, it's important that the family continue with their individual lives as much as possible. Not only is it important for the caregivers, but the patient will feel like less of a burden if everyone can maintain their normal routine.

The Power of Support

Research indicates that the impact of social support is among the most important factors linked to a cancer survivor's quality of life in that it can help change the patient's outlook. Support can come from spouses, family members, friends, individual therapy, or support groups.

Though not everyone will benefit, many cancer patients derive an enormous sense of relief and comfort when they join a group of other cancer patients (see discussion in Chapter 12). Meeting regularly with other people who have similar problems can dramatically reduce one's sense of isolation, loneliness, and fear. Such group settings allow patients to share their experiences and feelings, and hear those of others; they can empower patients by providing additional emotional support, companionship, and information as well as a sense of connection and perhaps meaning. Many patients also find that support groups help them find the strength to regain their fighting spirit.

Many hospitals, physicians, and local branches of the American Cancer Society can offer referrals to local support groups.

When Depression Persists or Is Severe

When a patient becomes so anxious or depressed that negative moods are constant, or if excessive feelings of guilt, sadness, anxiety, worthlessness, helplessness, and hopelessness override all else and don't pass with time, then a major psychiatric illness is brewing. Professional help may be appropriate to try to cut short the spiral of negative emotions that can severely compromise the patient's quality of life and may even lead to thoughts of suicide. The power of depression over suicidal thoughts is so strong that people who are depressed are much more likely to feel suicidal than even patients in pain.

Although severe pain or other symptoms can trigger depression and thoughts of suicide, the opposite should never be assumed. That is, pain should never be viewed solely as a result of a patient's psychological state. Although there is no such thing as a "pain detector"—no blood tests or X-rays that disclose how much pain a patient experiences—a patient's own report should be the last word. Many studies show that self-reports are more reliable than the observations of nurses, physicians, and family members. As a rule, then, it should be assumed that a patient's pain is just as he says it is, even if he is depressed.

When pain and depression do occur together, they both need to be carefully assessed and treated. In most cases, relieving the pain will relieve the majority of psychiatric symptoms.

Interestingly, depression is not an inevitable aspect of cancer, as many people believe. According to the National Cancer Institute, many cancer patients experience some sadness and grief, but only 15 to 25 percent suffer from clinical depression.[2] The distress is largely related to pain, disfigurement, dependence, and financial concerns. It is more common among patients with pain, advanced cancer, physical disability, or a history of depression or major psychiatric illnesses.

However, cancer specialists rarely refer patients for mental health evaluation. It's up the family to do so. *Consult a professional if depressive symptoms (see above) last more than two weeks.*

Depression and Cancer

Depression can compromise health, not only by affecting sleep, appetite, and mood but by inducing biochemical changes in the body that researchers suspect may compromise the immune system and may even stimulate tumor growth. Some studies have suggested that cancer patients with symptoms of depression, such as feelings of helplessness and hopelessness, recover more slowly and don't live as long as those with a positive outlook. Researchers have found that breast cancer patients who felt helpless and hopeless, or who just accepted their disease with stoicism, were more likely to die within ten years than women who displayed a fighting attitude. Similarly, other women with breast cancer who looked at the brighter side and who didn't attribute their discomfort to progressive disease not only were less psychologically stressed but exhibited lower levels of anxiety and depression and also were less likely to report pain. In fact, how the women viewed the meaning of the pain—whether it meant the disease had advanced or not—was a much better predictor of how intense the pain was than where the tumors were located. And although it's difficult to extrapolate from animal studies, research in which rats and other animals learn that they are helpless to escape shocks or other negative experiences (feelings of helplessness are a symptom of depression) demonstrated depressed immune function and faster growth of cancer. Indeed, many studies have shown that stress not only can make pain worse but can trigger changes in the levels of a host of hormones that may suppress the immune system, and that feelings of helplessness and powerlessness increase the deleterious effects of stress.

Cancer is often associated with depression and anxiety. Women with breast cancer who have had mastectomies, for example, have a 50-percent chance of developing depression, anxiety, and sexual problems. When they also receive chemotherapy, their rate of depression and other psychiatric problems may soar to 80 percent. Knowing this in advance should spur patients and their families to take a proactive approach and to look for help early. Like pain, depression is not good for a healthy recovery.

With psychiatric illnesses in particular, the role of the family is extremely important. One of the insidious features of depression and other psychiatric disorders is that the person who is suffering may not recognize the signs and, because he is feeling low, may not be motivated to seek help. Families need to play a vital role here (see next section).

With counseling and support, however, cancer patients can be greatly helped in changing their outlook, which not only vastly improves their quality of life but also can have a dramatic effect on their illness. Thus treating depression is a vital part of any comprehensive treatment for cancer pain.

Depression and Pain

People in pain and in the advanced stages of cancer have a greater chance of being depressed or of suffering from other mood disorders than those not in pain and those in earlier stages of the disease. Likewise, those who are depressed or who were in pain before their illness are at greater risk for experiencing more intense pain than the nondepressed patient. Studies show, for example, that pain thresholds are lower (meaning that patients are uncomfortable and distressed by pain more easily) in pain patients suffering from major depression than those with milder depression; similarly, patients with mild depression have lower pain thresholds than those who showed no symptoms of depression. Patients who are depressed also report that their pain interferes with their lives more often than patients who are not depressed, despite similar intensities of pain. Breast cancer patients, for example, who join support groups had lower rates of depression and experienced 50 percent less pain.[3] Researchers suspect that there are similarities in the biochemistry of chronic pain and depression. Thus, on one hand, relieving pain can often help relieve depression and other mood disturbances, and successfully relieving depression can, on the other hand, help reduce the pain.

How to Help the Depressed or Anxious Patient

Families can help ease a loved one's depression or anxiety in important ways. Here are some suggestions:

- Help the patient sort out genuine losses from imagined ones, guiding the patient to acknowledge and mourn those losses. The genuine losses might include dwindling independence, loss of a positive self-image, and in some cases the end of certain dreams and goals. Encourage the patient to talk about these issues and, in response, try to express an understanding of those thoughts. Don't try to deny them. Statements that begin with "Don't be silly" or similar phrases discount what the patient is feeling. On the other hand, "How does that make you feel?" and "That must be so hard for you" are expressions of empathy and understanding.
- Support the patient in reframing feelings of helplessness by developing, in concert with the patient, small achievable goals that are realistic and practical. Help the patient maintain a sense of control by empowering him with choices related to care and comfort.
- Try to engage the patient in more positive thinking that involves active loving, laughing, looking on the bright side, and focusing on positive thoughts, even in the face of serious illness.
- Help the patient separate his or her identity and personality from the illness and a sick body; the patient's body may be impaired or weakened, but he or she is still the person others love and respect.
- Help the patient cope with fears of pain by reassuring them that aggressive pain management strategies are available and will be

used and pursued if they are needed. To address feelings of loneliness and meaninglessness, reassure the patient that he is a highly valued and loved member of the family and community, and that he is not alone either physically or emotionally—you are in it together. Patients may tend to view their glass as half empty rather than half full and may need to be reminded of their blessings, although without minimizing the seriousness of their illness and concerns.

- The patient may lament what he can't do if the illness is debilitating or life-threatening; he may regret what he didn't do in his life. In a loving, supportive manner, help him focus instead on what he *can* do and what he *has* achieved. For example: "I know how disappointing it is for you not to be able to go to Billy's games now, but isn't it great that you have more time to help him with his homework?" Or "I hear what you re saying, Mom, but you have been a wonderful mother/friend/ neighbor/artist, and that counts for a lot. I'm proud of you."

- Help the patient distinguish between realistic fears and exaggerated, distorted ones. For example, if the patient believes that he is dying when it is clear that his prognosis is good, challenge his belief with statistics, pointing out that averages mean that as many people live longer as shorter, and that a positive attitude can help. If he is truly dying and is frightened that it will be a painful, lingering, agonizing experience, challenge this in a loving but factual manner, assuring him that the pain and discomfort can be greatly relieved and controlled these days.

- When someone believes the worst, it is understandable that irrational fears will surface. Accurate, factual information is essential to reassure the patient in these instances.

- Acknowledge that sadness is a legitimate emotion and a normal response. Feeling appropriately sad, though, is different from depression, which is psychologically immobilizing and physically draining. Don't minimize a patient's (or your own) expressions of sadness, or try to change the subject. Crying together can create a strong and loving bond between you. Yet remember to introduce thanks and joy for what the person has offered and still offers to those around him. At this time, patients may feel more despair if they see a long recovery or period of dependence ahead of them. Acknowledge that the illness is unexpected and unfortunate, but help the patient focus on small goals for today or for the week— whatever is appropriate at the time.

- If the patient is terminal and frightened, acknowledge his or her fears; don't minimize them or brush them off with simple reassurances. Convey that you really hear what he is saying. For example: "I know what you're saying, and you're right, dying is scary because you don't know what's beyond." Yet reassure him that those around him will help him live life to its fullest for as long as possible. Help him accept and mourn his losses. Focus on past accomplishments, what has been meaningful in the patient's life, and how he can strive to live each day as fully as possible until the very end.
- Don't allow the patient to feel that he has failed the family by getting ill or by not getting better. The patient also shouldn't be made to feel that tears, grief, and acknowledgment of losses are weaknesses. Rather, courage can be emphasized—courage to face the losses and the grief and to express the sadness and the struggles associated with serious illness. Patients need to grieve these losses, so denying them may be harmful. Whenever possible, reassure the patient that he is not alone and is not to blame.

Don't worry about not saying the "right thing." These are difficult issues, and you don't have to give any answers. The important thing for the patient is to know he is listened to and loved; you can help by providing understanding and encouragement.

Treating Depression with Medication

The primary physician may suggest a medication to ease depressive symptoms. At major cancer centers, patients are often started on a stimulant such as an amphetamine, followed a few days later by a tricyclic antidepressant such as amitriptyline (Elavil), imipramine (Tofranil), doxepin (Sinequan, Adapin), or nortriptyline (Pamelor, Aventyl) to prolong the short-term benefits of the amphetamine. Those benefits include improved attention, concentration, and appetite as well as an improved sense of well-being while diminishing fatigue and weakness. Amitriptyline is particularly useful for relieving insomnia, anxiety, or agitation, while imipramine may be chosen if the patient is having slowed physical reflexes and showing fatigue. But because tricyclics carry a range of side effects, such as dry mouth, nausea, constipation, and blurred vision, a newer generation of antidepressants (such as Zoloft, Prozac, Wellbutrin, Paxil, Celexa, Effexor, Lexapro) may be prescribed.

When both anxiety and depression are problems, some doctors prefer using an antianxiety medication such as alprazolam (Xanax).

Treating Anxiety with Medication

Although many patients are somewhat anxious during exams, treatments, and other procedures, a person's anxiety sometimes may become so severe that it interferes with his ability to function, comprehend, and take an active part in what's going on.

When the anxiety is linked to acute pain, a painkiller usually helps; if it's linked to trouble with breathing, then oxygen, morphine, or a mild sedative should help. When the patient is on corticosteroids, side effects may include insomnia and signs of anxiety, in which case a tranquilizer such as oxazepam (Serax), lorazepam (Ativan), diazepam (Valium), or alprazolam (Xanax) can usually help. An antipsychotic drug such as haloperidol (Haldol), chlorpromazine (Thorazine), or prochlorperazine (Compazine) may be useful when the patient doesn't respond to minor tranquilizers or is suffering from a more serious mood disturbance. A tranquilizer may also be useful if a patient develops panic attacks (see "The Typical Distress of Cancer Patients," above), which is not uncommon. Side effects of the tranquilizers may include drowsiness, confusion, and uncoordinated movements. Sudden alcohol withdrawal can also trigger anxiety, and families should be sure to tell the doctor if a patient was dependent on alcohol prior to being hospitalized or becoming bedridden.

All of these drugs—antidepressants, antipsychotics, tranquilizers, and antianxiety medications—are commonly used with the opioids because they have in many cases been found to heighten the pain-relieving effects of the opioids (see Chapter 8). In addition, most of the therapies described in Chapter 12 (such as relaxation techniques, biofeedback, supportive counseling, psychotherapy, and hypnotism) have also been found useful in easing depression or depressive moods and in relieving anxiety and panic; these therapies can play a significant role in reducing pain and suffering while enhancing quality of life. Especially useful is cognitive psychotherapy, which targets the specific thoughts and silent assumptions that may generate and maintain painful emotional responses (described more fully in Chapter 12).

Sustaining Hope

More and more studies are showing that positive feelings—such as hope, optimism, and a sense of control over one's life—can have a powerful effect on a patient's health and quality of life. As we discussed in Chapter 12, how people view their adversity, how they explain bad things to themselves, can influence their health. People who blame themselves or who generalize one unfortunate event and apply its outcome to many events in their lives are pessimists compared to those who can view a bad event in perspective, and pessimists seem to have higher rates of depression and illness. Studies at the University of Pennsylvania, for example, have looked at a possible link between overall perspective—that is, pessimism or optimism—and the activity of the immune system. Optimists were found to have a greater ability to ward off disease; pessimists were found to be under more stress and showed reduced immune functioning. Similarly, studies have found that people who feel as if they have more control over their lives are happier and healthier than those who feel passive and helpless.[4] As we saw in Chapter 12, researchers have studied optimism and pessimism and feelings of control and helplessness, and have developed concrete ways that people can improve their coping skills and outlook. In other words, we can learn and acquire an optimistic and hopeful attitude.

Many patients can look forward to full recovery and many healthy and productive years ahead of them. Although treatment and recovery may be difficult, families and caregivers can help by focusing on goals and hopes for the day or week—a day of no pain, a day of enjoying a visit with a loved one, a meal of favorite foods, and so on. When a full recovery may no longer be possible, maintaining hope is still essential because hope restores meaning to life. Those facing a terminal illness should know that a peaceful, pain-free death is not only a hope but a reality for most cancer patients. Other patients may find it beneficial to join a clinical trial and try experimental anticancer treatments. Doctors tell of a famous case in which a patient with huge tumors and an enlarged spleen and liver was given two weeks to live. When given an experimental drug he improved enormously, and in ten days' time he was released from the hospital and even flew his own plane. But when the patient read that the drug he took was ineffective, his faith waned, and in two months he was back on his deathbed. His doctor tried a "double-strength, superrefined" dose of the medication, and the tumors receded again, after which he was symptom-free for two months. Then the man read again that the drug was worthless. In a few days he was back on his deathbed and died soon thereafter.

Pain, Depression, and Thoughts of Suicide

It is not unusual for patients with advanced cancer or uncontrolled pain to state that they wish to die, to ask that something be done to hasten their death, or to talk about wanting to commit suicide. In fact, a recent Canadian study found that the will to live among hospitalized terminal cancer patients varied by as much as 30 percent in a twelve-hour period and 60 to 70 percent over several weeks, depending on how much pain the patients were in.[5]

It is quite common for patients with advanced disease to want assurances that if the disease gets too bad, they will have "a way out." Many patients have an intense need to know that, if necessary, they could have control over their life—and death. Such talk should be taken seriously and communicated to the patient's doctor, and may even warrant professional help. Nevertheless, suicide among cancer patients is rare. For many, talking about potential suicide is often more a bid to regain control than a real threat.

Debate in many countries is ongoing about whether there ever is a time when the wish to die is a rational request, especially when a disease is terminal, painful, and the patient wishes to hasten death so he can die with dignity. (For a fuller discussion of suicide or assisted suicide, see Chapter 15.)

While actually rare among cancer patients, suicide is a potential threat since the symptoms of cancer put these patients at a somewhat higher risk. What is known is that patients who believe themselves to be totally helpless, who despair at their fate, who are clinically depressed, or who experience unrelieved pain are many times more likely to want to commit suicide. Those who have histories of major depression and other psychological mood disorders (such as severe panic or anxiety disorders) as well as past drug or alcohol abuse are also at greater risk for suicidal tendencies.

Families need to be aggressive and vocal about ensuring that their loved ones are not suffering uncontrolled pain by working closely with the patient and the medical team. If pain persists, the primary doctor may recommend consultation with a pain specialist or a visit to a pain clinic (see Appendix 1). For the depressed patient, professional counseling may help. Often discussing the option of suicide in a calm, nonjudgmental manner may be enough to determine what is really bothering the patient the most, so it can be attended to. Often such a discussion dissipates thoughts of suicide simply because the patient is assured that his distress is being taken seriously. If the main problem is pain or fear of pain, once it is relieved most patients will stop talking about wanting to end their lives.

Studies of cancer patients who have actually committed suicide show that about half were suffering from major depression. And since about one-quarter of all cancer patients suffer from the symptoms of depression at one time or another, and up to 75 percent of those with advanced cancer suffer from depression, cancer patients should be considered at risk for suicide. Recent studies, in fact, have shown that up to 73 percent of people living with advanced cancer want assisted suicide or euthanasia to at least be a legal option. However, when patients who are treated for physical pain or depression, the vast majority change their mind. About 5 percent, however, still want euthanasia or physician-assisted suicide.[6]

It is essential to discuss such thoughts with the patient openly. A doctor or mental health professional can help initiate this discussion if it is too difficult for the family member.

What is most important to keep in mind is the fact that both pain and depression lead many patients to thoughts of suicide. If we manage pain and depression adequately, we will dramatically reduce the number of terminally ill patients who wish for premature death.

Coping with a Terminal Illness

Dealing with the disability of cancer is one thing; dealing with the knowledge that you are dying is another. If a patient is terminal, he may experience a series of emotions, sometimes in stages, as he comes to terms with the realization that he is going to die. These emotions are similar to those associated with other losses, such as the loss of a breast, a child, a job, and so forth; they are normal psychological reactions that help buffer the patient temporarily from a harsh reality. Patients, and their families for that matter, need time to experience this process, and while the stages listed here are typical, each person is different. Below is a pattern that is typical. Not everyone will follow these particular stages in the order listed here, and not everyone will experience each stage. The transition from one stage to another is often not smooth; people can get "stuck" in one or another stage. The characteristics of each stage, however, are recognizable, if not to the patient, certainly to the family.

1. *Denial and avoidance.* Upon first learning that the cancer is terminal, the patient typically denies it to himself, refusing to accept the reality, claiming or believing that there must be some mistake. He may even avoid the whole issue, acting as if he didn't even hear the bad news.
2. *Anger.* Upon facing the fact that he is dying, the patient may express anger—anger that life isn't fair, that someone else who is a nasty person is still fine but he (the patient) is going to die; anger at God for the illness and impending death.
3. *Depression.* Depression typically follows the anger stage and is characterized by feelings of loss on all levels—loss of life and dreams, loss of family, loss of health and a positive self-image, declining self-esteem, and so on. This type of reactive depression is not unexpected.
4. *Bargaining.* In this stage, the patient may try to bargain with God, or whatever divine being the patient believes in. Bargaining is

just that; the patient says, "I'll do this if you'll do that." For example, a patient may say to God: "If you just let me live until my daughter's wedding, I'll be a better person. I'll go to church every day; I'll donate more to charity." Or "If I could just live until the holidays, I'll die peacefully." Interestingly, cancer patients often make it to the important date up ahead, be it a birthday, a holiday, or a wedding. In fact, studies of Jewish patients in Los Angeles have found that the death rate falls just before Passover and then increases afterward before returning to normal.

5. *Acceptance.* The final stage is acceptance—a relatively peaceful state in which the patient accepts that he is going to die and is psychologically and emotionally ready to prepare for it as best he can.

No two people are the same, and we each move through or get stuck in these stages in our own unique way. While some may reach acceptance rather quickly, others may remain stuck in depression. A supportive, open environment can do much to facilitate this process.

The Taboo of Discussing Death

Unfortunately, some families don't talk about dying, especially with the person who is dying. In our society, it is not uncommon for people to simply deny the existence of death. The family and the patient both act as if the patient is going to get well and live forever. These attitudes end up leaving the dying patient feeling shunned and isolated, alone at a time when he needs love and support the most. He may feel guilty, frustrated, and angry inside but may be unable to show it. Families that deny a dying cancer patient the opportunity to talk about his dying or what will happen to his loved ones after he dies are denying the patient the chance to discuss issues of vital importance to him. Some patients will need to engage in such discussions to feel more at peace as they are dying.

To some of us, perhaps to most of us, however, the act of dying forces us to face our most basic fear. For some family members and friends, the dying person may stop being a person and become a symbol of something they fear. As a result, some of us distance ourselves from the dying person at a time when a parting loved one needs us more than ever. Far more of what isn't said to a dying patient has to do with the fears of living individuals.

If the family cannot cope with communicating openly about the course of the disease, they should seek the help of a hospice nurse, social worker, or other mental health professional. Of course, some patients choose not to discuss these matters. Families can help by taking any leads they hear from the patient, asking questions that encourage them to elaborate, such as "What do you mean?" or "I don't know [or I don't understand]. Help me understand." Some families may be comfortable about having an experienced hospice nurse or a mental health professional try to talk to the patient about dying. At a time like this there may be a far greater disservice done because of what isn't said than what might be said, and family members should try to bring up the subject if they can. The threat of death offers a remarkable opportunity for family members to come together and share their fears, even if they have never done this before.

Family Burnout

At the same time the patient is experiencing a wide range of distressing emotions, families and loved ones are going through their own emotional upheaval—feeling depressed, guilty about what they could have done or can't do, worried over finances, children, and jobs, concerned over the patient's illness and disability, and in some cases overwhelmed by impending death. These concerns, combined with the physical and emotional exhaustion of caring for someone who is ill, can take a great toll.

Families should he aware that depression in spouses of cancer patients is very common, especially among wives, among those who are less satisfied with their marriages, and among those whose spouse expresses anger or reports pain. Studies show that 20 to 50 percent of spouses report symptoms of depression and feelings of helplessness. Interestingly, however, a spouse's symptoms of depression do not seem linked to the patient's feelings of depression and disability.

It is important for caregivers to continue their own lives, to give themselves breathing space to do what they enjoy—to go to a movie, exercise, visit friends. If the patient declines, it may become increasingly difficult for caregivers to sustain their constant care and vigilance. (See Chapter 15 for discussions about home and hospice care.) Families may consider seeking further help from the health care team to step up interventions with medications for pain, shortness of breath, nausea, and other distressing symptoms. And as they shift their attention from feelings of helplessness to activities that focus on making their loved one as comfortable and as free of pain as possible, families may feel more empowered. Ensuring that the loved one has a comfortable death is a major victory; fretting about the past or the future takes on less importance when the focus is on the present.

Families may also find themselves experiencing anticipatory grief, which means experiencing symptoms of grief even before death occurs. In fact, sometimes the living may go through the grieving process so effectively that they emotionally prepare themselves before the death occurs. If family members find they are detaching themselves from their loved ones, they may wish to discuss these feelings with other family members, a hospice nurse, or a professional counselor.

Tending to the Spirit

Whether religion is involved or not, humans throughout the ages have thought of themselves as being more than mind and body. That third dimension is often referred to as spirit. Most of this book has addressed the body and the physical changes that may occur with cancer. We have also discussed the mind as we have tried to broaden our concept of pain to include the larger concept of suffering, which encompasses more than pain and takes into consideration the powerful interplay between the mind and the body: how depression or anxiety can exacerbate pain and further debilitate the body; how distraction and relaxation techniques can use the mind to calm the body; how a loving hand and caring concern can ease the suffering and soothe the pain.

The Spiritual Dimension of Being Human

The spiritual dimension is that characteristic of our lives that many philosophers define as the essence of being human. Whether they have led a traditionally religious life or not, patients and family members often find themselves exploring these questions from a new perspective when dealing with a life-threatening illness. When a person is facing impending death, he becomes acutely aware of the finite nature of his life, his vulnerability, his temporal existence. It may be a terrifying realm, and many of us spend our lives avoiding it and building walls around it. Or it may be a source of calm, comfort, and peace—a "coming home" or a completion of a well-spent life. In considering our mortality and humanity, especially when death seems near, we may ponder issues of meaning, values, unity, and how we humans connect with that which is greater than ourselves, be it nature and its harmony, the universal mind, or God.

Many religious traditions embrace this stage of life as a reminder that we are not alone—that in death, we lose our separateness and become part of a greater whole. Perhaps through worship, ceremony, song, or dance, a sense of unity and oneness may free us, our spirit, to be truly human. This may be unfamiliar territory to some, even to those with deep religious beliefs. Death offers us the opportunity to explore these questions and approach life in new ways. When the time comes, let us hope we will be a willing partner in such explorations.

Caring for the Whole Person

Dr. Balfour Mount, professor of surgery, surgical oncologist, founder of the first hospital-based inpatient/outpatient hospice program in the world and of palliative care in Canada, and director of the palliative care unit at McGill University, talks about addressing the whole person—looking beyond the patient's physical needs and psychosocial needs. Mount suggests that we need to understand all the dimensions of an individual's personhood and refers to the model proposed by Eric Cassell, an internist, humanist, bioethicist, and professor of public health at Cornell University Medical College and author of *The Nature of Suffering*. Cassell views human nature as having many domains—personality, character, a past, roles with others, views of life, an unconscious life, a secret life, perceived future, and a physical body. Humans also have what Cassell calls the transcendent dimension—the need to identify with what is larger than ourselves.

"Who Are We?"

Spoken or not, the question "Who are we?" is an example of the kind of issue that comes up for people who find themselves seeking meaning in their life as it draws to a close. Since it is a question without a simple and obvious answer, engaging in an exploration of all it implies may have unexpected and beneficial results.

Regrettably, contemporary society emphasizes the physical—superficial—you. Think of all the commercials that emphasize looking good. The implicit message is that you are your body and your image. But obviously, a person's core goes beyond image.

When an illness results in some physical decline, it doesn't take too much time to begin to reject this superficial notion. The internal dialogue may go something like this: "If I am my body—if that is what defines me—how come even though my body's not working so well right now, I still feel like me? There must be something more." Another possibility is that what we are is a mind—that as long as we're still thinking straight and clearly, our loved ones will identify the person they have known and loved as being intact. Over time, most people will also reject this notion as being far too simple. Just think back to a time spent with a loved one who is now no longer as sharp as he once was. Perhaps he is now forgetful or unable to follow a conversation quite as well. And yet there is a sense that the person you knew and loved is still before you—perhaps changed in some ways but, at least from one perspective, in ways that are not important enough to detract from his personhood. Recognition of a human being as something more than a body and mind is what keeps us loving each other during the aging process—often loving more profoundly, even though the body and mind become less fit. It can be argued that one of the ways to establish meaning in the face of serious illness is to work at continuing to relate to the component of the person that is more than just his body or mind.

Caregivers who view the patient as a whole person will consider these varied domains of personhood and how the illness affects, or doesn't affect, each one. They can help the patient transcend the illness by exploring the larger picture—the sources of meaning in life and of the larger human family.

As the body deteriorates, eroding a person's mastery and control over his life, independence, and autonomy, more and more power is given up to others. As the body changes and our abilities to smile, laugh, touch, or gesture diminish, the way the world sees us and how we relate to those closest to us changes as well.

The Search for Grace

In embracing the whole person and acknowledging the reality of progressive and inevitable physical decline, the caregiver may help the person transcend the body and embrace a dimension of grace. Balfour Mount talks about giving the person an opportunity to express his unique essence, the core of his personhood, by focusing on the person's "otherness." By doing so, one can avoid depersonalizing someone whose body and face may sometimes become almost unrecognizable. There's no one right way of approaching this opportunity, and, in fact, loving intention is often enough. Just consciously focusing one's attention on all the domains of the person will go a long way. The person may have lost his roles, but he has not lost the essence of his selfhood, which makes him unique.

What can help the patient express that selfhood? Perhaps a discussion of the meaning of life and what that person's creations and accomplishments have been. Or perhaps expressing to that person how grateful others are to have been his children, friends, and coworkers will awaken the dignity and integrity of someone who is close to death. Or mentioning how things learned from him will be passed on to grandchildren or students will make him feel his work lives on beyond his own life. Mount suggests asking about the places, people, music, things, and ideas that the patient has loved; of keying into the person's memory to recall a life of purpose and involvement, to talk about what hopes can be shared that day.

To help the patient talk about the meaning of his life, the listener might also ask the patient questions about his childhood, turning points in his career, the most exciting and the best of times, the worst and the hardest of times, as well as lessons that he learned along the way and would want to pass on, or the best and worst things he ever did. Would he change anything about his life or past? Does he need to forgive himself or others for things that have been said or done in the past? What is the hardest thing now or the longest part of the day now? What does he think about most these days? Can he talk about how he feels about what is happening to him now? Is there unfinished business with loved ones, with God, with himself?

"To see that hope is not the way out, it's the way through" is for Mount a healing lesson. He continues: "The healing of spirit may be accompanied by an awareness of quietness, a sense of solidity, a broadness, a security or a sense of being held. The most and the least we can do is to accompany them [the dying] on their journey."

15

If Death Approaches

How people die remains in the memories of those who live on.
—Dame Cicely Saunders

Our lives are time travel, moving in one direction only. We accompany one another as long as we can; as long as time grants us.
—Joyce Carol Oates

There may come a time when patients and their families start doubting the benefits of further treatment or intervention, wondering whether it will do more harm than good. At some point it may be necessary to accept that the cancer can no longer be treated and that a loved one is dying. Rather than focusing on beating the cancer or buying time, the focus shifts to enhancing the quality of whatever precious time is left. The goal of palliative care is to make the person as comfortable as possible, satisfying his physical, psychological, emotional, and spiritual needs. Families focus on how to help their loved one die as dignified, peaceful, and tranquil a death as possible.

Deciding When to Stop Treatment

Treatments ideally should do good and preserve life while doing no harm. In almost all cases, though, potentially beneficial medical treatments have the potential to do harm via side effects or complications. Doctors always have to assess the potential benefit versus risk in making recommendations. With cancer, there often comes a point, especially among those who have become weak, when conventional treatment is clearly more potentially toxic than beneficial.

Deciding when this time has come, however, can be difficult. Although many doctors will identify the critical turning point for families, other doctors may not readily do so, continuing to treat the illness, assuming that is what the patient wants. Legally, doctors need to offer continuing treatments, however tiring or uncomfortable. A family may need to initiate a dialogue with the doctor about what is the kindest and most humane approach at this time.

Often, though, this critical point isn't so clear-cut. When will further therapy no longer be useful? The many difficult decisions at this time involve when to consider palliative (noncurative) radiotherapy or chemotherapy, blood transfusions, platelet transfusions, antibiotic therapy, intravenous feeding, and so on. Each decision can be difficult, with no accepted and clear guidelines for each individual case.

Interestingly, African Americans are twice as likely as whites to ask for life-sustaining treatments at all costs and tend not to use living wills or hospice programs because these are seen as implying the abandonment of hope or the failure to show adequate caring.

Questions to Ask

To assess potential benefit versus risk, ask:

- How might the treatment help?
- How might it hurt?
- Does the treatment have a chance of curing the cancer? Some people will choose to make extreme sacrifices for even a small chance at beating the cancer.
- How likely is it that the treatment will prolong life and for how long—how many days, weeks, or months?
- What are the chances that the treatment will shrink the tumor or slow its growth? In other words, what are the chances that symptoms can be reduced?
- How likely are side effects? What will their impact be on the time that remains?
- Is the person's quality of life sufficient to warrant attempts to extend it, especially when the proposed treatment may make him feel worse?

With advanced cancer, even simple diagnostic tests (chest X-rays, blood tests, CAT scans, etc.) are often avoided unless they are likely to change the treatment plan, not only because they are expensive but, more important, because of their demands on limited energy.

Even when conventional therapies are no longer useful, some families may want to explore experimental drugs and procedures, if they haven't already done so. Doctors can make referrals to major cancer centers where experimental treatments are offered. If seeking unconventional or unortho-dox therapies, discuss them with the doctor and keep him informed about decisions. Guard against pursuing a "miracle cure" to the bitter end at the sake of a potentially soothing, peaceful, and pain-free end of life.

The Hospice Concept

Despite impassioned conversations about last-ditch treatment efforts, ul-timately the patient and even family members will often express surpris-ing relief when a realistic viewpoint is reached and the focus shifts to viewing dying as a process and a milestone in the journey of life.

From its inception in England in 1967, hospice care, which focuses on promoting and supporting a comfortable, dignified life and death during terminal illness, has mushroomed. The word itself—*hospice*—is a catchall term to describe either a homelike, inpatient facility staffed by palliative care experts or community health organizations that offer their expertise to families who wish to keep a dying loved one at home. Hospice is more of a philosophy of care that transcends settings.

The basis of hospice is comfort care devoted to relieving pain and the physical, emotional, social, and spiritual suffering of both the patient and family unit without trying to cure the cancer or prolonging or shortening life. The goals are to help the dying and their loved ones maintain control over their lives, to provide support and information about state-of-the-art techniques that ensure that the patient remains as free as possible from suffering due to pain and other symptoms, to help promote open commu-nication and coping strategies, and to avoid feelings of isolation as death approaches. It's been described as "low-tech and high-touch." Although people tend to associate hospice care with less costly care (perhaps be-cause of the hospice Medicare benefit available in the United States), low cost care isn't its fundamental feature, just a fortunate coincidence.

Dying at Home

As a loved one moves into the terminal phase of his illness, choices for care typically include a hospital (which insurance companies will try to limit), a nursing home or other long-term skilled-care or rehab facility (for which placements may be difficult to arrange), a residential hospice (rela-tively rare), or home. By far, dying patients prefer to be in the comfort of their own home with loved ones around. Although in England hospice is common as an institutional setting, the easiest option in the United States is for patients to remain at home, especially since they can receive almost all hospital services to maintain comfort at no personal expense. Some communities have small backup units in their hospitals to provide short stays where terminal patients can get stabilized or to provide some respite for families. Also, many nursing homes have a hospice option managed by experienced hospice providers. More and more, insurance companies, including Medicare, support at-home or hospice-centered care. Some will even cover part of the costs of community, hospital, or home health care units that provide palliative care for the dying.

At home, patients are in familiar and private surroundings and have more autonomy than in a hospital. Home care allows the family to more gradually adjust to the fact that the person is dying and usually reduces stress since their daily routine of having visitors, cooking, shopping, watching TV, and so forth can be maintained. It avoids constant visits to a hospital room where visitors and loved ones may sit around for hours, feeling helpless and useless. Dying at home allows loved ones to actively help in the care of the patient without abandoning their personal routines. Helping to provide care often helps family members experience less guilt and a more complete grieving process after the death than when a family member dies in the hospital. Dying at home also means there's a far greater chance that a family member will be present at the actual moment of death.

Keeping a loved one at home, though, requires specialized resources and support, so families feel adequately prepared for various eventualities. Caring for an ill family member requires tremendous energy, attention, and loving care. It can at times be stressful, exhausting, and difficult, because the patient's condition may change rapidly and small emergencies may arise unexpectedly. Caregivers must be able to help with daily activities, including bathing, feeding, toilet care, medication, pain relief, and so on. And since most patients need full-time care, often more than one caregiver is necessary to ensure that the primary caregiver is adequately rested.

Although this may sound terrifying, especially for someone who is not a nurse or doctor, countless people have done it and find it rewarding and gratifying because it enhances closeness. With good support, family members can look back at their involvement with pride.

While coping with the patient's fragile emotional and physical condition, caregivers need to deal with their own grief, anxiety, and depression. Family members often neglect themselves as they become absorbed in the job of doing all they can for the patient. They need to be reminded that if they don't tend to their own needs, they may ultimately let the patient down, for the patient would never have wanted them to neglect themselves.

Experienced professionals are increasingly available to help families ensure that the dying process is as peaceful and free of pain as possible.

Families often can accept palliative and supportive care at home more than electing hospice, which may be interpreted as "giving up," even though such care is quite similar to hospice care.

Families who will be caring for a loved one at home need to consider the following issues:

- How is the disease expected to progress, and what type of symptoms might occur?
- What kind of support services are available? Who will be the main medical professional with whom the family can have frequent contact and who will respond to the patient's diverse needs?
- Are there hospice nurses, hospice volunteers, home health aides, social workers, mental health professionals, or clergy available? The last three of these can help with personal or emotional matters, home health aides can help bathe and care for the patient, and volunteers or respite workers can provide needed temporary relief for the caregiver. How much of these services will insurance cover?
- Is there twenty-four-hour help available by phone or to visit and assess the patient at home? Is there an inpatient backup unit available if things ever seem overwhelming?
- What kinds of equipment should be considered and when— walker, wheelchair, bed cushions, commode, pump for pain medication, hospital bed, and other items? What is provided by the program and covered by insurance? What can be rented rather than purchased? Are there programs sponsored by the local chapter of the American Cancer Society or a community church or synagogue that offer this equipment on loan if required?
- Who will help teach the family how to provide hands-on care for the patient and answer practical, day-to-day questions—for example, how to move or bathe the patient, how to administer or change pain medication, and so forth?
- What is likely to happen as the patient's condition worsens? Is the family member or caregiver emotionally and physically prepared to cope? Although not always necessary, some families may consider using a supplemental private nurse or aides to help out if they can afford the service. Does the family wish to consider making advance arrangements with a funeral home to respond when needed?

If such resources are in place, caring for a dying loved one will not seem so overwhelming and can more easily be viewed as part of the natural cycle of loving, living, and dying that we all participate in.

Dying in a Hospital or Care Facility

According to recent polls, although seven out of ten Americans would prefer to die at home, more than seven out of ten still die in health care facilities—often in pain and surrounded by strangers.

Many families do not have the emotional or physical stamina or the resources to care for a dying person. Many patients have no reliable caregiver for home care, and some people don't want to die at home—they don't want to be a burden to their family, they may not have confidence that the family can cope well, or they may feel the family will be unable to provide the services needed. Others feel that, in their deteriorated condition, they do not want to be cared for or treated by the family, especially when young children are around. Many families lack the flexibility and means to add to their responsibilities the care of a sick relative, even when that person is unquestionably loved.

Dealing with these issues can be difficult. The family may feel inadequate because they are not up to the challenge of caring for a loved one at home. A patient may fear hurting loved ones if he spurns offers of home care. Hospital social workers are trained to help families work through such difficult issues.

If hospital or long-term care is needed, a residential hospice or palliative care unit at a nearby hospital or long-term skilled-care facility is a good option. Many insurance plans will help pay for such care. Again, hospital social workers will know which doctors are experienced in palliative care and what options exist.

A combination of home and hospital care is common, with the patient hospitalized briefly during stressful times but the primary care setting at home.

Living Wills, Do-Not-Resuscitate Orders, and No-Code Status

Legislation increasingly acknowledges patients' rights to exert control over health care decisions, including the right to refuse unwanted or invasive medical intervention. State and federal courts support the right of an incompetent or comatose patient to have his or her wishes respected if there is good evidence that those wishes are known. Most states require clear and convincing evidence of what the patient would want. Living wills, do-not-resuscitate (DNR) orders, and health care proxies (naming a person who can make decisions if the patient cannot) are common ways to honor these rights.

Living wills spell out the desires of the patient to accept and to refuse certain medical interventions, such as feeding tubes, respirators, or cardiac resuscitation, when hopes for a cure or quality long-term survival are futile. A do-not-resuscitate (DNR) order directs health care professionals to avoid efforts at resuscitation for patients in crisis. Resuscitation can be very painful and intrusive and often is not justified in the terminally ill. A health care proxy allows the patient to appoint a family member or close friend to make health care decisions in the patient's best interest if the patient cannot.

Although these rights are available, most people (well or not) still do not have such paperwork in order. Whether ill or not, discuss these issues as early as possible and keep the appropriate documents both at home and in the hands of the primary doctor. (See Appendix 4 for sample documents.)

Ethics of Pain Control

Pain generally diminishes as death approaches; despite this general rule, a small proportion of patients may experience worsening pain and distress (crescendo pain) near death, in which case controlling pain remains one of the highest priorities.

Despite some strongly held opinions to the contrary, adequately treating pain rarely hastens a death that is already imminent. Recent studies, in fact, find that there's no significant connection between how high opioid doses are in the last weeks of life and the timing of death. Many patients and families opt for freedom from pain whether it makes the patient sleepier or weaker or not. Many doctors will increase medication doses to relieve a dying patient's suffering, even if they believe this may hasten death. This practice is argued to be ethically justified by the principle of "double effect," which excuses these actions as long as their motivation is the relief of pain and suffering. Thus, using adequate doses of painkillers in a patient who is already severely weakened by illness is *not* the same as overdosing a patient and has nothing to do with suicide or euthanasia.

The World Health Organization asserts: "Any hastening of death that is linked to adequate pain control measures simply means that the patient could no longer tolerate the therapy necessary for a bearable dignified life."[1]

Further guidance on this difficult subject comes from David J. Roy of the Center for Bioethics, Clinical Research Institute of Montreal: "Spare no scientific or clinical effort to free dying persons from twisting and racking in pain that invades, dominates, and shrivels their consciousness, that leaves them no psychic or mental space for the things they want to think and say and do before they die."[2]

Estimating Life Expectancy

Even the most experienced oncologists have difficulty accurately predicting the exact life expectancy of patients with cancer. An experienced physician can usually predict whether a patient has six months or less to live, or when a patient may just have a few weeks or less to live, but more exact predictions are difficult.

Often physicians will use one of two performance scales to assess cancer patients. The ECOG (an abbreviation for the Eastern Cooperative Oncology Group) and Karnofsky (named after the physician who developed it) scales provide standards to assess disability, progress, or decline and to help predict life expectancy. Family members can use these scales to assess a patient themselves and to allow them to communicate more effectively with health care professionals by phone.

Letting Go

Some cancer patients who have had long periods of illness and are very close to death still linger despite prolonged suffering. As hard as it may be for family members when a cancer patient hovers near death for days, the patient may need reassurance that it is all right to die, that though the family will grieve their loss, they will be able to manage and take care of themselves. A child may need to hear from her mother that it is okay to "leave"; an elderly husband may need to hear from his wife that she will be all right after he dies; an elderly woman may need reassurance from a daughter that she will take care of her grandmother and that her mother doesn't have to hold on anymore; a pet owner may need reassurance that his pets will be cared for. Although it may sound cruel to tell someone it is okay to die, many doctors attest that it is what some patients need to hear to let go and die peacefully. As strange as it may seem, many patients cling desperately to life until they are given "permission" to let go, to stop fighting, and to let the natural order of things take its course.

Similarly, some patients seem to put off their death until an important event, such as a graduation, birthday, or wedding, takes place. This has even been studied and dubbed the "Passover phenomenon." Researchers looking carefully at the dates of death certificates among Jews in Los Angeles found that mortality rates fell consistently before Passover, an important Jewish holiday, and rose above normal just after the holiday, before finally returning to the normal or average rate of death.

Many patients at this time have dreams and visions related to dying that they may or may not readily share with those around them. Such visions often involve travel metaphors (especially "going home") and contacts with deceased family members.

Performance Scales (ECOG and Karnofsky)

Grade	ECOG	Grade	Karnofsky
0	Fully active, able to carry on all predisease performance without restriction.	100	Normal, no complaints, no evidence of disease
		90	Able to carry on normal activity; minor signs or symptoms of disease
1	Restricted in physically strenuous activity but ambulatory and able to carry out work of a light or sedentary nature (e.g., light housework, office work).	80	Normal activity with effort, some signs or symptoms of disease
		70	Cares for self; unable to carry on normal activity or to do active work
		60	Requires occasional assistance, but is able to care for most of his or her needs
2	Ambulatory and capable of all self-care but unable to carry out any work activities. Up and about more than 50% of the time.	50	Requires considerable assistance and frequent medical care
		40	Disabled, requires special care and assistance
3	Capable of only limited self-care, confined to bed or chair more than 50% of waking hours.	30	Severely disabled, hospitalization indicated; death not imminent
		20	Very sick, hospitalization necessary, active supportive treatment necessary
4	Completely disabled. Cannot carry on any self-care. Totally confined to bed or chair.	10	Moribund, fatal processes progressing rapidly
5	Dead.	0	Dead

Difficult Decisions

If the end seems to be drawing near, families may need to tackle some very difficult decisions. At what point should the patient no longer be strongly encouraged to take certain medications or to eat? Should a feeding tube or intravenous tube be considered?

Ideally, families have discussed these issues with the patient before these decisions must be made. Yet these conversations are difficult and uncomfortable, so many families put them off. To allow a terminally ill person to die peacefully, families may choose to withhold or to stop interventions such as respiratory support, chemotherapy, surgery, and assisted nutrition. The physician's team is accustomed to these situations and should be regarded as an essential source of guidance, support, and information.

In considering these decisions, consider these generally accepted guidelines:

- *Follow the patient's desires.* When possible, families should know ahead of time what their loved one would desire if such decisions ever have to be made.
- *When to simplify medications.* At some point, taking medication for a chronic medical condition, like high blood pressure or mild diabetes, may simply no longer make sense or justify the associated cost and effort. Families should be attentive to the patient's refusals to comply with medication schedules. With the advice of their physician, families will need to assess when may be the right time to simplify medications, maintaining only those absolutely necessary to make the patient comfortable.
- *Is the treatment prolonging life or prolonging death?* Will the proposed treatment (such as using a respirator or feeding tube) enhance the person's life or merely prolong the process of dying? Will the patient's suffering be eased by the intervention or be prolonged by it?

Take advantage of discussing these difficult issues with physicians, nurses, and other health care providers, clergy, and hospital ethicists, as they have experience with them.

Allowing a body that is riddled with cancer to die is a far cry from suicide or murder, even if it means refusing treatments or intervention. Instead, it is accepting a fact of life: that we all die, and that we have the right to choose how we die, with whatever kind of dignity and self-determination we prefer.

Feeding tubes and intravenous liquids are rarely needed. As a person's body begins to shut down—that is, begins to actively die—patients tend to dramatically cut down on food and drink. Sometimes the tastes or smells of even favorite foods become unpleasant or nauseating; others find it too painful to have food in their mouths or can't swallow easily. Caregivers may find themselves constantly trying different ways to get the patient to take small amounts of liquids or food, perhaps by only offering liquid food, by medicating mouth sores with a local anesthetic, offering medication for nausea, offering food through a straw or syringe or squirting liquids into the patient's mouth, offering little sponge pops, or allowing the patient to suck on a water-soaked washcloth. As discussed in Chapter 11, we feed those dear to us to show our love—sometimes even when they need love more than food.

As the body stops digesting and processing food, there may come a time when the patient cannot take any nourishment or water. Should patients be given liquids through intravenous means? Most hospitals routinely take this approach, while it is not customary practice for patients being cared for at home. Many doctors feel that intravenous infusions should be avoided if at all possible in patients with advanced cancer. Although they may make the family feel better that "something is being done," many doctors assert that such intravenous nutrition may merely encourage tumor growth, that the tubes are uncomfortable, and that terminally ill people who are given artificial nutrition and hydration often experience distressing symptoms, such as congestive heart failure, nausea, vomiting, swelling, and diarrhea. Just the need to urinate can trigger a painful episode as the person tries to move onto a portable toilet or get on a bedpan.

Studies that assess whether dehydrated people die sooner or more uncomfortably than terminal patients who were artificially (intravenously) fed or hydrated find that comfort levels and longevity were not influenced by a person's hydration state. The consensus is that dehydration is not painful, and that dehydrated people who are dying rarely experience hunger or thirst. In fact, dehydrated dying people tend to experience less difficulty breathing and produce fewer respiratory secretions.

Rather than force liquids or nutrition into a dying person, doctors generally recommend that you respond to the patient's wishes. Keep the mouth moist (see Chapter 11) and give only what the patient wants. Remember, the ill person has the right to make his own decisions and refuse intervention, including food or water.

Sedating the Dying Patient

Despite all best efforts, some terminally ill patients may continue to experience extreme pain. There may come a time when the doctor or family decides that the pain cannot be adequately relieved and that deeply sedating the person to unconsciousness—known as "terminal sedation"—is the best option. The person will remain unconscious until death and is believed to be free of suffering. When adjusted properly, the drugs used to sedate (usually a benzodiazepine such as midazolam, or a barbiturate) do not cause death, but death eventually occurs within days or perhaps weeks because of the underlying illness and other factors such as dehydration, starvation, pneumonia, or other complications.

Whereas the majority of doctors do not support euthanasia or physician-assisted suicide, most support terminal sedation as a morally legitimate step, and it is now openly practiced by hospice units and palliative care groups. In 1997 the U.S. Supreme Court asserted that while it does not support assisted suicide, it strongly endorses the aggressive use of opioids even if they make the person unconscious or hasten death. Since the sedation does not cause death, some physicians would prefer that the term "terminal sedation" be replaced with an alternative, such as "sedation for intractable distress in the dying."

"Rational" and Assisted Suicide

In recent years, debate about whether physician-assisted suicide or even socially approved euthanasia should ever be permitted has become more prominent and heated. Dr. Jack Kevorkian, the retired pathologist who helped several terminally ill patients die, brought the issue of doctor-assisted suicide to national attention in 1989 and 1990, and it's been highly controversial ever since. In 1992 Derek Humphries' book *Final Exit* became a national best-seller with its complete instructions for how to commit a suicide without the help of a doctor.

Unfortunately, we tend to view assisted suicide, suicide, and euthanasia as part of a dichotomy, with the only other option leaving our loved ones to suffer a prolonged and agonizing death. But there is a large middle ground that offers a humane and scientific approach, and it is the premise of this book that patients need *not* suffer in pain and agony, that modern pain management tools are available that can ease and perhaps totally eliminate the physical pain and suffering many still endure today. In tandem with psychological support and counseling to manage anxiety and depression, patients can be in the last stages of disease and be free of pain and depression—the two primary causes of suicide in patients. Today it is unthinkable that patients may beg to die because their pain or depression is not being treated effectively. Once pain and depression are treated properly, the desire to hasten death diminishes, as quality of life improves. This is a realistic goal for every cancer patient.

In the meantime, as this debate rages, health care providers are legally restricted from engaging in any medical practice that is specifically intended to shorten a patient's life. If thoughts of assisted suicide have been voiced by a patient, most health care providers will listen with a sympathetic ear, but because of these legal and ethical concerns they are unlikely to take any direct action. If this is an issue, however, it is very important to *tell the health care team*, because it sends an important signal to the team that something is very wrong. Such a discussion may offer an opportunity to determine the underlying problems that make the continuation of life seem intolerable. After such a conversation, the team may pursue more aggressive management of pain, depression, and other symptoms, seek additional support for caregivers at home, recommend consultation with a social worker, clergy, pain specialist, or psychiatrist, or whatever seems to be needed. Suicidal thoughts, however, are a clear indication to the family to make absolutely certain that do-not-resuscitate orders have been instituted so that unnecessary suffering will not be prolonged.

Here are proposed criteria for a policy that would address assisted suicide:

- Does the patient clearly suffer from an incurable condition, and is he likely to experience severe and unrelenting suffering?
- Is the patient receiving appropriate medication for the suffering? Is he benefiting from the best that science has to offer in relieving suffering?
- Is the patient lucid and alert, with no psychological illness or severe emotional problems, including untreated depression?
- Does the patient have a realistic and accurate view of the situation? Has he clearly and continually asked for suicide to avoid suffering? Efforts should be made to avoid having to force the patient to beg. Would even uninvolved outsiders view the patient's desires as understandable? Can the patient's physician agree that the situation is hopeless and the patient is likely to suffer severely? Can an uninvolved physician concur and the three (patient and two doctors) sign a document of informed consent?

Of course, all efforts to treat pain and depression should be made before any consideration of assisted suicide. Those who endorse assisted suicide under the conditions described above assert that the patient should not be abandoned at the time of death and that if an overdose is prescribed, the physician must be present at the time the patient takes the overdose. It is tragic, many assert, that terminally ill patients are so often forced to die alone because they are fearful they would place their families or caregivers in legal jeopardy if they were present.

The World Health Organization's Guidelines on Euthanasia

When patients are not lucid and competent, some families wonder whether to take a more active role. Should they wait for death passively, or should they help promote a less painful, quicker death? What is humane? What is the right thing to do? These are among the most difficult decisions anyone will have to make in life. The World Health Organization has drawn up the following guidelines:

- It is ethically justifiable to withhold or discontinue life support interventions when, as desired by the patient, doctors cannot reverse the dying process and instead merely prolong it.
- Painkillers and other drugs should be used in whatever doses are needed to relieve pain and discomfort, even if that means shortening the patient's life.
- Family members can make these decisions when the patient is unconscious, is incompetent, or can no longer make these decisions himself.

As Death Approaches: What to Expect and How to Help

Just as every birth is dramatically different, so is every death. Some patients will experience only a few of the following symptoms. The most typical symptoms of a dying patient are dry mouth, loss of appetite (anorexia), confusion, and weakness all over. We list many symptoms here as a means to prepare the family or to help them cope should these symptoms occur. How to cope with these and other symptoms are discussed in detail in Chapter 11.

- *Dehydration.* Many patients become dehydrated and may experience thirst, low blood pressure, drowsiness, confusion, weakness, and perhaps even coma. Yet most doctors assert that the condition of dehydration is not uncomfortable as long as the mouth is kept moist; in fact, some conditions such as breathlessness, cough, urinary incontinence, and pain may be relieved when water intake is reduced.
- *Nausea.* As discussed more fully in Chapter 10, antinausea medication is very effective. If the patient cannot swallow easily, it may be administered rectally, through a skin patch (scopolamine), or by injection.
- *Difficulty swallowing.* Do not force any liquids or foods. If swallowing is very difficult, small amounts of liquids may be given

with an eyedropper, with a syringe, or from a wet washcloth that the patient sucks. When swallowing is difficult, make sure all medications are administered in ways other than by mouth (subcutaneously, rectally, etc.).

- *Confusion, restlessness, agitation, and delirium.* If patients seem confused, restless, agitated, or delirious, the family may wish to consult the health care team. Patients will need to be reassured if they become confused and, should hallucinations occur, even encouraged to maintain a sense of humor. Close (even constant) supervision is preferable to using any restraints, although these may sometimes be necessary to remind the patient to avoid pulling at dressings and other equipment. If symptoms persist, haloperidol or other antipsychotic medications can calm a patient; benzodiazepines are helpful for the restless and agitated patient, particularly to promote sleep and rest. Drugs may be administered in the mouth through an eyedropper next to the patient's cheek (when patients can no longer swallow) or through subcutaneous pumps.

- *Shortness of breath.* Breathlessness is a common symptom, often made worse by panic. Patients should be sat up and reassured. Allowing cool air into the room, either through an open window, with air-conditioning, or with a fan, can offer relief. Cool air directly into the nose can also help. Doctors may change the morphine levels (usually upward) to relieve the shortness of breath or may prescribe a benzodiazepine, such as Xanax.

- *Incontinence.* Catheters, tubes that directly empty the bladder through the urethra, can collect urine directly into a bag. If the patient is very close to death, however, and incontinence is a new problem, catheters may be avoided. Patients may well expel so little urine that an underpad on the bed may be sufficient. Males may use an external catheter or portable urinal; females may be given a pad in their underwear. Sometimes patients may have stool they can't expel—a suppository, an enema, or its removal with rubber-gloved hands can deal effectively with the problem.

- *Muscle twitching or jerking.* These involuntary movements (myoclonus) may be due to a variety of causes, including high doses of pain medications. A health care provider should be consulted to exclude a seizure disorder. But most often, although their appearance may be disturbing, they usually are not uncomfortable for the patient. The administration of a benzodiazepine, especially clonazepam, can often relieve the twitching.

- *Noisy, wet breathing.* About half of cancer patients begin to breathe noisily in the last few days of life, usually due to accumulations of mucus in the back of the throat. Although not particularly distressing to the patient, the noisy breathing may be hard for the family and caregivers to endure. A drug such as scopolamine (called hyoscine in Britain) usually can relieve the symptom, especially if the throat has been cleared first. Changing the patient's position and reassuring him may also help. Suctioning, which can be unpleasant, is only sometimes necessary.

- *Sweating and feeling hot.* In addition to a fan, steroids, acetaminophen, or an NSAID can usually help if sweating is unpleasant and uncomfortable. Bedlinens may need to be changed more often to ensure the patient's comfort, assuming that doing so does not produce much pain. Consider the use of analgesics prophylactically before activities that may be otherwise painful.

- *Pain.* Studies show that pain *usually* does not suddenly escalate near death. Pain, of course, may fluctuate at any time, but usually once intense pain has been relieved, most patients can be sustained at relatively steady levels of pain medication until death. In a smaller proportion of patients, pain either gradually diminishes (especially with increased acceptance that the end is near) or may mount steadily (crescendo pain). Regardless, patients and families should have access to extra or "escape" doses of narcotics to administer as needed. Even if they are never needed, having them available (like a seat belt) will help ease everyone's anxiety.

When Death Is Very Close

As death nears, stay with the patient—if at home, a baby monitor may be used so the caregivers can hear when the patient is awake, and may sit with him. Just the presence of another person helps the dying person be less apprehensive. Touching or holding the patient can do a lot to diminish feelings of fear, loneliness, and despair for the patient and loved ones.

Patients may need to be encouraged to turn frequently to prevent too much pressure on the same spots. Patients who are weak or unresponsive will need to be turned by their caregivers.

Although deaths vary as widely as do individuals, there are some signs that death is drawing very close:

- Fingertips and toes develop a dusky or bluish hue as circulation slows down; the skin on the arms and legs may feel cool to the touch. If tolerated, keep the patient covered with a sheet or light blanket.

- The person may sleep more or may be unresponsive. This does not mean that he is entirely unaware of his surroundings or that he might not become more wakeful.
- Intermittently, the person may become very confused about where he is, who the people are around him, and why things are happening. He may become agitated and may hallucinate about people and places, especially from the past. It can be helpful to calmly explain to the patient that the disease or medications are responsible and that he's not going crazy. Again, at such times, the proximity and touch of family and loved ones can be reassuring.
- Although the dying person can usually continue to hear well, responsiveness and vision may gradually fail. Keep the patient turned toward a window or the light with people close by, near the patient's head. Even if you are uncertain whether the patient can hear you, speak as if he or she is listening; talk to the patient as if he or she can understand every word, and don't say anything that the patient shouldn't hear.
- Urine may darken, its volume may decrease, and at times the patient may lack control of his bladder or bowel. Underpads from a drugstore may be placed under the patient to absorb wastes; these can be easily replaced.
- Mucus may accumulate in the back of the throat, causing noisy breathing or even choking. Keeping the patient's head elevated on several pillows and turned to the side may help, but be prepared to either clear mucus with a washcloth or suction tube or to do nothing.
- Keep the mouth moist with a sponge stick (available from nurses), a wet washcloth (allowing the patient to suck on it), or ice chips. If it doesn't startle the patient, a straw can be used to gently place several drops of water on the patient's lips or in the mouth. Cotton swabs dipped in olive oil can be used to moisten the tongue. Do not force anything in the mouth.
- When death is very close, breathing may seem delayed or irregular, and the patient may make rattling noises in the back of the throat. If the patient is distressed, the physician may prescribe scopolamine, usually in the form of a skin patch placed behind the ear.

During this time, caregivers may wish to play soothing music and have soft light in the room. Remain close to the patient, speaking reassuringly, indicating that loved ones are close by, and that the patient should try to relax and should not be afraid. Any agitation can usually be soothed with prescribed medications. Holding the patient's hand and talking softly can be reassuring for the dying patient. Make sure the patient is not in pain, and if in doubt, administer escape doses of pain medication according to your doctor's instructions. When pain levels are uncertain, it is better to err by overmedicating than by undermedicating.

Grief

After a loved one's death and its associated grief there may also be a sense of relief that the ordeal is over, which is often coupled by feelings of guilt for having that relief. Things may seem more bearable just after a death occurs, because there is so much to do and many relatives and friends are around the household. Although there may be a delayed response, characteristically grief soon washes over the lives of survivors.

People experiencing grief may feel just about anything, from mild pangs to severe, deep upset—even of a physical nature. There is no "right" way to grieve or "right" schedule for grieving. It is one of the most personal of life's events. The following reactions occur commonly and, although unpleasant or even intolerable, are relatively normal.

- Mental pain and tension
- The need to sigh
- Empty feeling in the pit of the stomach
- Frequent crying spells
- Muscular weakness and fatigue or exhaustion
- Tightness in the throat
- A choking feeling with shortness of breath
- A feeling of being "removed" from one's own body
- Waves of physical distress, often lasting twenty minutes to an hour

Those who are grieving sometimes experience a sense of unreality or may feel emotionally distant from others. Crying should be encouraged to relieve stress. Sometimes those grieving are preoccupied with visions of the dead person or are plagued by feelings of guilt—that they could have done better for the person who died, that they were somehow inadequate, even negligent or inattentive. When a person is experiencing such feelings of guilt, he may be irritable and seem angry with others, emotionally pushing them away even at a time when others come to sympathize or make a special effort to connect. Other features of grieving include restlessness, feelings of aimlessness, hostility, passiveness in actually doing anything or taking action, and an almost neurotic desire to stick to usual routines even when all zest and vitality are sapped. Family members in grief may experience more exaggerated responses and begin to take on personality traits or idiosyncrasies of the deceased—walking or talking like him, picking up a special interest of his, enshrining or even worshiping the deceased, and so on.

Working through these feelings has been characterized by some as "grief work." Goals of this work include:

- Freeing the living from feeling in bondage to the dead person
- Adapting to the environment without the deceased person
- Forming new relationships and moving ahead with life

However, part of the process of grief work is to express pent-up emotions that are otherwise avoided at all costs in order to minimize distress. Those experiencing grief may stay tense and tight as a way to prevent breaking down, and may react with hostility to those who mention the dead person. People grieving in this way need to be helped and should be encouraged to accept the distress of active grief, which allows the one feeling left behind to move forward.

Beyond Normal Grief

Not uncommonly, people get stuck in the grieving process. Unable to move through it, someone who is grieving may:

- *Delay it* by acting as if nothing happened or as if the person has accepted the death easily. It may be years before the person becomes preoccupied with the death and images of the one who died; it will be at that time that the grieving process must be worked through.
- *Distort his reactions,* perhaps by exaggerating his activities and sense of well-being, keeping very busy and overly cheerful.
- *Develop an illness, either physical, psychological, or both,* sometimes even in a way that is similar to the loved one's illness. Psychosomatic illnesses are those that can be caused or aggravated by psychological factors, such as an ulcer, asthma, or rheumatoid arthritis.
- *Persistently reject social relationships by* distancing himself from others. As the bereaved person becomes increasingly isolated from family and friends, he becomes overcritical or merely disinterested in others and events.
- *Experience feelings of rage or fury,* especially against specific people, such as a doctor who treated the dead person.

- *Act cold and formal* with old friends or family members. The person may go through the motions of daily living, but with a demeanor that is stilted, formal, and without warmth.
- *Be socially passive*, with the grieving person unable to initiate new activities or relationships because he believes that it will all be unrewarding anyway.
- *Be overgenerous*, with the grieving person appearing not to care anymore about money or belongings and perhaps willingly giving them away, possibly hurting family and business associates in the process.
- *Be chronically depressed or have ideas of suicide* as a reaction to grief. Suicide may be considered an option if anxiety, panic, or a major depression persist. Sometimes the depressed or anxious person becomes agitated, feeling tense, restless, and worthless, unable to sleep well, and perhaps even accusing himself of all kinds of mistakes for which he should be punished. Those with obsessive traits and histories of depression are most likely to develop this agitated form of depression.

Getting Through the Grieving Process

The process of grieving involves the living person's freeing himself from the "hold" the departed person has over him and finding new and rewarding patterns in daily living and social interactions. The grieving individual must work through in his own way the pain he feels. True acceptance usually involves expressing expected feelings of sadness and loss, and even unexpected feelings of hostility and guilt that may linger. Mental health professionals have specific short-term strategies (usually requiring eight to ten sessions) for helping people work through the mourning process. By working through a process of allowing the deceased back into our lives, thoughts, and feelings, by making our loved one a part of our lives, rather than apart from them, we can learn to accept our loss, as hard that may be, and move through the process of grieving to acceptance.

Dying is a natural and inevitable part of living. To ease a loved one's passage may be one of the most profound and generous gifts we can offer. Both individually and as a culture, learning to make that passage as easy and comfortable as humankind knows how is a most worthy goal. As Michelangelo said, "Death and love are the two wings that bear the good man to heaven."

Appendix 1

Where to Find More Information

Note: Many of these organizations can also help you locate a cancer specialist or a pain specialist near you. The listings here are meant to serve as a resource guide only and not necessarily as an endorsement of an organization.

On Cancer Pain

For a free copy of *Managing Cancer Pain* (AHCPR Publication No. 94-0595, March 1994), a 22-page document by a panel of experts sponsored by the Agency for Health Care Policy and Research (AHCPR), contact:
AHCPR Publications Clearinghouse
P.O. Box 8547
Silver Spring, MD 20907
800-4 CANCER (800-422-6237)

For a free copy of *Cancer Pain Treatment Guidelines for Patients* and other information online from the National Comprehensive Cancer Network, go to www.nccn.org or call 888-909-NCCN (6226), or call the American Cancer Society at 800-ACS-2345.

A summary of *Management of Cancer Pain* is available online at http://www.ahrq.gov/clinic/epcsums/canpainsum.htm
For a printed copy, contact:
AHRQ Publications Clearinghouse
P.O. Box 8547
Silver Spring, MD 20907-8547
800-358-9295

The American Alliance of Cancer Pain Initiatives (AACPI)

A national organization dedicated to promoting cancer pain relief nationwide by supporting the efforts of state and regional pain initiatives. Initiatives are voluntary, grassroots organizations composed of many kinds of professionals. Initiatives work to disseminate accurate pain management information, educate health care professionals, raise public and patient awareness of the cancer pain problem, promote institutional change, and advocate for the removal of regulatory and legislative barriers to pain management.

American Alliance of Cancer Pain Initiatives
1300 University Avenue, Suite 4720
Madison, WI 53706
608-265-4013
Fax: 608-265-4014
www.aacpi.wisc.edu

For information about cancer pain initiatives around the world:
Cancer Control Programme
World Health Organization
1211 Geneva 27
Switzerland

The Association of Cancer Online Resources

Developed by an online community of cancer patients, the Web site covers the causes of cancer pain and lists medications, treatment options, and tools to help patients communicate with their physicians. The site also allows patients and caregivers to exchange knowledge.

http://www.cancer-pain.org

Cancer Information Service

For a referral to the closest pain control clinic, or for other cancer-related information, call the Cancer Information Service (CIS), supported by the National Cancer Institute, a nationwide toll-free telephone inquiry system.

800-4 CANCER (800-422-6237)
http://www.nci.nih.gov or http://cancer.gov

Childcancerpain.org

Sponsored by the Texas Cancer Council, this Web site has a lot of basic information on cancer pain in children.
For a free copy of *Making Cancer Less Painful,* an online handbook for parents who have children with cancer, see

http://www.dal.ca/~pedpain/mclp/mclp.html

Clinical Trials on Cancer Pain

http://clinicaltrials.gov
http://www.centerwatch.com/patient/studies/cat303.html

A List of Links Related to Cancer Pain Resources

National Cancer Institute Information Resources
http://oesi.nci.nih.gov/RELIEF/RELIEF_MAIN.htm

Pain Control Program from Cancer Supportive Care
http://www.cancersupportivecare.com/pain.html

Pain Management in Children with Cancer Handbook
Available free at http://www.childcancerpain.org/
frameset_nogl.cfm?content=handbook.html

Patt Center for Cancer Pain and Wellness
Based in Houston, Texas, this Web site provides medical care for patients
suffering from cancer pain or chronic pain.
http://www.cancerpain.org

Persistent Pain After Breast Surgery
http://www.cancerlynx.com/breastpain.html

WebMD/Lycos
Includes articles about cancer pain, discussion boards, and Ask the Expert.
http://webmd.lycos.com/condition_center?doi=pnm

World Health Organization
Publishes *Cancer Pain Relief,* second edition (1996), available in English, Spanish, and French, and *Cancer Pain Relief and Palliative Care in Children.*
WHO Publications Center USA
49 Sheridan Ave
Albany, NY 12210
518-436-9686
Fax: 518-436-74 33

Interdisciplinary Clinics in the United States

The following is a brief list of some of the leading programs in the country that
focus on pain management:

The Cleveland Clinic Pain Management Program
W. O. Walker Building/C25
Cleveland, OH 44195
800-392-3353 or 216-444-PAIN (7246)
For general information, questions, or to make an appointment: 216-445-7370 or
800-223-2273 ext. 57370
Hearing-impaired (TTY) assistance: 216-444-0261
http://www.clevelandclinic.org/painmanagement

Rosomoff Comprehensive Pain and Rehabilitation Center
Southshore Hospital
Miami, FL 33139
305-532-PAIN (7246)
Fax: 305-534-3974
http://www.rosomoffpaincenter.com
E-mail: painrelief@rosomoffpaincenter.com

Department of Pain Medicine and Palliative Care, Beth Israel Medical Center
First Avenue at 16th St.
New York, NY 10003
877-620-9999
www.stoppain.org

Johns Hopkins Cancer Pain Service
Baltimore, MD
410-955-8964
http://www.hopkinscancercenter.org/programs/pain.cfm
Includes an interactive Web site for solving the problems of cancer pain.

Mayo Clinic's Pain Management Center
St. Mary's Hospital
Rochester, MN
507-284-2511
http://www.mayoclinic.org
A separate Mayo Clinic Web site also has information about drugs, diseases,
and much more: http://www.mayoclinic.com

Mensana Clinic
1718 Greenspring Valley Road
Stevenson, MD 21153
866-653-2403 or 410-653-2403
Fax: 410-653-3633
http://www.mensanaclinic.com
E-mail: info@mensanaclinic.com

Multidisciplinary Pain Center, University of Washington
1959 N.E. Pacific
Seattle, WA 98195
206-598-4282
http://www.washington.edu/medicine/patients/specialty/uwmc/mpc/
index.html

**Pain Clinic at M. D. Anderson Hospital and Tumor Institute,
University of Texas System Cancer Center**
1515 Holcombe Blvd, Houston, TX 77030
800-392-1611 or 713-792-6161
http://www.mdanderson.org/topics/paincontrol

Pain Service at Memorial Sloan-Kettering Center
1275 York Avenue
New York, NY 10021
212-639-2000 or 800-525-2225 or 888-675-7722
Pediatric patients: 212-639-5954
International patients: 212-639-4900
http://www.mskcc.org/mskcc/html/474.cfm

Pain Treatment Center, University of Rochester Medical Center
Rochester, NY 14642
585-275-2141
http://web.anes.rochester.edu/ptc/index.htm

On Pain in General

American Academy of Pain Medicine
4700 W. Lake Avenue
Glenview, IL 60025
847-375-4731
Fax: 877-734-8750
http://www.painmed.org
E-mail: aapm@amctec.com

For referrals to pain specialists:
American Chronic Pain Association
P.O. Box 850
Roclilin, CA 95677
800-533-3231

American Pain Foundation
A nonprofit information resource and patient advocacy organization serving
people with pain.
201 North Charles Street, Suite 710
Baltimore, MD 21201-4111
888-615-PAIN (7246)
http://www.painfoundation.org

American Pain Society
The American Pain Society (APS) is a nonprofit educational and scientific
organization that is the national chapter of the International Association for the
Study of Pain. Composed of specialists from diverse fields, the APS is devoted
to promoting education and training in the field of pain.
4700 W. Lake Avenue
Glenview, IL 60025
847-375-4715
Fax: 877-734-8758
http://www.ampainsoc.org
E-mail: info@ampainsoc.org

American Society of Addiction Medicine
4601 North Park Avenue, Upper Arcade #101
Chevy Chase, MD 20815
301-656-3920
Fax: 301-656-3815
http://www.asam.org
E-mail: email@asam.org

The American Society of Interventional Pain Physicians
An association of physicians dedicated to promoting the development and
practice of safe, high-quality, cost-effective interventional pain medicine
techniques for the diagnosis and treatment of pain and related disorders, and to
ensure patient access to these interventions.
2831 Lone Oak Road
Paducah , KY 42003
270-554-9412
Fax: 270-554-5394
http://www.asipp.org

For a list of accredited pain programs, contact:
Commission on Accreditation of Rehabilitative Facilities
4891 E. Grant Road
Tucson, AZ 85712
520-325-1044
Fax: 520-318-1129

Committee on Pain Therapy
American Society of Anesthesiologists
520 N. Northwest Highway
Park Ridge, IL 60068-2573
847-825-5586

International Association for the Study of Pain
An international, multidisciplinary, nonprofit professional association dedicated to furthering research on pain
http://www.iasp-pain.org

National Chronic Pain Outreach Association
This organization has local branches which might sponsor support groups for
patients with chronic pain. They can also make referrals and offer newsletters.
P.O. Box 274
Millboro, VA 24460
540-862-9437
http://www.chronicpain.org

Pain.com
This Web site has interviews with cancer pain specialists as well as articles on
the topic, a list of cancer pain clinics by state, forums on cancer pain, and
several hundred abstracts from articles on cancer pain online.
http://www.pain.com

Pain Management
>http://www.cancerlynx.com/pain_management.html

Partners Against Pain
>http://www.partnersagainstpain.com

Pediatric Pain Education for Patients, Families and Nurses
The University of Iowa College of Nursing
>http://pedspain.nursing.uiowa.edu

Physical Medicine Approaches to Pain Relief
Focuses on how pain comes from movement, lack of movement, position of limbs, position of the entire body, or such sources as muscle tension.
>http://www.cancersupportivecare.com/relief.html

In the United Kingdom:
CancerBACUP, a cancer information service, launched the National Pain Relief Campaign in 2000.
>http://www.cancerbacup.org.uk/

On Cancer in General

The American Cancer Society
This national, nonprofit organization has more than 3,500 offices in the United States and Puerto Rico that provide accurate, up-to-date information on cancer to patients and their families, health professionals, and the general public. Some of their booklets include the following: "Questions and Answers About Pain Control: A Guide for People with Cancer and Their Families" and "Living with Cancer." It also offers booklets for patients concerning diet and nutrition, treatments, emotional support, symptom control, and dying at home. In addition, the ACS can provide information about local support groups and educational programs. Check with a local office.
>1599 Clifton Road
>Atlanta, GA 30329
>800-ACS-2345 (800-227-2345)

CancerNet
Information for health professionals, patients, and the public, including information from PDQ about cancer treatment, screening, prevention, supportive care, and clinical trials, and CancerLit, a bibliographic database.
>http://cancernet.nci.nih.gov

Cancer Trials
NCI's comprehensive clinical trials information center for patients, health professionals, and the public. Includes information on understanding trials, deciding whether to participate in trials, finding specific trials, plus research news and other resources.
>http://cancertrials.nci.nih.gov

Cancer Care
A national organization providing comprehensive support information for patients with cancer and their families and caregivers, including toll-free one-to-one counseling over the phone and referrals to services in local areas. Spanish-language services available.
> 800-813-HOPE (4673)
> www.cancercare.org

Candlelighters Childhood Cancer Foundation
For information and support specifically about children with cancer.
> P.O. Box 498
> Kensington, MD 20895-0498
> 301-962-3520 or 800-366-2223
> E-mail: info@candlelighters.org
> http://www.candlelighters.org

Look Good . . . Feel Better
When cancer affects one's appearance, it can be devastating to one's body image and self-esteem. Free consultations and group meetings help women resume normal lives after cancer.
> 800-395-LOOK
> http://www.lookgoodfeelbetter.org

MedlinePlus Health Information
This service of the National Library of Medicine provides a guide to more than 9,000 prescription and over-the-counter medications, 11 million articles, and links to medical dictionaries, directories, libraries, and databases.
> http://www.nlm.nih.gov/medlineplus/pain.html
Many of the listings have short summaries of the article (abstracts) and some have links to the full articles.
> http://www.ncbi.nlm.nih.gov/pubmed/
Another way to access the medical databases (known as MEDLARS, an umbrella database comprised of about forty specific databases, including Medline and CancerLit) is through a public library or medical library. Reference librarians will do a search for you, but usually for a fee. Call the reference desk and ask if they can access Medline or MEDLARS. All these searches will result in a bibliography with citations and abstracts of journal articles on specific topics published in the medical literature.

Information specialists translate the latest scientific information into understandable language and respond in English or Spanish at 800-227-2345, or on TTY equipment at 800-332-8615.
> http://www.cancer.org/

An advocacy group for cancer survivors:
The National Coalition for Cancer Survivorship
> 1010 Wayne Avenue, Suite 770
> Silver Spring, MD 20910
> 301-650-9127 or 877-NCCS-YES (622-7937)
> http://www.canceradvocacy.org

National Health Information Center
For information on some one hundred hotlines for specific diseases:
800-336-4797
> http://www.health.gov/nhic

Groups that provide support and information for people who have had cancer treatment are:
Post-Treatment Resource Program
> Memorial Sloan-Kettering Cancer Center
> 1275 York Avenue
> New York, NY 10021
> 212-717-3527
> http://www.mskcc.org/mskcc/html/5667.cfm

The Wellness Community
> 919 18th Street, NW, Suite 54
> Washington, DC 20006
> 888-793-WELL
> 202-659-9709
> http://www.thewellnesscommunity.org

This group has branches in cities throughout the country.

Y-ME National Organization for Breast Cancer Information and Support
> Breast cancer hotline
> 800-221-2141
> http://www.y-me.org

On Medications

In addition to checking the drug insert, you can research a medication online at http://www.rxlist.com/

Whole-Body Approaches

The Fetzer Institute
For general information on mind-body research.
> 9292 West KL Avenue
> Kalamazoo, MI 49009
> 269-375-2000
> E-mail: info@fetzer.org
> www.fetzer.org

Acupuncture

To obtain referrals close to your area, contact:
> American Academy of Medical Acupuncture
> 800-521-2262
> http://www.medicalacupuncture.org

American Association of Oriental Medicine
  5530 Wisconsin Avenue, Suite 1210
  Chevy Chase, MD 20815
  301-941-1064 or 888-500-7999
  Fax:: 301-986-9313
  E-mail: info@aaom.org
  http://www.aaom.org

British Acupuncture Council
  http://www.acupuncture.org.uk

British Medical Acupuncture Society
  http://www.medical-acupuncture.co.uk

National Certification Commission on Acupuncture and Oriental Medicine
  703- 548-9004
  www.nccaom.org or www.acupuncture.com

National Acupuncture Foundation
  P.O. Box 2271
  Gig Harbor, WA 98335-4271
  253-851-6538
  Fax: 253-851-6883

Biofeedback

Association for Applied Psychophysiology and Biofeedback (formerly the Biofeedback Society of America) and the **Biofeedback Certification Institute of America**
May provide information and referrals:
  10200 W. 44th Avenue, Suite 304 (AAPB) or Suite 310 (BCIA)
  Wheatridge, CO 80033-2840
  303-422-8436 or 303-420-2902
  Fax: 303-422-8894
  http://www.aapb.org or http://www.bcia.org
  E-mail: bcia@resourcenter.com

International Society for Neuronal Regulation
An international organization of professionals from various disciplines doing neurotherapy, neurofeedback training, and research. Supports education and excellence in the field of neurofeedback training and neurotherapy and seeks the validation and acceptance of this discipline by a broad spectrum of society.
  394 Road 34
  Merino, CO 80741
  E-mail: office@snr-jnt.org

Hypnosis

The American Council of Hypnotist Examiners
Has 7,400 members and may be able to recommend a certified hypnotist
700 S. Central Ave.
Glendale, CA 91204
818-242-1159
Fax: 818-247-937
http://www.sonic.net/hypno/ache.html
E-mail: hypnotismla@earthlink.net

American Society of Clinical Hypnosis
140 N. Bloomingdale Road
Bloomingdale, IL 60108-1017
630-980-4740
Fax: 630-351-8490
http://www.asch.net
E-mail: info@asch.net

Society for Clinical and Experimental Hypnosis
An international organization of nurses, social workers, dentists, psychologists, psychiatrists, and other physicians who are dedicated to applying hypnosis in the clinical setting.
Washington State University
P.O. Box 642114
Pullman, WA 99164-2114
Fax: 509-335-2097
E-mail: sceh@pullman.com

Support Groups

In addition to the American Cancer Society, the **American Self-Help Clearing-house** can help locate a group for specific medical programs.
http://mentalhelp.net/selfhelp

Counseling and Psychotherapy

For a referral to a counselor, ask your doctor for a psychiatrist, clinical psychologist, or psychiatric social worker. National organizations that might have local branches or can offer referrals include:

American Psychiatric Association
888-357-7924
E-mail: apa@psych.org

American Psychological Association
800-374-2721 or 202-336-5510
TDD/TTY: 202-336-6123
http://www.apa.org

Center for Cognitive Therapy
215-898-4102
http://www.uphs.upenn.edu/psycct

National Association of Social Workers
800-638-8799 or 202-408-8600
http://www.naswdc.org

Caring for Dying Patients

Children's Hospice International
Provides medical and technical assistance, research and education for children with life-threatening conditions and their families.
901 North Pitt Street, Suite 230
Alexandria, VA 22314
800-2-4-CHILD or 703-684-0330
Fax: 703-684-0226
http://www.chionline.org
E-mail: info@chionline.org

Hospice Foundation of America
Sponsors an annual Living with Grief teleconference series, a monthly bereavement newsletter, and other publications.
2001 S Street, NW, Suite 300
Washington, DC 20009
800-854-3402
http://www.hospicefoundation.org

National Hospice Foundation
1700 Diagonal Rd., Suite 625
Alexandria, VA 22314
703-516-4928
Fax: 703-837-1233
http://www.hospiceinfo.org
E-mail: nhf@nhpco.org

Living Wills/Right to Die

The following association will provide standard living will forms and information about them. To be sure that they are valid in a particular state, check with an attorney or a hospice nurse or professional. See Appendix 4 for sample living wills and health care proxies.

Partnership for Caring: America's Voices for the Dying
A national nonprofit organization devoted to raising consumer expectations for excellent end-of-life care and increasing demand for such care. Provides

information about advance directives (living wills and durable powers of attorney for health care). Call for state-specific forms.
1620 I Street, NW, Suite 202
Washington, DC 20006
800-989-WILL (9455)
http://www.choices.org/

Grief

To obtain a referral or information about grief, contact:
Association for Death Education and Counseling
342 North Main Street
West Hartford, CT 06117-2507
860-586-7503
Fax: 860-586-7550
http://www.adec.org
E-mail: info@adec.org

Bereavement Publishing, Inc.
Publishes the magazine called *Bereavement: A Magazine of Hope and Healing.*
4765 North Carefree Circle
Colorado Springs, CO 80917-2118
888 60-4HOPE (4673)
http://www.bereavementmag.com
E-mail: grief@bereavementmag.com

The Compassionate Friends
A self-help organization offering friendship and understanding to parents and siblings following the death of a child. They have 580 chapters nationwide.
P.O. Box 3696
Oak Brook, IL 60522-3696
630-990-0010 or 877-969-0010
Fax: 630-990-0246
http://www.compassionatefriends.org

GriefNet
A comprehensive gateway to bereavement and grief-related resources on the Web, including a support community for people dealing with death, grief, and major loss, including life-threatening and chronic illness.
http://griefnet.org
E-mail: griefnet@griefnet.org

Grief Recovery Institute
P.O. Box 6061-382
Sherman Oaks, CA 91413
818-907-9600
Fax: 818-907-9329
http://www.grief-recovery.com
E-mail: usinfo@grief.net

In Canada:
RR #1
St. Williams, Ontario
Canada N0E 1P0
519-586-8825
Fax: 519-586-8826
http://www.grief-recovery.com/
E-mail: info@grief.net

The International THEOS Foundation

An international support network for recently widowed men and women, to sponsor programs and provide services to help participants work through their immediate grief and cope with day-to-day practical concerns of widowhood.

332 Boulevard of the Allies, Suite 105
Pittsburgh, PA 15222-1919
412-471-7779

Appendix 2

Common Drugs Used for Cancer Pain and Foreign Names for the Drugs

GENERIC	United States	Australia	United Kingdom	Canada, South Africa, and other NSAIDs
Acetaminophen	Tylenol; Panadol; Aminophen; Phenaphen; Tenol; Valadol; Valorin; Aceta; Genepap; Panex	Panadol; Panamax; Dymedon; Tylenol; Tempra; Paralgin	(generic name: paracetamol) Panadol; Medinol; Calpol; Disprol; Paldesic	Atasol; Exdol; Robigesic (Can.)
Aspirin	Empirin; Bayer; Norwich	Solprin; Disprin; Aspro; Winsprin	Aspro; Caprin; Disprin; Phensic	Apo-Asa; Apo-Asen; Riphen
Choline/magnesium trisalicylate	Arthropan; Tricosal; Trilisate; Magan; Mobidin; Doan's			Trilisate; Back-Ese
Ibuprofen	Advil; Motrin; Haltran; Trendar	Nurofen; Actiprofen; ACT-3; Brufen; Rafen; Codral Period Pain	Brufen; Apsifen; Ebufac; Fenbid; Motrin; Paxofen; Librofem; Lidifen	Apo-Ibuprofen (Can.); Algofen, Brufort (Italy); Anco, Ibufug, Mensoton (Ger.); Antarene (France); Betaprofen, Antiflam, Inza, Ranfen (South Africa)

GENERIC	United States	Australia	United Kingdom	Canada, South Africa, and other NSAIDs
Naproxen	Naprosyn		Synflex	Novonaprox, Naxen, Apo-Napro-NA, Apo-Naproxen (Can.); Proxen, Naproflam (Ger.); Naprius, Xenar, Primeral, Prexan (Italy); Traumox (South Africa)
Piroxicam	Feldene	Feldene; Candyl; Fensaid; Mobilis; Pirox	Feldene; Larapam; Piroflam, Flamatrol	Roxicam, Xycam (South Africa)
Nabumetone	Relafen		Relifex	Relisan
Diclofenac	Voltaren	Voltaren; Fenac	Voltarol; Rhumalgan; Diclomax; Motifene	Fortfen, Flexagen, Panamor, Sodiclo (South Africa)
Ketoprofen	Orudis; Oruvail	Orudis; Oruvail	Orudis; Oruvail, Ketovail; Ketocid; Alrheumat	Rhodis (Can.)
Sulindac	Clinoril	Clinoril; Aclin; Clusinol; Saldac	Clinoril	
Mefenamic acid	Ponstel	Ponstan; Mefic		Ponstan; Meflam; Dysman; Opustan
Flurbiprofen	Ocufen; Froben; Ansaid		Froben	Apo- Sulin (Can.); R-Flex (South Africa)

Combination products for mild to moderate pain ("weak opioids")

Aspirin + codeine	Aspalgin; Codiphen; Solcode; Veganin	Aspalgin; Veganin	Co-codaprin; Codis 500; Cojene;	
Aspirin + more codeine	Emcodeine; Empirin	Codral Forte		Coryphen with codeine
Acetaminophen + codeine	Panadeine; Dymadon Co; Codalgin; Mersyndol Daystrength; Codapane; Codiphen	Co-codamol 8/ 500; Panadeine; Neurodyne; Paracodol; Parake; Codanin		

GENERIC	United States	Australia	United Kingdom	Canada, South Africa, and other NSAIDs
Propoxyphene	Darvon; Dolene; Doraphen; Doxaphene; Profene; Pro Pox; Propoxycon	Doloxene	Doloxene	642, Darvon-N (Can.)
Acetaminophen + oxycodone	Percocet; Roxicet			Oxycocet, Percocet-Demi, Percocet-5 (Can.)
Tramadol	Ultram	Tramal	Zydol; Zamado	Tramal (South Africa); Topalgic (France); Trabar (Israel); Tramagetic, Tradol-Puren, Tramagit (Ger.); Tramal (New Zealand)

"Strong opioids" for severe pain

GENERIC	United States	Australia	United Kingdom	Canada, South Africa, and other NSAIDs
Morphine—oral (immediate release)	MSIR; Roxanol	Anamorph	Oramorph; Sevredol	Statex (Can.)
Morphine—oral (slow release)	MS Contin; Roxanol SR	MS Contin; Kapanol	Morcap SR; MST Continus; Oramorph SR	MS Contin (Can.)
Morphine injections	Astramorph; Duramorph; Infumorph	DBL Morphine	Morphine sulphate	Epimorph (Can.)
Methadone	Dolophine; Methadose	Physeptone	Physeptone	
Oxycodone	Roxicodone; OxyContin (SR)	Endone; OxyContin; Proladone (supp)	Oxycodone	Oxygesic (Ger.); Supeudol (Can.); OxyContin, Oxycod (Israel)
Levorphanol	Levo-Dromoran		Dromoran	
Buprenorphine	Buprenex	Temgesic		Buprenex; Temgesic

Adjuvant medications

Antidepressants

GENERIC	United States	Australia	United Kingdom	Canada, South Africa, and other NSAIDs
Amitriptyline	Elavil; Endep; Emitrip	Tryptanol; Elavil; Endep; Amitrol Tryptine	Trytizol; Domical; Lentizol	Levate, Novotriptyn, Apo-Amitriptyline (Can.); Trepiline, Saroten (South Africa); Adepril, Amilit (Italy); Amineurin, Novoprotect, Saroten, Syneudon (Ger.); Amitrip (New Zealand); Amyline (Ireland); Adepril (Europe); Elatrol, Elatrolet (Israel); Domical (Hong Kong)

GENERIC	United States	Australia	United Kingdom	Canada, South Africa, and other NSAIDs
Doxepin	Sinequan; Adapin; Zonalon	**H R** Sinequan; Deptran	Sinequan	Triadaprin (Can.)
Desipramine	Norpramin	Pertofran	Pertofran	Pertofrane (Can.); Nortimil (Europe)
Imipramine	Janimine; Norfranil; Tofranil; Tipramine	Tofranil	Tofranil	Tofranil; Nova-pramine (Can); Ethipramine; Panpramine; Miprilin (SA)
Nortriptyline	Aventyl; Pamelor	Allegron	Allegron; Aventyl	
Trazadone	Desyrel; Trazon; Trialodine		Molipaxin	
Sertraline	Zoloft	Zoloft	Lustral	
Paroxetine	Paxil	Aropax, Lumin	Seroxat	
Mirtazapine	Remeron	Avanza, Remeron		
Fluoxetine	Prozac	Prozac; Lovan; Zactin; Erocap	Prozac	Lorien (SA)
Anticonvulsants				
Gabapentin	Neurontin	Neurontin	Neurontin	
Carbamazepine	Tegretol	Tegretol; Teril	Tegretol; Epimaz; Epita	
Valproic acid	Depakote; Depakene; Myproic Acid; Dalpro		Convulex	Depakene, Epival (Can.)
Phenytoin	Dilantin; Phenytex; Dilantin Kapseals; Diphenylan	Dilantin	Epanutin; Pentran	
Clonazepam	Klonopin	Rivotril; Paxam	Rivotril	

GENERIC	United States	Australia	United Kingdom	Canada, South Africa, and other NSAIDs
Tranquilizers				
Fluphenazine	Prolixin; Permitil	Modecate; Anatensol	Moditen	
Haloperidol	Haldol	Serenace	Serenace; Haldol; Dozic	Cereen
Chlorpromazine	Thorazine; Ormazine	Largactil	Largactil	Chlorpromanil (Can.)
Prochlorperazine	Compazine; Cotranzine; Ultrazin	Stemetil; Compazine	Stemetil	Prorazin (South Africa)
Antianxiety medications				
Diazepam	Valium; Vazepam	Valium; Ducene; Propam; Antenex	Valium; Rimapam; Tensium; Atensine; Dialar; Diazemuls	Vivol, Novodipam, Apo-diazepam (Can.); Noan (Italy); Novazam (France); Benzopin, Pax, Doval (South Africa)
Alprazolam	Xanax	Xanax; Kalma; Ralozam	Xanax	Apo-Alpraz, Novo-Alprazol (Can.); Alzam (South Africa)

List of brand names is not exhaustive
Sources: http://homepage.powerup.com.au/~rmottare/drugs.htm
http://www.genrx.com/genrxfree/Top_200_2000

Appendix 3

Detailed Relaxation Instructions

There are three sets of relaxation instructions that follow. The first set has both a tension phase and a relaxation phase. The second uses imagery and the third is a breathing exercise.

These types of relaxation are appropriate for adults and children ten years or older. The relaxation instructions should be spoken in a slow, quiet voice. It is best to learn the instructions so that they flow smoothly. It is OK to vary the instructions to suit the patient. The instructions can be tape recorded and then played back at a convenient time. Children and adults can learn relaxation and then apply it when needed.

What to Do

Find a comfortable place for you and the patient to relax. Ensure that you will be free from interruption or distraction. If the patient fidgets or feels uncomfortable, stop and try again at some other time. Do not try to force the patient to follow the instructions. You can't make someone relax.

Loosen any tight clothing or shoes and make sure you have a light blanket (in case the patient gets cold during relaxation). Make sure the patient does not cross his or her legs or arms (they might "fall asleep"). It is fine if their body twitches during the relaxation. If he or she feels uncomfortable, you should stop the relaxation exercise. If the patient laughs or seems self-conscious, just continue and the feeling will probably pass.

What to Say

Relaxation with Imagery

Let's use your imagination to help you relax. Start by imagining being in a very pleasant and happy mood. Imagine that you are doing something you really like. Imagine what you can see, what you can feel, and what you are doing. You can close your eyes if you wish.

Breathe in deeply and then breathe out slowly relaxing your lower arms and your hands. Your arms and hands may be kind of heavy and tingly. You feel peaceful and relaxed. Allow your arms and hands to loosen and relax more and more. Let your arms and hands relax from your elbows to your fingers. Just let go. Enjoy the calm, relaxed feeling.

Now pay attention to relaxing your upper arms and shoulders. Notice where there is some tension. Let the muscles become loose and relaxed. Try to smooth out and calm the muscles in your imagination. Be calm and peaceful. Notice how pleasant it is to relax your muscles. Just let go of any tension in your arms and shoulders.

Pay attention to the muscles in your neck and face. Relax these muscles. Let them become loose and heavy. If you can, you may want to rest your head on the pillow or couch. As you relax your face, your mouth may open. That is fine. Breathe slowly and calmly. Now pay particular attention to your forehead. Relax and smooth the muscles of your forehead. Relax your forehead as much as you can. Relax your jaw. Let all the muscles in your head and face relax and loosen. Let these muscles become heavy and calm.

Think again of the very pleasant thing you were thinking about at the beginning of this exercise. Imagine you are totally relaxed and happy. Enjoy this memory.

Now, focus attention on the muscles of your chest. Loosen the muscles of your chest. Try and make your breathing smooth and slow, calm and peaceful. Breathe in relaxation, breathe out tension.

Relax your stomach and abdomen. Notice the difference between tension and relaxation. Imagine all of your tension escaping as you relax.

Let the muscles in your upper legs become relaxed and peaceful. Feel that your legs are relaxed. Allow your legs to sink into the chair or bed. Your legs are becoming calm and relaxed. Relax your lower legs and feet. Let the muscles become calm and peaceful. Let them become very relaxed.

Imagine the warm peaceful feelings of relaxation gradually moving through your body and loosening all your muscles. Allow all your tension to disappear. Breathe in relaxation, breathe out tension.

Let the warmth move through your head. Relax all the muscles in your head and face. Allow the warm feeling of relaxation move through your neck and shoulders. Relax your shoulders. Allow the warm feelings of relaxation to move throughout your back muscles. Let the warm feelings of relaxation move down your spine. Let the warm relaxing feeling fill your legs and move into your feet. Imagine that the tension is just gradually draining away. Let the tension disappear gradually as you relax. Breathe slowly and deeply. Allow yourself to be calm and peaceful, warm and relaxed. Let all your muscles become heavy and loose. Enjoy the calm gentle feelings of relaxation.

You are calm and relaxed and feel very confident and peaceful. Just enjoy these feelings for a few moments. Gradually come out of this relaxation as I count backwards from 5. Five, four, three, two, one. You will feel good as you open your eyes. Open your eyes, stretch if you wish. Good, now just enjoy the pleasantness of the situation. Relax. Enjoy every moment of it.

Tension and Relaxation

Move so that you are as comfortable as you can be. Take a deep breath and exhale slowly. Now do it again, breathe in and slowly breathe out.

Relax all of your muscles as best you can. Focus your attention on your right hand. Squeeze the hand into a fist. Tighten all the muscles and hold the tension for five seconds. Notice the tension. Study the tension. Now relax. Relax your hand as much as you can. Notice the difference between tension and relaxation.

Now create tension in your left hand. Tight, tight (hold for five seconds). Notice the tension; study it. Now relax, release the tension in the hand. Let go and release the muscles in your hands. Let your hands become totally relaxed.

Tense your right arm by pushing it down on the chair or bed. Hold it for five seconds and study the difference between tension and relaxation. Now relax. Loosen the muscles and enjoy the warm relaxing feeling.

Now tense your left arm by pushing it down on the chair or bed. Hold it for five seconds and study the contrast between tension and relaxation. Relax. Calm and loosen the muscle in your arms. Enjoy the peace and tranquillity of relaxation.

Tense your shoulders by thrusting them forward. Hold the shoulders in this position for five seconds and notice the muscles in your back and shoulders stretching and tensing. Release and relax. Loosen your muscles and allow your shoulders to drop. Allow the tension to leave your shoulders and allow the warm pleasant feeling to move into your arms and shoulders.

Tense your shoulders by thrusting your shoulders back and noticing the tension. Hold the tension and then release and relax. Finally tense your shoulders by moving and lifting them up and holding them for five seconds. Release, relax, deepen the relaxation by breathing deeply and slowly. Your hands, arms, and shoulders now will form a ring of relaxation.

Concentrate now on your face. Create tension by scrunching up your face and hold it for five seconds. Notice the tension spreading throughout your face and scalp. Relax and let all the tension disappear.

Clench your teeth and notice tension in your jaw. Hold it and study how the tension and tightness spreads. Loosen, relax, and let go. Let your jaw go slack. You can let your mouth open if that is comfortable. Breathe slowly and deeply. Relax.

Now create tension in your neck. Be careful not to cause yourself any pain. Turn your head to the left as far as the tension in your neck and back. Hold it for five seconds and then return your head to the resting position. Next turn your head in the other direction. Hold the tension for a few moments and then relax. Finally, create tension by pushing your head onto your chest. Hold the tension and then relax.

Focus attention on your breathing. Create tension by taking a deep breath and holding it. The tension will spread gradually. Allow the tension to build until it is mildly uncomfortable. Then breathe out. Breathe deeply and slowly for three breaths. Imagine that you are breathing in through the bottom of your feet. Breathe out through your mouth or nose. If you begin to feel dizzy, breathe more slowly.

Now create tension by exhaling all your breath. Hold it for a few moments and then breathe in. Resume normal breathing and breathe deeply and slowly. Each time you exhale, try to breathe out any tension.

Cause tension in your abdomen by pulling in the muscles and holding them. This will curtail your deep breathing and tension will increase. Relax, loosen the muscles, and enjoy slow and relaxing breathing. Create tension by pushing your stomach out and holding it for five seconds. Relax, loosen your stomach muscles, allow the muscles to become calm and peaceful. Enjoy the calm feeling.

Tense your right leg by pushing it down on the bed or chair. Study the tension in your upper and lower leg. Do not tense your foot. Hold the tension for five seconds and then let go. Relax, let go, enjoy the feeling of relaxation spreading through your leg.

Now repeat the same procedure with your other leg. Tense your left leg by pushing it down on the bed or chair. Study the tension in your thigh and your calves. Do not tense your foot. Hold the tension for five seconds and then let go. Relax, let go, enjoy the feeling of relaxation spreading through your leg.

Finally, make some tension in both of your feet by pointing your toes towards your head. Do not cause too much tension or you may cause cramping and pain in your feet. Relax your feet, legs and thighs. Let the relaxation move into your abdomen and back. Notice the warm pleasant feelings of relaxation. Breathe deeply and slowly. Allow the relaxation to move into your lungs and chest. Relax your shoulders and neck. Relax your arms and hands. Now deepen your relaxation by trying to loosen any remaining tense areas.

Now, let's use your imagination to deepen the relaxation. Create in your mind a very pleasant and relaxing scene. Perhaps it would be lying on a beach or walking through a forest. Imagine the calmness in your body as you enjoy the sounds and smells of your created scene. Feel the refreshing air and enjoy the calm relaxed peaceful feeling that you have throughout your body. Feel the warmth of the sun on your head and allow the warmth to spread throughout your upper body. Feel the warm relaxing feeling spread throughout your entire body. Imagine that your body is actually a bag of sand and allow it to totally relax and mould to the chair or bed.

You are calm and relaxed and feel very confident and peaceful. Just enjoy these feelings for a few moments. Gradually come out of this relaxation as you count backwards from 5. Five, four, three, two, one. You will feel good as you open your eyes. Open your eyes, stretch if you wish.

Good, now just enjoy the pleasant feelings. Relax. Enjoy every moment of it.

Relaxation by Deep Breathing

Just relax and if you wish close your eyes. Now, take a deep breath, try to breathe in as much air as possible. Hold it for a few seconds. Now, let your breath out very, very slowly. As you let out your breath, relax all of your muscles.

Now, breathe in again, slowly and deeply. Breathe in relaxation. Slowly, breathe out and let tension flow outwards. Relax your face, arms and shoulders. Enjoy the warmth of the relaxation.

Take another deep slow breath. Fill your lungs. Relax and breathe out. Relax your chest and tummy. Allow calm and peacefulness to replace any tension.

Now breathe in again as if you are breathing in through the bottom of your feet. Slowly. Slowly. Slowly. Relax your legs and feet. Pause for a few moments and then breathe out slowly. If you begin to get dizzy breathe more slowly.

Breathe in again, deeply and slowly. Try and relax some part of your body that is a bit tense. Breathe out slowly. Release all tension. Relax and enjoy being peaceful.

Begin breathing normally but continue to increase your relaxation with every breath. Open your eyes and enjoy how you feel.

© Copyright 1992

Reprinted with permission by Dr. Pat McGrath. These instructions are also available at http://is.dal.ca/~pedpain/mclp/mclpn-re.html or on audiotape from McGrath, Department of Psychology, Dalhousie University, Halifax, Nova Scotia, B3H 4J1, for $5.00.

Appendix 4

Planning for Your Mental and Physical Health Care and Treatment

The following is reprinted with permission of
> The Advance Directive Training Project
> 291 Hudson Avenue
> Albany, New York 12210
> Phone: 800-811-1175, 518-463-9242
> Fax: 518-463-9264
> E-mail: advance@nycap.rr.com

Note: These directions and forms are not intended to constitute legal advice. You may wish to consult with your own attorney for advice specific to your situation. They have been adapted to be non-state-specific.

What is an Advance Directive?

An Advance Directive is a type of written or verbal instruction about health care to be followed if a person becomes unable to make decisions regarding his or her medical treatment. Because you prepare an Advance Directive when you are competent, it will be followed during periods of time when you lack capacity to make medical treatment decisions. There are several different types of Advance Directives, including a *health care proxy*, a *living will*, and a *do not resuscitate (DNR) order*. Each one of these is described in this pamphlet.

Why should I create an Advance Directive?

Sometimes, because of illness or injury, people are not able to decide about treatment for themselves. You may want to plan in advance and create an Advance Directive to appoint a health care agent and/or make your wishes and instructions known regarding your mental and physical health care, so that these wishes may be followed if you become unable to decide for yourself for a short or long term period. If you don't plan ahead, family members or other people close to you may not be allowed to make decisions for you or follow your wishes, and/or no one will know what treatment choices you may have preferred.

How do I create an Advance Directive?

You can use the form and directions in this pamphlet or have an attorney create an alternative form for you. Your state's health department can provide you with forms and information regarding Advance Directives as well.

Can anyone refuse to provide me with mental or physical health treatment because I have created an Advance Directive?

No. It is against the law for treatment providers to discriminate against someone because he or she has an Advance Directive.

On what basis will a physician determine that I am incapable of making mental and physical health care decisions?

Your capacity to consent to mental and physical health care is determined by your ability to understand the nature and consequences of health care decisions, including the benefits, risks, and alternatives to proposed treatment, and then to make an informed choice.

If I wish to use the attached form as my Advance Directive, must I complete the entire form?

If you choose to use the attached form, you should make sure that your name is stated at the beginning of each form and that the section regarding signatures and witnesses is completed as necessary. However, you can choose whichever other sections within the form regarding your treatment decisions that you wish to complete. It is your choice whether to fill out this form and what provisions to include in it.

To whom should I give copies of my Advance Directive?

You should give copies of your Advance Directive to your health care agent and alternate agent (if you have appointed them), to the treatment providers and health care professionals who routinely provide care to you, and to your family or friends. You may also want to give a copy to the hospital where you are likely to be treated if the need arises, and to keep a copy with your important papers.

Health Care Proxies

What is a Health Care Proxy?

Many states have a Health Care Proxy Law that allows you to appoint someone you trust and who knows you well, such as a family member or close friend, who will agree to act in your best interests regarding your health care if you lose the ability to make decisions about treatment for yourself. The document in which you appoint this person as your health care agent is called a Health Care Proxy.

What is the purpose of a Health Care Proxy?

The Health Care Proxy Law gives you the power to ensure that health care professionals know your wishes regarding medical treatment. Your health care agent can also decide how your wishes apply as your medical condition changes. Hospitals, doctors, and other health care providers must follow your agent's decisions as if they were your own.

If I appoint a health care agent, how much authority does he or she have to make treatment decisions on my behalf?

You can give your agent as little or as much authority as you want. You can allow your agent to decide about all health care or only certain treatments. For example, you may appoint a health care agent to make decisions only about your mental health care. However, you may not appoint more than one health care agent to act at a given time (e.g., you cannot appoint one for physical health care decisions and one for mental health care decisions).

If your health care agent is not aware of your wishes about artificial nutrition and hydration (nourishment and water provided by feeding tubes), he or she will not be able to make decisions about these measures.

You may also give your agent instructions that he or she has to follow. Your agent must follow your verbal and written instructions, as well as your moral and religious beliefs. You may include a living will and/or a statement of your preferences and desires regarding medical treatment with your health care proxy, which can provide a useful resource for your health care agent. If your agent does not know your wishes and beliefs, your agent is legally required to act in your best interests.

How does appointing a health care agent empower me?

Appointing an agent lets you control your medical treatment by:

- allowing your agent to stop treatment when he or she decides that is what you would want or what is best for you under the circumstances; and

- choosing one person to decide about treatment because you think that person would make the best decisions or because you want to avoid conflict or confusion about who should decide.

What are the advantages of creating a Health Care Proxy?

The purpose of the Health Care Proxy law is to give a person of your choice the authority to speak for you when you are incapacitated to ensure that decisions regarding your medical treatment are made in accordance with your wishes, including your religious and moral beliefs if known to your agent, or, if your agent does not know your views, in accordance with your best interests. Therefore, a major advantage in appointing a health care agent through a Health Care Proxy is that you do not have to know in advance all the decisions that may arise. Instead, your health care agent can interpret your wishes as medical circumstances change and can make decisions you could not have known would have to be made. The Health Care Proxy is just as useful for decisions to receive treatment as it is for decisions to stop treatment.

What are the disadvantages of creating a Health Care Proxy?

It is very important that the person you choose to be your health care agent be an adult that you trust to protect your wishes and interests. If there is no such adult in your life, you may wish to consider a Living Will to provide guidance about your attitudes and preferences regarding your medical care.

Who should I choose to be my health care agent?

The health care agent must be an adult 18 years of age or older. It is not necessary that he or she reside in your state. You should choose a person you trust to protect your wishes and interests.

An operator, administrator or employee of a general hospital, nursing home, mental hygiene facility, or hospice cannot serve as an agent for you if you are a patient at the facility, unless you are related to the person you wish to appoint, or you created the Health Care Proxy before being admitted to, or applying for admission to, the facility.

You can appoint your physician as your agent, but the physician will not be able to serve both as your agent and your attending physician after his or her decision-making authority as your agent begins. Furthermore, if you appoint a physician as your agent, that physician cannot determine your capacity to make health care decisions.

How can I appoint a health care agent?

All competent adults can appoint a health care agent by signing a form called a Health Care Proxy. You don't need a lawyer, just two adult witnesses.

You can use the form in this pamphlet, but you don't have to.

When would my health care agent begin to make treatment decisions for me?

Your health care agent would begin to make treatment decisions after doctors decide that you are not able to make health care decisions. If you regain capacity to make health care decisions, the health care agent's decision-making authority ends. *As long as you are able to make treatment decisions for yourself, you will have the right to do so.*

Will my agent's decisions be honored?

All hospitals, doctors, and other health care facilities are legally required to honor the decisions by your agent, unless they obtain a court order overriding the decision.

What if my health care agent is not available when decisions must be made?

You can appoint an alternate agent to decide for you if your health care agent is not available or able to act when decisions must be made. Otherwise, health care providers will make treatment decisions for you that follow instructions you gave while you were still able to do so. Any instructions that you write on your Health Care Proxy form will guide health care providers under these circumstances.

What are the requirements for signing and witnessing a Health Care Proxy?

You must sign and date a Health Care Proxy in order for it to be enforceable. You must include the name of your agent and state that you intend the agent to make health care decisions for you.

You must sign the Health Care Proxy in the presence of two witnesses who are 18 years of age or older. Neither witness can also be the person who you are appointing as your health care agent. The witnesses must also sign the document and state their belief that you are personally known to them, you appear to be of sound mind, and you are acting of your own free will.

How long is a Health Care Proxy valid?

The Health Care Proxy will be valid unless and until you cancel it. In addition, you can require that the Health Care Proxy expire on a specified date or if certain events occur. If you choose your spouse as your health care agent and you get divorced or legally separated, the appointment is automatically canceled.

Living Wills

What is a Living Will?

A Living Will is a written document in which you, as an adult who is now competent, can express your wishes regarding your future health care in the event that you are unable to make health care decisions. You can also include a statement of your preferences and desires regarding medical treatment with your Living Will, which can provide a useful resource for your treatment providers.

*What is the difference between a Living Will and a
Health Care Proxy?*

A Living Will is a document in which you can give specific instructions about your health care treatment, as well as express your attitudes and wishes about your health care.

A Health Care Proxy is different because it allows you to choose someone you trust to make treatment decisions on your behalf in case you lose your decision-making capacity. With a Health Care Proxy, you don't need to know in advance what will happen to you or what your medical needs might be in the future.

How does creating a Living Will empower me?

A Living Will serves to make your wishes and instructions known regarding your mental and physical health care, if you become incapable of making treatment decisions. Treatment providers should follow your specific instructions. The instructions you write in this document would be evidence of your expressed wishes in the event that your wishes are challenged in court.

What are the advantages of a Living Will?

If you have no one you can appoint to be your health care agent, or you do not wish to appoint one, yet you still want to make your wishes about your health care preferences known, a Living Will is a legally valid way of recording these instructions. This information will provide evidence of your wishes should you become incapable of making treatment decisions.

What are the disadvantages of a Living Will?

General instructions about refusing treatment, even if written down, may not be effective if they do not meet the "clear and convincing proof" test. Further, expressions of intent regarding unforeseen circumstances or new developments in technology cannot be reflected in a Living Will unless it is routinely updated.

Can I create both a Health Care Proxy and a Living Will?

Yes. If you complete a Health Care Proxy form, but also have a Living Will, the Living Will provides instructions for your health care agent, and will guide his or her decisions. Copies of your Living Will should be given to your health care agent. You will want to have your health care agent share the views expressed in the Living Will with your health care providers to make sure your wishes are understood. With both documents, if you include a statement of your preferences regarding your medical treatment, it will provide additional useful guidance.

What are the requirements for signing and witnessing a Living Will?

Because there is not a specific law that governs Living Wills, there are no exact requirements with regard to signatures and witnesses. However, it is recommended that you follow the requirements for signing and witnessing a Health Care Proxy when executing a Living Will.

What if I change my mind?

You should review your Living Will from time to time to ensure that the document you signed still represents your current wishes. You can change or revoke your Living Will by making a new one, destroying it, or simply stating that it is revoked. You should be sure to tell your treatment providers and your family and/or friends that you have revoked your Living Will.

How long is a Living Will valid?

The Living Will should be valid unless and until you revoke it.

Do-Not-Resuscitate (DNR) Orders

What is a Do-Not-Resuscitate (DNR) Order?

Cardiopulmonary resuscitation (CPR) refers to the medical procedures used to restart a person's heart and breathing when the person suffers heart failure. CPR may involve simple efforts such as mouth-to-mouth resuscitation and external chest compression. Advanced CPR may involve electric shock, insertion of a tube to open the patient's airway, injection of medication into the heart and, in extreme cases, open chest heart massage.

A do-not-resuscitate (DNR) order tells medical professionals not to perform CPR. This means that doctors, nurses, and emergency medical personnel will not attempt emergency CPR if the patient's breathing or heartbeat stops. A DNR order is only a decision about CPR and does not relate to any other treatment

Can I request a DNR Order?

Yes. All adult patients can request a DNR order.

If you have not requested a DNR order and have not appointed a health care agent to decide for you, a family member or close friend can consent to a DNR order when you are terminally ill, permanently unconscious, CPR would not work (would be medically futile), or CPR would impose an extraordinary burden on you given your medical condition and the expected outcome of CPR. Anyone deciding for you must base the decision on your wishes, including your religious and moral beliefs, or if your wishes are not known, on your best interests.

How can I make my wishes about DNR known?

During hospitalization, an adult patient may consent to a DNR order verbally or in writing, if two adult witnesses are present. When consent is given verbally, one of the witnesses must be a physician affiliated with the hospital. Prior to hospitalization, consent must be in writing in the presence of two adult witnesses. In addition, the Health Care Proxy law allows you to appoint someone you trust to make decisions about CPR and other treatments if you become unable to decide for yourself.

What if I lose the ability to make decisions about CPR and do not have anyone who can decide for me?

A DNR order can be written if two doctors decide that CPR would not work or if a court approves of the DNR order. It would be best if you discussed your wishes about CPR with your doctor in advance.

What if I change my mind?

You or anyone who consents to a DNR order for you can revoke consent for the order by telling your doctor, nurses, or others of the decision.

ADVANCE DIRECTIVE
FOR MENTAL & PHYSICAL HEALTH CARE

I, _____, hereby make known my desire that, should I lose the capacity to make health care decisions, the following are my instructions regarding consent to or refusal of medical treatment, and if I choose, the designation of my health care agent. I intend that all completed sections of this advance directive be followed.

PART I. HEALTH CARE PROXY

A. Appointment of a Health Care Agent: I hereby appoint the following individual as my health care agent to make any and all health care decisions for me, except to the extent that I state otherwise. This health care proxy shall take effect when and if I become unable to make my own health care decisions.

_____

(Agent's Name)

_____

(Agent's Home Address)

_____

(Agent's Telephone Number)

B. Authority of Health Care Agent: My health care agent may make decisions regarding* (choose ONE):
    ☐   All mental and physical health care
    ☐   Mental health care ONLY
    ☐   Physical health care ONLY
    ☐   The following health care decisions ONLY

_____

_____

_____

*Note: While you may limit your health care agent's decision-making authority, you cannot appoint more than one health care agent at a time. For example, you cannot appoint one health care agent to make only physical health care decisions and another one to make only mental health care decisions.

C. Alternate health care agent *(optional)*: If the person appointed above is unable or unwilling to serve as my health care agent, I hereby appoint the following individual to act as my alternate health care agent.

_____

(Agent's Name)

_____

(Agent's Home Address)

_____

(Agent's Telephone Number)

D. Duration of proxy: Unless I revoke it, this health care proxy shall remain in effect indefinitely, or until the date or conditions stated below. This proxy shall expire (specify date or conditions, if desired):

_____

_____

_____

PART II. STATEMENT OF DESIRES AND INSTRUCTIONS REGARDING MENTAL AND PHYSICAL HEALTH CARE AND TREATMENT

I direct my agent to make health care decisions in accordance with my wishes and limitations as stated in this Advance Directive, or as he or she otherwise knows. If I have not appointed a health care agent, I wish my health care providers to act in accordance with my instructions as stated below.

[Note: Unless your agent knows your wishes about artificial nutrition and hydration (tube feeding), your agent will not be allowed to make decisions about artificial nutrition and hydration.]

A. Special Instructions Regarding My Mental Health Care and Treatment

1. Medications for Psychiatric Treatment: If it is determined that I am not legally capable of consenting to or refusing medications relating to my mental health treatment, my wishes are as follows:

   (a) I prefer to be given the following medications:

   Medication Name:

   _____

   _____

   _____

(b) I prefer not to be given the following medications, for the following reasons:

Medication: _____

Reason: _____

Medication: _____

Reason: _____

2. Treatment Facilities: If my psychiatric condition is serious enough to require 24-hour care and I have no physical conditions that require immediate access to emergency medical care the following are my instructions.

(a) I would prefer to receive this care at the following hospitals or programs/facilities, if possible:

_____

_____

_____

_____

(b) I prefer not to receive this care at the following hospitals or programs/facilities, if possible, for the reasons I have listed:

Facility: _____

Reason: _____

Facility: _____

Reason: _____

(c) My choice of treating physician, if possible, is:

_____ Phone # _____

OR

_____ Phone # _____

OR

_____ Phone # _____

(d) I do not wish to be treated by the following physicians, if possible, for the reasons stated:

Dr.'s Name: _____

Reason _____

Dr.'s Name: _____

Reason _____

3. Additional Instructions Regarding My Mental Health Care (e.g., individual psycho-therapy, group therapy, electroconvulsive therapy, self-help services, research):

_____

_____

_____

B. Special Instructions Regarding My Physical Health Care and Treatment

1. These wishes should be followed if: *(choose one of the following)*

_____ I am terminally ill, in a coma or unconscious, or in an irreversible condition from which there is no reasonable hope of recovery, OR

_____ the following medical conditions exist:

_____

_____

_____

2. Medical treatment about which you may wish to give your agent or health care providers special instructions include the following treatments. Write instructions for each treatment you choose on the lines provided.

Artificial respiration: _____

_____

Artificial nutrition and hydration: _____

_____

Cardiopulmonary resuscitation: _____

_____

Antibiotics: _____

_____

Dialysis: _____

_____

Transplantation: _____

_____

Blood transfusions or blood products: _____

_____

Invasive diagnostic tests: _____

_____

Other physical health treatments or medications: _____

_____

_____

_____

Additional instructions regarding physical health care and treatment: _____

_____

_____

_____

_____

PART III. IMPORTANT INFORMATION IF I AM HOSPITALIZED

(You may choose to complete this section to provide additional guidance to your health care agent and/or providers.)

I wish to provide the following information regarding my current mental health care and treatment and to state my preferences regarding mental health care and treatment, in the event I am hospitalized. I strongly hope that my stated preferences will be honored to assist me in having more control over my life and to aid in my recovery.

A. My physician and/or psychiatrist's name and address:

_____

_____

_____

B. My outpatient mental health care provider(s):

_____

_____

_____

C. Approaches that help me when I'm having a hard time:

If I am having a hard time, the following approaches have been helpful to me in the past. I would like the staff to try to use these approaches with me:

_____ Voluntary time out in my room	_____ Listening to music
_____ Voluntary timeout in quiet room	_____ Reading
_____ Sitting by staff	_____ Watching TV
_____ Talking with a peer	_____ Pacing the halls
_____ Having my hand held	_____ Calling a friend
_____ Going for a walk	_____ Calling my therapist
_____ Punching a pillow	_____ Pounding some clay
_____ Writing in a journal	_____ Deep breathing exercises
_____ Lying down	_____ Taking a shower
_____ Talking with staff	_____ Exercising

Other: _____

_____

_____

_____

D. Actions that are not helpful:

In the past, I have found that the following actions make me feel worse. I prefer that staff not do the following:

_____

_____

_____

E. Preferences regarding physical contact by staff:

_____

_____

F. Hospital and community treatment programs (outpatient clinics, community-based residential facilities, community support programs, self-help programs, etc.)

Upon my discharge, if possible, I would like to receive treatment from the following hospitals and community treatment programs:

_____

_____

_____

Upon my discharge, if possible, I do not want to receive treatment from the following hospitals or community treatment programs for the reasons listed:

Provider: _____

_____

Reason: _____

_____

Provider: _____

_____

Reason: _____

_____

G. Additional preferences regarding my mental health care and treatment:

_____

_____

_____

_____

_____

PART IV. SIGNATURE AND STATEMENT OF WITNESSES

A. Your Signature: _____

    Address: _____

    Date: _____

B. Statement by Witnesses (must be age 18 or older)

    I declare that the person who signed this document is personally known to me and appears to be of sound mind and acting of his or her own free will. He or she signed (or asked another to sign for him or her) this document in my presence.

Witness 1: _____
              (Name)

              _____
              (Address)

Witness 2: _____
              (Name)

              _____
              (Address)

Sample Health Care Proxy

HEALTH CARE PROXY

(1) I, _____

hereby appoint _____

as my health care agent to make any and all health care decisions for me, except to the extent that I state otherwise. This proxy shall take effect when and if I become unable to make my own health care decisions.

(2) Optional instructions: I direct my agent to make health care decisions in accord with my wishes and limitations as stated below, or as he or she otherwise knows. (Attach additional pages if necessary.)

_____

_____

_____

_____

_____

(Unless your agent knows your wishes about artificial nutrition and hydration [feeding tubes], your agent will not be allowed to make decisions about artificial nutrition and hydration. See instructions for samples of language you could use.)

(3) Name of substitute or fill-in agent if the person I appoint above is unable, unwilling, or unavailable to act as my health care agent.

_____

_____

_____

(4) Unless I revoke it, this proxy shall remain in effect indefinitely, or until the date or conditions stated below. This proxy shall expire (specific date or conditions, if desired):

_____

_____

_____

(5) Signature _____

_____

Address _____

_____

_____

Date _____

Statement by Witnesses (must be 18 or older)

I declare that the person who signed this document is personally known to me and appears to be of sound mind and acting of his or her own free will. He or she signed (or asked another to sign for him or her) this document in my presence.

Witness 1

_____

Address

_____

_____

Witness 2

_____

Address

_____

_____

(Name, Home address, and Telephone number)

Call your state health department with questions.

Notes

Preface

1. Bernabei R, Gambassi G, Lapane K, et al. Management of pain in elderly patients with cancer. JAMA 1998;279:1877–1882.
2. Foley KM. Testimony before Senate Committee on the Judiciary on H.R. 2260 (106th Congress), Pain Relief Promotion Act, April 25, 2000. Available at: http://judiciary.senate.gov/oldsite/42520kf.htm.

Chapter 1

1. Staats PS. Pain, depression and survival. Am Fam Physician 1999;60:38. Available at: http://www.aafp.org/afp/990700ap/editorials.html.
2. American Cancer Society. Cancer facts and figures. Atlanta: ACS; 2003. p. 1. Available at: http://www.cancer.org/docroot/STT/content/ STT_1x_Cancer_Facts__Figures_2003.asp. Associated Press. UN Reports Cancer Rates to Soar Worldwide. April 3, 2003.
3. American Cancer Society. Cancer Facts and Figures. Atlanta: ACS; 2003. p. 1–3. Available at: http://www.cancer.org/docroot/STT/content/ STT_1x_Cancer_Facts__Figures_2003.asp.
4. Texas Cancer Pain Initiative. Available at: http://www.texascancercouncil.org/tcpi/problem.html.
5. American Cancer Society. Cancer facts and figures. Atlanta: ACS; 2003. p. 2. Available at: http://www.cancer.org/docroot/STT/content/ STT_1x_Cancer_Facts__Figures_2003.asp.

6. Stephenson J. Researchers hope techno-teaching will improve cancer pain treatment. JAMA 1996;276:1783.

7. Bernabei R, Gambassi G, Lapane K, et al. Management of pain in elderly patients with cancer. JAMA 1998;279:1877–82. Foley KM. Testimony before Senate Committee on the Judiciary on H.R. 2260 (106th Congress), Pain Relief Promotion Act, April 25, 2000.
Available at: http://judiciary.senate.gov/oldsite/42520kf.htm.

8. Bernabei R, Gambassi G, Lapane K, et al. Management of pain in elderly patients with cancer, JAMA 1998;279:1877–82. Foley KM. Testimony before Senate Committee on the Judiciary on H.R. 2260 (106th Congress), Pain Relief Promotion Act, April 25, 2000.
Available at: http://judiciary.senate.gov/oldsite/42520kf.htm.

9. Foley KM. Testimony before Senate Committee on the Judiciary on H.R. 2260 (106th Congress), Pain Relief Promotion Act, April 25, 2000.
Available at: http://judiciary.senate.gov/oldsite/42520kf.htm.

10. Cleeland CS, Gonin H, Baez L, Loehrer P, Pandya K. Pain and pain treatment in minority outpatients with metastatic cancer. Ann Intern Med 1997;127:813–6.

11. Pain: must people suffer? Harvard Mahoney Neuroscience Institute Letter 1995 4(3). Available at: http://www.med.harvard.edu/publications/On_The_Brain/Volume4/Number3/Pain.html. World Health Organization. Cancer pain relief, with a guide to opioid availability. 2nd ed. Geneva: WHO; 1996.

12. World Health Organization. Cancer pain relief and palliative care. Technical Report Series 804. Geneva: WHO; 1990. (Revised in 1996.)

13. Joranson DE, Ryan KM, Gibson AM, Dahl JL. Trends in medical use and abuse of opioid analgesics. JAMA 2000;283(13):1710–4.

14. American Cancer Society. New guidelines aim to improve communication, patient care. 2001 Apr 3.
Available at: http://www.cancer.org/docroot/NWS/content/NWS_1_1x_New_Guidelines_Aim_To_Improve_Communication__Patient_Care.asp.

Chapter 12

1. Redd WH, Montgomery GH, DuHamel KN. Behavioral intervention for cancer treatment side effects. J Natl Cancer Inst 2001;93(11):810.

2. Peterson C, Seligman ME, Vaillant GE. Pessimistic explanatory style is a risk factor for physical illness: a thirty-five-year longitudinal study. J Pers Soc Psychol 1988;55:23–7. Schulz R, Bookwala J, Knapp J, et al. Pessimism and mortality in young and old recurrent cancer patients. Paper presented at the American Psychosomatic Society annual meetings, 1994 Apr 15, Boston. Seligman M. Optimism, pessimism and mortality. Mayo Clin Proc 2000;75:133–43.

3. Longer-lasting pain relief—without pills. Facts of Life: Issue Briefings for Health Reporters 1998;3(6), Center for the Advancement of Health.
Available at: http://www.cfah.org/factsoflife/vol3no6.cfm.

4. Keefe FJ. (1996). Cognitive behavioral therapy for managing pain. Clinical Psychologist 1996;49(3):4–5.

5. Blanchard EB. Psychological treatment of benign headache disorders. J Consult Clin Psychol 1992;60(4):537–51. Blanchard EB, Diamond S. Psychological treatment of benign headache disorders. Wheat Ridge (CO): Association for Applied Psychophysiology and Biofeedback; 1996.

6. Maclean CRK, Walton KG, Wenneberg SR, Levitsky DK, Mandarino JV, Waziri R, Schneider RH. Altered responses of cortisol, GH, TSH, and testosterone to acute stress after four months' practice of Transcendental Meditation (TM). Ann N Y Acad Sci. 1994;746:381–4.

7. See, for example: http://content.health.msn.com/content/article/11/1668_50519. Eckert RM, Understanding anticipatory nausea, Onc Nurs Forum 2001;28(10). Molassiotis A. A pilot study of the use of progressive muscle relaxation training in the management of post-chemotherapy nausea and vomiting. Eur J Cancer Care 2000;9(4):230–4. Barnett RA. Working up an appetite. Touch 2000;2(2).

8. Spiegel D, Moore R. Imagery and hypnosis in the treatment of cancer patients. Oncology (Huntingt) 1997;11:1179–89; discussion 1189–95.

9. Marchioro G, Azzarello G, Viviani F, Barbato F, Pavanetto M, Rosetti F, Pappagallo GL, Vinante O. Hypnosis in the treatment of anticipatory nausea and vomiting in patients receiving cancer chemotherapy. Oncology 2000;59(2):100–4.

10. Liossi C, Hatira P. Clinical hypnosis in the alleviation of procedure-related pain in pediatric oncology patients. Int J Clin Exp Hypn 2003;51(1):4–28.

11. National Institute of Nursing Research News Release. Relaxation and music significantly reduce patients' postoperative pain. 1999 May 7. Bethesda, Maryland. Available at: http://www.nih.gov/ninr/news-info/press/relaxation.html.

12. Syed IB. Music therapy. Islamic Research Foundation International, Inc. Available at: http://www.irfi.org/Islamic%20Articles%20Folder/music_therapy.htm.

13. Magill L. The use of music therapy to address the suffering in advanced cancer pain. J Palliat Care 2001;17(3):167–72. Cassileth, BR. Music from the soul, for the body. 2000 Sep 4. Available at: http://www.mult-sclerosis.org/news/Sep2000/MusicTherapy.html.

14. Martinez M. Acupuncture helps ease symptoms of many chronic illnesses. Associated Press Newswire 2000 Nov 22.

15. Acupuncture curbs chemo nausea. Fam Pract News 1997;15 Jul.

16. Acupuncture reduces nausea, pain of breast surgery. Duke University Medical Center news release 2001; Oct 15. Available at: http://dukemednews.duke.edu/news/article.php?id=4698.

17. Johnstone PA, Polston GR, Niemtzow RC, Martin PJ. Integration of acupuncture into the oncology clinic. Palliat Med 2002;16(3):235–9.

Chapter 14

1. Derogatis LR, Morrow GR, Fetting J, Penman D, Piasetsky S, Schmale AM, Henrichs M, Carnicke CL Jr. The prevalence of psychiatric disorders among cancer patients. JAMA 1983;249(6):751–7.

2. National Cancer Institute. Depression PDQ. 2002 Aug. Available at: http://cancer.gov/cancerinfo/pdq/supportivecare/depression/healthprofessional.
3. Spiegel D, Bloom J. Group therapy and hypnosis reduce metastatic breast carcinoma pain. Psychosom Med 1983;45(4):333–9.
4. Seligman M. Learned Optimism. New York: Pocket Books; 1990.
5. Chochinov HM et al. Will to live in the terminally ill. Lancet 1999;354(9181):816–9.
6. Daly R. Pioneers in palliative care remaining cool to euthanasia—dying a natural process, sedation can treat worst pain, they say. Toronto Star; 2000 Sep. 27.

Chapter 15

1. World Health Organization. Cancer pain relief and palliative care. World Health Organization. Geneva, 1990 (WHO Technical Report Series, No. 804).
2. David J. Roy. "Need They Sleep Before They Die?" Journal of Palliative Care 6:3, 1990, 3–4.

Glossary 1

Pain and Cancer Terms

absolute alcohol, phenol—Also called neurolytic drugs. Medicines usually injected for destructive or neurolytic blocks; intended to relieve certain pains for a period of months. They may injure all nerves indiscriminately, so they must be used carefully to avoid complications.

a.c.—An abbreviation for instructions to take a medication before meals.

acute pain—Pain of short duration that directly follows an injury (or surgery); it's usually sharp and its source is usually easy to identify. Its features are in contrast to those of chronic pain (*see* **chronic pain**).

addiction—The psychological craving for a drug; the need to obtain and use a drug for nonmedical reasons completely overwhelms and controls the addict's life, and persists despite the presence or threat of physiologic or psychological harm. Extremely rare in the cancer patient, but still feared by patient and doctor alike.

adjuvant medications—Also known as co-analgesics. Usually medications developed for purposes other than pain relief but are later recognized to control specific types of pain. They are usually mechanism-specific (that is, they are not effective for all types of pain), and often are only effective after regular use for a period of weeks has been established; also refers to medications prescribed to help enhance the effects of painkillers or to relieve the side effects of medications

alopecia—A condition in which one's hair fall out. Sometimes associated with chemotherapy or radiation therapy.

analgesics—Medications that relieve pain.

anesthesia dolorosa—A painful numbness occurring in a small proportion of patients after a destructive nerve block, especially after peripheral nerve blocks.

anorexia—A condition in which one has a reduced appetite.

antiemetic—Any drug that helps relieve vomiting and nausea.

asthenia—Weakness.

ATC—A directive to take a medication at scheduled intervals, around-the-clock, as opposed to as-needed (prn).

b.i.d.—An abbreviation for instructions to take a medication two times over a twenty-four-hour day, usually implying at regularly spaced intervals (about every twelve hours).

biopsy—A procedure to remove a small bit of tissue from a growth to have it analyzed to determine whether the growth is harmless or cancerous. May be done as a surgical procedure or with a needle. The patient may need general anesthesia or just local anesthesia depending on its location.

bolus—The same as an escape or rescue dose: an extra dose of medication to take as needed to relieve pain that breaks through despite medication given at regularly scheduled intervals.

breakthrough pain—Brief but frequently severe flare of pain that a person may experience despite taking pain medication regularly. *See* **escape dose**.

bradycardia—A condition in which the heart beats slowly, under 50–60 beats per minute. Opposite of tachycardia.

cachexia—Significant weight loss; usually but not always accompanied by loss of appetite and reduced oral intake.

cancer—Any of one hundred or so different diseases in which a mass of abnormal tissue grows uncontrollably and has the potential to spread throughout the body.

catheter—A Foley catheter is a small tube passed into the bladder to make urination easier; an epidural or spinal catheter is a tiny tube inserted into the spinal canal between two bones of the back, passed either through a needle or under minor surgery, with or without X-ray (fluoroscopic) guidance. It is required to provide a means to repeatedly administer intraspinal morphine and other pain killers.

ceiling dose—The dose above which a drug will do no further good; aspirin and acetaminophen, for example, have ceiling, or maximum doses; morphine and other opioids do not. Ceiling doses differ from patient to patient and can even increase or decrease in the same patient over time.

central nerve block—An injection within the spinal canal, between two of the spinal bones. May be an epidural or spinal (also called intrathecal or subarachnoid) injection. The dura is a membrane that forms a sac containing the spinal cord and the cerebrospinal fluid (CSF) in which it floats. An epidural injection deposits medication in the epidural space, just outside the dural sac. In a spinal injection, the dura is pierced and an injected medication mixes freely with the CSF.

chemotherapy—Cancer treatment with toxic drugs (including hormones) administered usually through needles or orally.

chronic pain—Established pain that has persisted despite diagnostic tests and treatment, usually for longer than three to six months or so; having already been investigated, the pain has outlived its warning function and can only be harmful. Rather than being sharp and easy to locate, chronic pain tends to be dull and achy and often can't be pinpointed. Treating this kind of pain often needs a combination of medical and psychological approaches.

cingulotomy – One of the least risky forms of psychosurgery or functional neurosurgery, which aims to pinpoint and destroys a small part of the brain (with minimal if any surgery) to relieve pain, often by interfering with the interpretation of its meaning. The risk of personality change remains a formidable barrier to more widespread use. Much safer than the most extreme treatment of this type, frontal lobotomy.

controlled-release morphine—Also referred to as sustained-release, extended-release, or long-acting morphine. A morphine preparation specially formulated to deliver eight to twelve hours of steady pain relief. Use is associated with a reduction in wide swings of drug blood levels, making this and similar treatments (administered around-the-clock) a cornerstone of treatment. A controlled-release formulation of oxycodone (OxyContin) is an alternative, and more controlled-release opioids are on the horizon. Most are in tablet form and should not be broken, crushed, or chewed; a few preparations are available in capsule form and the contents may be sprinkled on applesauce for patients who cannot swallow medication.

debulking—Surgery that reduces the size of a tumor, as opposed to removing the entire tumor. It may render certain tumors more responsive to chemotherapy or radiation.

deep brain stimulation, thalamic stimulation—A procedure in which one or more tiny electrodes are placed within the brain to relieve pain. It is still considered experimental, so the procedure is available in only a limited number of cancer centers.

dependence—A vague term; addiction is regarded as a form of psychological dependence, which is not to be confused with physical dependence, which is a common and natural result of the body growing used to a medication, particularly an opioid such as morphine. If the drug were suddenly stopped, the patient would experience symptoms of withdrawal (also called abstinence syndrome), which are easily avoidable by reducing drug doses gradually, when treatment is no longer needed.

destructive block, neurolytic block, neuroablation—Names for semipermanent nerve blocks, usually performed with alcohol, phenol, extreme heat, or freezing. Pain relief results from the destruction of a portion of the nerve.

diaphoresis—A condition characterized by excessive perspiration.

diagnostic nerve block—A temporary or local anesthetic block (injection) that is performed specifically to help understand the cause of the pain and which nerves are involved in its transmission.

diuretic—A medication that helps the body rid itself of excess fluids. It may help breathing difficulties and swelling. Regular use may also alter blood levels of potassium and sodium, which may be dangerous unless monitored with blood work.

dose titration—Upward and downward adjustments in medication doses usually performed under medical supervision to achieve the optimal balance between favorable medication effects and side effects.

drug receptors—Microscopic sites on the walls of individual cells that recognize specific drugs and which trigger their effects. Receptors for morphine and other opioids are concentrated in discrete parts of the brain (periaqueductal gray) and spinal cord (substantia gelatinosa). Like a lock and key, the receptor recognizes only a specific type of drug based on its unique structure.

dura—The sac or membrane that contains the spinal cord and surrounding spinal fluid (cerebrospinal fluid or CSF).

dysphagia—Difficulty in swallowing.

dysphoria—An unpleasant mental state that can arise from drugs that affect the brain. The opposite of euphoria (a state of elation). May or may not be accompanied by confusion.

dyspnea—Labored breathing.

elixir—An oral solution containing drug, water, and some alcohol. *See* **tincture.**

epidural injection—An injection within the bony vertebral column and spinal canal, but outside the sac (dura) that contains the spinal cord and its surrounding fluid (cerebrospinal fluid or CSF). Temporary or local anesthetic injections are used commonly to treat labor and surgical pain. Steroid injections may be recommended for chronic back pain. Alcohol and phenol are injected occasionally here to achieve an intermediate duration of relief from cancer pain (neurolytic block). *See* **epidural morphine.**

epidural morphine—One type of intraspinal opioid therapy. Morphine (or another opioid) is administered into the epidural space, usually continuously, to induce profound relief with few side effects, which is possible because of the low drug doses needed when medications are administered so close to their sites of action (receptors).

equianalgesic dose— The adjusted dose of one drug that is required to achieve a similar level of pain relief obtained from another drug. Adjustments to achieve an equianalgesic effect are required when switching from one drug to another as well as when using the same drug but switching from one route to another (IV instead of oral, etc); doctors refer to equianalgesic tables to identify the approximate starting dose of the new drug, after which small adjustments (titrations) are made based on reported and observed effects.

escape dose—Also called a rescue dose. *See* **bolus.**

external pump—The type of pump used to give morphine and other pain medications intravenously, subcutaneously, or intraspinally; can be hooked to a temporary or implanted catheter for home use. Usually portable and battery-driven; family can operate it, but it requires supervision by a nurse or doctor.

externalized catheter—A permanent catheter with one end that leaves the skin of the abdomen to be connected to an external pump.

gate control theory of pain—An explanation of how electrical stimulation and other nonpainful stimuli (e.g., heat, massage) can sometimes block or reduce pain.

IM—An abbreviation for intramuscular , i.e., to take a medication by a shot in the muscle.

immediate-release morphine—An opioid that will relieve breakthrough pain rapidly.

infusion—A method of giving pain medication into a vein, subcutaneously or intraspinally via gravity or a mechanical pump rather than pushed in by a syringe.

intraspinal opioid therapy—Pain relief techniques, including epidural and intrathecal/subarachnoid, in which morphine (or other opioid) is given directly near receptors in the spine. Only tiny amounts are needed, and usually pain relief is very good with few side effects.

intrathecal, subarachnoid, or spinal morphine—A procedure in which the drug is mixed with the spinal fluid. Since it is even closer to the receptors, even less pain medication is needed than with the epidural route.

ischemia—The condition in which there is not enough blood getting to the tissue.

IV— The abbreviation for intravenous, i.e., taking medication or nutrition through a tube or injection in the vein.

local anesthetic nerve block—A procedure that relies on a numbing medication to provide temporary pain relief, although more lasting effects sometimes occur just from interrupting the cycle of pain. Analogous to injections performed in a dentist's office with novocaine. However, longer-acting drugs are now more commonly used, such as lidocaine and bupivacaine.

malignancy—A growth of abnormal cells that have been determined to be cancerous, i.e., unless treated, the growth will continue to grow at the expense of healthy cells locally and/or distantly (metastases).

mcg—The abbreviation for microgram, a unit that many medications are measured in. Also abbreviated µg. One-millionth of a gram.

meningitis or epidural abscess—A serious infection near the spine that occasionally occur with intraspinal opioid therapy. Can usually be treated with hospitalization and intravenous antibiotics, but surgery may be needed to remove an infected catheter or to alleviate pressure from a deep infection or collection of blood.

metastasis—The process in which cancer cells spread to other areas of the body. Cancer growths that have spread from their original site are called metastases.

mg—The abbreviation for milligrams, a unit that many medications are measured in. One-thousandth of a gram.

ml—The abbreviation for milliliter, a liquid unit.; ml is the same as cc (cubic centimeter).

myelopathy—A disorder (infection, trauma, etc) involving the spinal cord

myoclonus—Sudden, brief, involuntary jerking movements, usually involving the entire body. A common but harmless side effect of opioid medications that can often be minimized by the addition of clonazepam. In other settings myoclonus may be a sign of an impending seizure or convulsion, and thus should be reported to the treating physician.

narcotics—Commonly used but outmoded term that is essentially the same as opiates or opioids. Use of the term is discouraged in the medical setting because of its historical connection to drug abuse and addiction. *See* **opioids.**

neoplasms—Abnormal growths comprised of cells that are different from normal cells. Neoplasms (meaning "new growths") may be harmless (benign) or cancerous (malignant). When cancerous, the condition is called cancer, a malignancy.

nerve block—A procedure involving an injection near a nerve or group of nerves to produce numbness and/or pain relief. There are many different types of nerve blocks.

neuroablation—*See* **neurolytic drugs**.

neurolytic drugs—Medicines usually used for destructive or neurolytic blocks. They injure all nerves indiscriminately, so they must be used carefully to avoid weakness and even paralysis. Those in common use today include alcohol and phenol.

neuropathic pain— Pain that stems from a damaged nerve and usually is burning, tingling, numbing or itching in character. Often treated with adjuvant analgesics, as well as with opioids.

neuropathy—Damage to nerves; may produce neuropathic pain.

nociception—The process of pain transmission, usually commencing with peripheral pain receptors that transmit impulses to the central nervous system.

nociceptor—A nerve receptor that responds to an injury, initiating signals or impulses that result in pain.

NPO—An abbreviation for instructions to take nothing by mouth, commonly a requirement at least eight hours before surgery. If instructed to remain NPO, ask whether this includes medications with a sip of water.

oncology—The study or science of cancer and its treatment. A person who specializes in the study of cancer is an oncologist. Subspecialties include medical oncology, radiation oncology, and surgical oncology.

opiate, opioids – Narcotic painkillers, the main medications used to relieve moderate to severe pain. A person taking them often develops physiological conditions known as physical dependence and tolerance, which can be easily treated and have nothing to do with addiction, an infrequent outcome of medical use of opioids.

pain threshold—The point at which a sensation or stimuli is perceived to be painful. Pain thresholds differ among individuals and even in the same individual over time.

pain tolerance—How much pain a person is willing or able to endure. Pain tolerance may be lowered by factors such as fatigue, anxiety, fear, depression, boredom, mental isolation, and anger and can be raised by symptom control, sleep, rest, compassion, understanding, medications, and diversions.

palliative care—Care that focuses on the comfort of the patient when a cure is not a realistic goal. Comes from the Latin root meaning "to cloak or cover up"; in the last few years, palliative care has emerged as a new but evolving medical specialty.

parenteral—Medication that is not taken by mouth. Includes alternate routes of medication delivery, such as intravenous, subcutaneous or intramuscular injection.

p.c.—An abbreviation for a directive to take a medication take after meals.

PCA—An abbreviation for patient-controlled analgesia, meaning that the patient may control when to get medication within parameters set by their doctor. Usually refers to a pump system in which the doctor has preprogrammed doses of painkiller.

percutaneous cordotomy—Similar to a nerve block but is usually performed by a neurosurgeon. A needle is advanced between two of the spinal bones directly into the spinal cord, where a small hole is burned. Very effective in relieving pain limited to one side of the body below the midchest level, with a duration of effect typically lasting six to twelve months or more.

peripheral nerve block—An injection of a nerve in the body's periphery, after the nerve has left the spinal cord.

permanent catheter—A more durable catheter implanted under the skin for long-term use; less chance of infection or falling out (migration).

permanent nerve block—Injections of neurolytic substances intended to destroy nerves involved with transmitting pain. There are no truly permanent nerve blocks because even after they are destroyed most nerves will grow back, usually within three to six months, or at most twelve months.

pituitary ablation—An injection of a small amount of alcohol into the pituitary gland to relieve bony pain, especially from breast or prostate cancer. Performed in only a few centers.

PO—An abbreviation for a directive to take a medication by mouth.

PR—An abbreviation for a directive to take a medication by rectum.

PRN—An abbreviation for a directive to take medication as needed, as opposed to at scheduled intervals (around the clock or ATC). Discouraged as the sole means to treat pain, especially when pain is constant.

prognosis—The doctor's determination of what the outcome of an illness will be. As related to cancer, this is an inexact science.

prognostic (predictive) nerve block—A temporary or local anesthetic block that is performed specifically to predict the results of a more permanent nerve block. Determining how much of the pain is relieved, whether there are side effects and if the patient prefers the numbness that comes with most injections versus the pain helps decide whether or not to recommend a more permanent (neurolytic) block.

pruritus—An itching condition; may be a side effect of some opioid medications.

pseudoaddiction—Drug-seeking behavior that is interpreted as a psychological craving for a medication, usually an opioid such as morphine, but which in fact is the result of undermedication and the desire for greater pain relief.

psychosurgery—Surgery in which brain pathways are disrupted so that even though pain persists, it is not bothersome. It has been almost abandoned because of undesirable personality changes and the greater availability and willingness to use pain medications. *See* **cingulotomy**.

q.a.m.—An abbreviation for instructions to take a medication in the morning upon awakening.

q.d.—An abbreviation for instructions to take a medication once each day

q.i.d.—An abbreviation for instructions to take a medication four times over a twenty-four-hour day, usually implying at regularly spaced intervals (about every six hours).

q.3h., q.4h.—An abbreviation for instructions to take a medication every three hours, every four hours, etc.

q.h.s.—An abbreviation for instructions to take a medication before bed.

radiation therapy—A treatment for cancer that uses high-energy beams to kill or shrink tumors. Such therapy is prescribed by a medical specialist, usually a radiation oncologist.

radiofrequency thermoablation, cryoablation—A neuroablative (destructive) block that involves the heating or freezing of the needle tip positioned near a nerve. Used less often than alcohol and phenol.

rescue dose—Also known as an escape dose. *See* **bolus**.

sequential drug trial—Treatment with a series of different analgesics administered over time, undertaken to determine the best medicine for a particular person. Should be conducted prior to trying more invasive treatments, but requires considerable patience and education.

singultus—Hiccoughs. May occur with brain tumors, stomach or chest tumors, and kidney problems.

spinal cord stimulation—An electrode is surgically placed in the epidural space to relieve pain; used mostly for pain due to causes other than cancer.

spinal injection—A needle is advanced through the epidural space and dura into the sac containing the spinal cord and fluid. Also called subarachnoid or intrathecal injection or spinal tap. Local anesthetics are used commonly here for cesarean section and other surgery. Other examples are lumbar puncture, for laboratory analysis of spinal fluid , and myelogram, which involves injecting dye into the spinal canal and which is then imaged with X-rays, both of which are diagnostic procedures. Alcohol and phenol may be injected here in special cases by a qualified doctor (anesthesiologist) to perform a neurolytic block to achieve more lasting relief of specific pain syndromes.

spinal port—Instead of a spinal catheter exiting from the skin of the abdomen, the end of this catheter is attached to a silicone dome left under the skin. A pump is then attached with a tiny needle that is changed weekly.

spinal pump—A special pump (usually computer-controlled) inserted under the skin to deliver morphine and other medications through a permanent (subcutaneously tunneled) catheter. It only needs to be refilled every one to two months, and many versions can be adjusted with a special laptop computer. It is initially very costly and cannot be reused, but care can be very economical over time, so its use is reserved for selected cases.

stat—An abbreviation used in health care settings meaning "immediately."

subcutaneous – Also SC, SQ, or sub-q. Refers to administering medications just below the surface of the skin, which has the advantages of (1) being less painful than a deeper intramuscular injection and (2) circumventing the need for an intravenous (IV) line or catheter. SC injections can be administered as needed or, depending on the circumstances, can be performed through a needle or catheter positioned under the surface of the skin, which requires maintenance but eliminates the need for repeated sticks.

tachycardia—A condition in which the heart beats rapidly. Usually applied to rates faster than 100 beats per minute. Opposite of bradycardia (slow heart beat).

thoracotomy—Surgery involving the chest.

t.i.d.—An abbreviation for instructions to take a medication three times over a twenty-four-hour day, usually implying at regularly spaced intervals (about every eight hours).

temporary catheter—Not everyone gets good relief from intraspinal morphine, so a temporary catheter may be inserted and taped to the back for a trial period of up to a week or so. If someone is very sick, the temporary catheter can be left in indefinitely, although there is some risk of infection.

temporary nerve block—An injection of a local anesthetic. The effect of the medication is usually temporary, although, by interrupting the pain cycle sometimes long lasting pain relief can result after one or several temporary blocks. Sometimes a steroid is added to reduce inflammation around an irritated nerve.

TENS (transcutaneous electrical nerve stimulation) unit—A simple, portable device the size of a beeper; gives gentle shocks to electrodes applied to the skin to relieve pain. It is not usually effective for severe pain. More sophisticated units are now available that also stimulate underlying muscle.

therapeutic nerve block—A nerve block that is not just diagnostic or prognostic, but is intended to provide lasting pain relief.

thrombocytopenia—A low platelet count; may cause bleeding episodes. If present, may increase the risk of bleeding from a nerve block or surgical procedure.

tincture—A solution containing a drug (usually highly concentrated) and a lot of alcohol. *See* **elixir**.

titration—Adjusting the dosage of a medication for a particular patient at a particular time.

tolerance—A condition in which a patient will need larger doses of a drug over time to achieve the same relief. It is an expected effect of using opioids, is manageable, and is totally unrelated to addiction.

Glossary 2

Terms Associated with End-of-Life Issues and Care

Advance care directives (or simply advance directives) are written documents meant to make explicit the conditions under which individuals expect to wish to receive certain treatment or to refuse or discontinue life-sustaining treatment, in the event that they are no longer legally competent to make their own decisions. (See Appendix 4 for specifics.)

A **durable power of attorney** (sometimes referred to as a **health-care proxy**) is a form of advance directive that designates an individual who can make decisions if the dying person is no longer competent to do so. (See Appendix 4 for specifics.)

A **living will** is a form of advance directive that specifies in writing what kinds of treatment are and are not wanted. (See Appendix 4 for specifics.)

Aggressive pain management is an essential component of palliative care intended to provide relief from physical suffering at the end of life.

The **double effect** is a term given to the practice of providing large doses of medication to relieve pain even if the unintended effect of such medication may be to hasten death.

Terminal sedation is the term given to the practice of administering sufficient pain medication to render a dying person who is suffering severe, intractable pain unconscious (i.e. to induce an artificial coma). Generally, artificial nutrition and hydration are also withheld or withdrawn, and the state of unconsciousness is maintained until death occurs.

Assisted suicide refers to the situation in which persons request the help of others, in the form of access to information or means, the means, and/or actual assistance, in order to end their own lives.

Physician-assisted suicide refers to cases in which a physician deliberately and knowingly helps an individual to die (American Association of Suicidology, 1996).

418

Euthanasia generally refers to situations whereby someone intentionally takes a person's life with stated intent to alleviate or prevent perceived suffering (American Association of Suicidology, 1996).

Active euthanasia is the practice of shortening an individual's life by taking a lethal action such as administering a lethal dose of medication with the intent to hasten death. It is illegal in the United States.

Passive euthanasia is an older name given to withholding or withdrawing life-sustaining treatment that could otherwise prolong life. The term is no longer in wide use in the United States.

Voluntary euthanasia occurs when a competent dying individual has given voluntary, informed consent to actions that will result in death.

Nonvoluntary euthanasia occurs when a person who is not currently capable of giving consent to actions that will result in death receives such actions. It applies to situations when death by euthanasia is believed to be consistent with the person's prior wishes.

Involuntary euthanasia occurs in situations in which the euthanasia is carried out without consent or against the will of the recipient. Active euthanasia of all kinds is illegal in the United States, and all involuntary euthanasia, whether passive or active, could lead to charges of homicide.

Hastened death is an inconsistently defined term meaning to end one's life earlier than would have happened without intervention. Some use it to refer to assisted suicide and euthanasia only. Others, however, include in this category withholding and withdrawing treatment, death caused by aggressive pain management, and voluntary cessation of eating and drinking.

Hospice refers to programs that focus on quality of life for dying persons. The first modern hospice, St. Christopher's Hospice in London, was founded by Dr. Cicely Saunders in 1967. The defining components of the hospice approach are as follows (Lattanzi-Licht & Connor, 1995, p. 145):

- The patients and family are the unit of care.
- A comprehensive, holistic approach is taken to meet the patient's physical, emotional, social, and spiritual needs, including major attention to effective symptom control and pain management.
- Care is provided by an interdisciplinary team, which includes medical supervision and use of volunteers.
- The patient is kept at home or in an inpatient setting with a homelike environment where there is coordination and continuity of care.
- In addition to regularly scheduled home care visits, services are available on a 24-hour, 7 day-a-week, on-call basis.
- The focus of care is on improving the quality of remaining life; that is, on palliative, not curative, measures.
- Bereavement follow-up services are offered to family members in the year after the death of their loved one.

Palliative care refers to the type of care an individual may receive at the end of life after it becomes obvious that no cure is possible. The World Health Organization (1990) stated that good palliative care:

- Affirms life and views dying as a normal process;
- Neither hastens nor postpones death;
- Provides relief from pain and other distressing symptoms;
- Integrates the psychological and spiritual aspects of patient care;

- Offers a support system to help patients live as actively as possible until death; offers a support system to help family members cope during a patient's illness and during their own bereavement.

The **Patient Self-Determination Act** (Omnibus Budget Reconciliation Act, 1990) is a bill passed by Congress that requires all hospitals, HMO's, hospice, and extended care nursing homes participating in Medicare or Medicaid to ask all adult inpatients if they have advance directives, to document their answers, and to provide information on related state laws and hospital policies.

Withholding or withdrawing life-sustaining treatment is an ethically and legally accepted practice that may be specified in advance care directives. It permits patients to forego or terminate life-sustaining equipment such as ventilators, dialysis machines, feeding tubes for artificial nutrition and intravenous fluids for hydration, and the sophisticated technology of the intensive care unit. In addition, it allows for aggressive treatments to be foregone or terminated (e.g. chemotherapy or radiation therapy except for comfort care, antibiotics, certain anti-seizure medications, or anti-inflammatory agents that control brain swelling).

The **Do Not Resuscitate** request is a form of withholding life-sustaining treatment that requires that no attempt be made to revive a person who has died.

Voluntary cessation of eating and drinking, sometimes referred to as voluntary stopping of eating and drinking, is a form of withholding or withdrawing life-sustaining treatment. Some individuals near the end of life who wish to die several days to a few weeks sooner than would happen naturally may choose it. During this time palliative care may be provided to keep the person comfortable during the time it takes for death to occur from the underlying disease (Miller & Meier, 1998).

Selected Bibliography

Part I

Agency for Health Care Policy and Research. Management of Cancer Pain Guideline Panel: Management of Cancer Pain. U.S. Dept. of Health and Human Services, Clinical Practice Guideline 9, AHCPR Publication 94-0592, Rockville, Md., 1994.

Agency for Health Care Policy and Research. *Managing Cancer Pain.* AHCPR Publication No. 94-0595, March 1994.

Agency for Healthcare Research and Quality. *Surprisingly large gaps found in cancer pain research.* Press release, February 28, 2001, Rockville, MD. Available at http://www.ahrq.gov/news/press/pr2001/canpainpr.htm.

AHRQ. *Management of cancer pain.* Summary, Evidence Report/Technology Assessment: Number 35. AHRQ Publication No. 01-E033, January 2001. Agency for Healthcare Research and Quality, Rockville, MD. Available at http://www.ahrq.gov/clinic/canpainsum.htm.

American Academy of Pain Management (AAPM) and the American Pain Society. "The use of opioids for the treatment of chronic pain." Consensus Statement. 1997.

American Cancer Society. "Cancer facts and figures 2003." Atlanta, Georgia. Available at http://www.cancer.org/docroot/STT/content/ STT_1x_Cancer_Facts__Figures_2003.asp.

American Cancer Society, "New guidelines aim to improve communication, patient care." April 3, 2001. Available at http://www.cancer.org/docroot/ nws/content/nws_1_1x_new_guidelines_aim_to_improve_ communication__patient_care.asp.

American Medical Association. "Promoting pain relief and preventing abuse of pain medications: A critical balancing act." Nov. 7, 2001. Available at http://www.ama-assn.org/ama/pub/article/1617-5459.html.

American Society of Clinical Oncology. "Cancer pain assessment and treatment curriculum guidelines." *J Clin Oncol* 10:1976–1982, 1992.

ASAM, "Public policy statement on the rights and responsibilities of physicians in the use of opioids for the treatment of pain," April 16, 1997.

Associated Press. "U.N. reports cancer rates to soar worldwide." April 3, 2003.

BBC News Online Cancer pain relief drive launched Tuesday, 21 November, 2000. Available at http://news.bbc.co.uk/hi/english/health/newsid_1032000/1032265.stm.

Bernabei R, Gambassi G, Lapane K, et al. "Management of pain in elderly patients with cancer." *JAMA* 279:1877–1882, 1998.

Burt, RA. "The Supreme Court speaks—not assisted suicide but a constitutional right to palliative care." *N Engl J Med* 337:1234–1236, 1997.

"Cancer pain facts." Available at http://www.cancerbackpain.com/cancer3.html.

"Cancer pain and chronic pain questions and answers." Available at http://www.cancerbackpain.com/cancer2.html.

Cassel EJ. "The nature of suffering and the goals of medicine." *N Engl J Med* 306, 11:639–645, 1982.

Cherny NI, et al. "Opioid pharmacology in the management of cancer pain: A survey of strategies used by pain physicians for the selection of analgesic drugs and routes of administration." *Cancer* 76:1283, 1995.

Cleeland CS. "Barriers to the management of cancer pain." *Oncology*; 1 (2 suppl.):19–26, 1987.

Cleeland CS, Syrjala KL. "How to assess cancer pain." In *Pain assessment*, ed. D Turk, R Melzack. New York: Guilford Press; 360–387, 1992.

Cleeland CS. "Factors influencing physician management of cancer pain." *Cancer* 58, 3:796–800, 1986.

Cleeland CS, Gonin R, Hatfield A, et al. "Pain and its treatment in outpatients with metastatic cancer." *N Engl J Med* 330:592–596, 1994.

Cleeland CS, Gonin H, Baez L, Loehrer P, Pandya K. "Pain and pain treatment in minority outpatients with metastatic cancer." *Ann Intern Med* 127:813–816,1997.

Cleeland CS. "Undertreatment of cancer pain in elderly patients." (Editorial) *JAMA* 279, 23:1914, June 17, 1998.

"Failure to ease pain brings large jury award." *Critical Care Alert* 9, 7:84, Oct 2001.

Foley KM. "Advances in cancer pain." *Arch Neurol* 56:413, 1999.

Foley KM, Hendin H. "Don't ask don't tell." *The Oregon Report* 29, 3:37–42, 1999.

Foley KM. "Competent care for the dying instead of physician-assisted suicide." *NEJM* 336:54–58, 1997.

Foley KM. "Controlling cancer pain." Available at http://www.hosppract.com/issues/2000/04/foley.htm.

Foley KM. "Management of cancer pain." In *Cancer: Principles and Practice of Oncology, 5th ed.*, ed. DeVita VT, Hellman S, Rosenberg SA, 2807–2841. Lippincott-Raven, Philadelphia, 1997.

Foley KM. "The relationship of pain and symptom management to patient requests for physician-assisted suicide." *JPSM* 6:289–297, 1991.

Foley KM. "H.R. 2260, Pain Relief Promotion Act, " Testimony before Senate Committee on the Judiciary. April 25, 2000. Available at http://judiciary.senate.gov/oldsite/42520kf.htm.

Freeman HP, Payne RP. "Racial injustice in health care." *NEJM* 342, 14:1045–1047, 2000.

Hill CS Jr. "When will adequate pain treatment be the norm?" *JAMA* 274, 23:1881–1882, December 20, 1995.

Hill CS Jr. "The barriers to adequate pain management with opioid analgesics." *Semin Oncol* 20 (suppl 1):1–5, 1993.

"Ignorance or incompetence leave cancer patients in pain." *Cancer Weekly Plus* 18(1), November 18, 1996.

Jacox A, Carr DB, Payne R, et al. "Management of cancer pain. Clinical practice guideline." Agency for Health Care Policy and Research. 257, 1994 (AHCPR publication no. 94-0592). No. 9. Rockville, MD.

Joranson DE, Ryan KM, Gibson AM, Dahl JL. "Trends in medical use and abuse of opioid analgesics." *JAMA* 283, 13:1710–1714, April 5, 2000.

"Living with cancer but not with the pain (Reports on failures to provide pain relief to cancer patients)" *Harvard Health Letter* 23, 12:6–12, October 1998.

Lindgren M. "Cancer patients die painfully." *Cancer Weekly Plus,* April 19, 1999.

Lindgren M. "Late-stage cancer patients may suffer from physicians' 'opiophobia.'" *Cancer Weekly Plus* September 27, 1999.

Lindgren M, Reidenberg M. "Poor Pain Assessment a Barrier to Good Pain Management." *Cancer Weekly Plus,* August 9, 1999.

Lynn J, Harrold J. *Handbook for mortals: guidance for people facing serious illness.* New York: Oxford University Press, 1999.

Marble M. "Physicians in outpatient oncology practice fail to identify or treat pain." *Cancer Weekly,* March 20, 2001.

Mayor S. "Cancer pain still undertreated." *British Medical Journal* 321, i7272:1309, November 25, 2000.

McGrath PA, ed. "Pain in children: nature, assessment, and treatment." New York: Guilford Press, 1990.

McGrath PA, de Veber LL, Hearn MT. "Multidimensional pain assessment in children." In Fields HL, Dubner R, Cervero F, ed., *Proceedings of the Fourth World Congress on Pain, Seattle. Vol. 9. Advances in pain research and therapy.* New York: Raven Press, Ltd.; 387–393, 1985.

McGrath PJ, Unruh AM. *Pain in children and adolescents.* New York: Elsevier Science Publishers, 1987.

McQuay H. "Opioids in pain management." *Lancet* 353:2229–2232, 1999.

Melzack R. "The tragedy of needless pain." *Sci Am* 262, 2:27–33, 1990.

Miaskowski C, Dodd MJ, West C, Paul S, Tripathy D, Koo P, Schumacher K. "Lack of adherence with the analgesic regimen: a significant barrier to effective cancer pain management." *J Clin Oncol* 19:4275–4279, 2001.

Morrison SR, Wallenstein S, Natale DK, Senzel RS, Huang LL. "We don't carry that—failure of pharmacies in predominantly nonwhite neighborhoods to stock opioid analgesics." *NEJM* 342, 14:1023–1026, 2000.

National Comprehensive Cancer Network (NCCN) and the American Cancer Society. *Cancer pain treatment guidelines for patients.* Available at http://www.nccn.org/patient_guidelines/pain_cancer/pain/glossary.htm. *How is cancer pain treated?* Available at http://www.nccn.org/patient_guidelines/pain_cancer/pain/8_pain-treated.htm

National Institutes of Health and National Cancer Institute. *Get relief from cancer pain*, adapted from *Cancer pain relief*, developed by P Kedziera, MH Levy. NIH Publication No. 94-3735, May 1994. Available at http://cancernet.nci.nih.gov/clinpdq/fulltext/GET_RELIEF_FROM_CANCER_PAIN.html.

"Pain—a conversation about cancer pain." *Harvard Women's Health Watch* 8, 9: May 2001.

"Pain: must people suffer?" *The Harvard Mahoney Neuroscience Institute* 4 (Summer 1995). Available at http://www.med.harvard.edu/publications/On_The_Brain/Volume4/Number3/Pain.html.

"Patient-reported pain has prognostic significance." *Cancer Weekly Plus,* March 15, 1999.

Rich B. "A physician's legal duty to relieve suffering." *The Western Journal of Medicine* 175, 3:151, September 2001.

Staats PS. "Pain, depression and survival." *American Family Physician* 60:38, July 1999. Available at http://www.aafp.org/afp/990700ap/editorials.html.

Stephenson J. "Researchers hope techno-teaching will improve cancer pain treatment." *Journal of the American Medical Society* 276:1783, 1996.

Stevens B. "Pain assessment in children—birth through adolescence." *Child Adolesc Psychiatr Clin N Am* 6, 4:725–744, 1997.

Twycross RG. *Pain relief in advanced cancer*. Edinburgh: Churchill Livingstone, 1994.

Twycross RG. *Therapeutics in terminal cancer*, 3rd ed. Oxford: Radcliffe Medical Press, 1995.

"UCSD Cancer Center launches pain relief unit." February 3, 2000. Available at http://ucsdnews.ucsd.edu/newsrel/health/PainNR2.htm.

U.S. Department of Health and Human Services. *Management of cancer pain*. Rockville, MD, 1994 (Clinical Practice Guideline, No. 9).

World Health Organization. *Cancer pain relief and palliative care*. WHO Technical Report Series, No. 804. Geneva: WHO, 1990.

World Health Organization. *Cancer pain relief and palliative care in children*. Geneva: WHO, 1998.

World Health Organization. *Cancer pain relief, second edition, with a guide to opioid availability*. Geneva: WHO, 1996.

Zech D, Grond S, Lynch J, et al. "Validation of World Health Organization guidelines for cancer pain relief: a 10-year prospective study." *Pain* 63,1:65–76, 1995.

Part II

Abrahm J. "Pain management for dying patients." *Post Graduate Medicine* 110, 2:99, August 2001.

Abrahm J. *A physician's guide to pain and symptom management in cancer patients*. Baltimore: Johns Hopkins University Press, 2000.

"Adjuvant analgesics: drugs that may not be officially classified as 'pain medicines' but are used for pain." University of Iowa College of Nursing. Available at http://coninfo.nursing.uiowa.edu/sites/pedspain/Adjuvants/index.htm.

Baines MJ. "ABC of palliative care. Nausea, vomiting, and intestinal obstruction." *BMJ* 315:1148–1150, 1997.

Body JJ, Bartl R, Burckhardt P, et al. "Current use of bisphosphonates in oncology. International Bone and Cancer Study Group." *J Clin Oncol* 16, 12:3890–3899,1998.

Berger AM, Portenoy RK, Weissman DE, eds. *Principles and practice of supportive oncology.* Philadelphia: Lippincott-Raven, 477–495, 1998.

Cherny NJ. "The management of cancer pain." *CA* 50, 2:70, March 2000.

Cherny NJ, Chang V, Frager G, et al. "Opioid pharmacotherapy in the management of cancer pain: a survey of strategies used by pain physicians for the selection of analgesic drugs and routes of administration." *Cancer* 76:1283–1293, 1995.

Christie JM, Simmonds M, Patt R, et al. "Dose titration, multicenter study of oral transmucosal fentanyl citrate for the treatment of breakthrough pain in cancer patients using transdermal fentanyl for persistent pain." *J Clinical Oncology* 16:2238–2246, 1998.

Foley KM. "Management of cancer pain." In: DeVita VT Jr., Hellman S, Rosenberg SA, eds. *Cancer: principles and practice of oncology.* 5th ed. Philadelphia: Lippincott, 2807–2841, 1997.

Hawkey CJ. "COX-2 inhibitors." *Lancet* 353:307–314, 1999.

Heiskanen T, Kalso E. "Controlled-release oxycodone and morphine in cancer related pain." *Pain* 73:37–45, 1997.

Jacox A, Carr DB, Payne R, et al. *Management of cancer pain.* Clinical practice guideline no. 9. Rockville, Md.: Agency for Health Care Policy and Research, US Department of Health and Human Services, 1994:52; AHCPR publication No. 94-0592.

Jeal W, Benfield P. "Transdermal fentanyl. A review of its pharmacological properties and therapeutic efficacy in pain control." *Drugs* 53:109–138, 1997.

Lichter I. "Nausea and vomiting in patients with cancer." *Hematol Oncol Clin North Am* 10:207–220,1996.

"Marijuana Use in Supportive Care for Cancer Patients." *Marijuana and Medicine: Assessing the Science Base*, 2000. Institute of Medicine (IOM), part of the National Academy of Sciences. Washington, D.C.: National Academy Press. Available at http://pompeii.nap.edu/books/0309071550/html/index.html.

McQuay H, Carroll D, Jadad AR, et al. "Anticonvulsant drugs for management of pain: A systematic review." *BMJ* 311:1047–1052,1995.

McQuay HJ, Tramer M, Nye BA, et al. "A systematic review of antidepressants in neuropathic pain." *Pain* 68:217–227,1996.

Orentlicher D. " The Supreme Court and physician-assisted suicide—rejecting assisted suicide but embracing euthanasia." *N Engl J Med* 337:1236–1239,1997.

Patt RB, Proper G, Reddy S. "The neuroleptics as adjuvant analgesics." *J Pain Symptom Manage* 9:446–453, 1994.

Patt RB, ed. *Cancer pain.* Philadelphia: Lippincott, 1993.

Patt RB. "Cancer pain." In Burchiel KJ, ed., *Surgical management of pain.* New York: Thieme, 469–484, 2002.

Patt RB. "Cancer pain management: An essential component of comprehensive cancer care." In Rubin P, ed., *Clinical oncology: a multidisciplinary approach,* 8th ed. New York: Saunders, 864–892, 2001.

Patt RB. "Oncologic pain management." In Abrams SE et al, eds., *The pain clinic manual.* Philadelphia: Lippincott Williams & Wilkins, 293–351, 2000.

Payne R, Patt RB, Hill CS Jr., eds. *Assessment and treatment of cancer pain: progress in pain research and management.* Seattle: ASP Press, 1998.

Portenoy RK, Lesage P. "Management of cancer pain." *Lancet* 353:1695–1700, May 15, 1999.

Portenoy RK. "Oral transmucosal fentanyl citrate (OTFC) for the treatment of breakthrough pain in cancer patients: a controlled dose titration study." *Pain* 79(2&3):303–312,1999.

Ripamonti C, Zecca E, Bruera E. "An update on the clinical use of methadone for cancer pain." *Pain* 70:109–115, 1997.

Schmeler K, Bastin K. "Strontium-89 for symptomatic metastatic prostate cancer to bone: recommendations for hospice patients." *Hosp J* 11:1–10, 1996.

Sykes J, Johnson R, Hanks GW. "ABC of palliative care. Difficult pain problems." *BMJ* 315:867–869, 1997.

Sykes N, Fallon MT, Patt RB, eds. *Cancer Pain.* London: Arnold, 2003.

"Topical Agents." University of Iowa College of Nursing. http://coninfo.nursing.uiowa.edu/sites/pedspain/Topicals/index.htm

Walling AD. "Principles of pain control in cancer patients." *American Family Physician*, 63, 4:765, February 15, 2001.

Watanabe S, Bruera E. "Corticosteroids as adjuvant analgesics." *J Pain Symptom Manage* 9:442–445, 1994.

Part III

"Acupuncture curbs chemo nausea." *Fam. Pract. News,* July 15, 1997.

"Acupuncture Reduces Nausea, Pain of Breast Surgery." Duke University Medical Center News Release. Oct. 15, 2001. Available at http://dukemednews.duke.edu/news/article.php?id=4698.

Arathuzik D. "Effects of cognitive-behavioral strategies on pain in cancer patients." *Cancer Nurs* 17:207–214, 1994.

Barnett RA. "Working up an appetite." *In Touch* 2:(2), March 2000.

Bernabei R, Gambassi G, Lapane K, et al. "Management of pain in elderly patients with cancer." *JAMA* 281:136, 1999.

Blanchard EB. "Psychological treatment of benign headache disorders." *Journal of Consulting and Clinical Psychology* 60:537–551, 1992.

Blanchard, EB, Diamond S. "Psychological treatment of benign headache disorders." Association for Applied Psychophysiology and Biofeedback 1996.

Campbell FA, Tramer MR, Carroll D, Reynolds DJM, Moore RA, McQuay HJ. "Are cannabinoids an effective and safe treatment option in the management of pain? A qualitative systematic review." *British Medical Journal* 323:13–16, 2001. Available at http://www.bmj.com/cgi/content/full/323/7303/13.

"Cancer and Depression." Available at http://www.cancerbackpain.com/cancer4.html.

Cassileth BR. "Music from the soul, for the body." September 4, 2000. Available at http://www.mult-sclerosis.org/news/Sep2000/MusicTherapy.html.

Carnarius, MM. "The smell of sweet success." *Nursing* 96, 24ii–24nn, April 1996.

Cassell E. *The nature of suffering.* New York: Oxford University Press, 2003.

Cavanaugh TA. "The ethics of death-hastening or death-causing palliative analgesic administration to the terminally ill." *JPSM* 12:248–254, 1996.

Chaters, S. "Terminal sedation." 11th International Congress on Care of the Terminally Ill. Montreal, September 10, 1996.

Cherny NI, Coyle N, Foley KM. *Guidelines in the care of the dying cancer patient.* In NI Cherny, KM Foley, eds., *Pain and palliative care.* Philadelphia: Saunders, 235–259, 1996.

Chochinov HM, et al. "Will to live in the terminally ill." *Lancet* 354:816, 1999.

Collins, JJ, Grier HE, Kinney HC, Berd CB. "Control of severe pain in children with terminal malignancy." *J Pediatr* 126, 4:653–657, 1995.

Crawley L, Payne R, Bolden J, Payne T, Washington P, Williams S. "Palliative and end-of-life care in the African American community." *JAMA* 284:2518–2521, 2000.

Daly R. "Pioneers in palliative care remaining cool to euthanasia—dying a natural process, sedation can treat worst pain, they say." *Toronto Star,* September 27, 2000.

Derogatis LR, Morrow GT, Fetting J, Penman D, Piasetsky S, Schmale AM, Henrichs M, Carnicke CL Jr. "The prevalence of psychiatric disorders among cancer patients." *JAMA* 249, 6:751–7, 1983.

Doyle D, Hanks GWC, MacDonald N. "Introduction." In D Doyle, GWC Hanks, N MacDonald, eds., *Oxford Textbook of Palliative Medicine,* 2nd edition. Oxford: Oxford Medical Publications, 1–8, 1998.

Eckert RM. "Understanding anticipatory nausea." *Oncology Nursing Forum Continuing Education* 28(10), November/December 2001. Available at http://www.ons.org.

"End-of-life issues and care; glossary of terms." American Psychological Association. Available at http://www.apa.org/pi/eol/glossary.html.

Ezekiel J, Emanuel L, Fairclough D, Emanuel L. "Attitudes and desires related to euthanasia and physician-assisted suicide among terminally ill patients and their caregivers." *JAMA.* 284:2460–2468, November 15, 2000. Available at http://jama.ama-assn.org/issues/v284n19/abs/joc01512.html.

Fallon M, O Neill B. "ABC of palliative care. Constipation and diarrhoea." *BMJ* 315:1293–1296, 1997.

Field MJ, Cassel EJ. *Improving care at the end of life.* Washington, DC: National Academy Press, 1997.

Foley KM. "Medical Issues Related to Physician-Assisted Suicide." Testimony, House Judiciary Subcommittee on the Constitution, Hearing on Physician-Assisted Suicide. April 29, 1996.

Foley KM. "The relationship of pain and symptom management to patient requests for physician-assisted suicide." *JPSM* 6:289–297, 1991.

Ganzini L, Nelson HD, Schmidt TA, Kraemer DF, Delorik MA, Lee MA. "Physicians' experiences with the Oregon Death with Dignity Act." *NEJM* 342, 8:557–563, 2000.

Higginson IJ, Hearn J. "A multicenter evaluation of cancer pain control by palliative control teams." *J Pain Symptom Manage* 14:29–35, 1997.

Home care guide to advanced cancer. Philadelphia: American College of Physicians, 1997.

Jared P. "Dealing with cancer: can alternatives help?" MSN.com. July 24, 2000. Available at http://content.health.msn.com/content/article/11/1668_50519.

Jay SM, Elliott CH, Katz E, Siegel SE. "Cognitive-behavioral and pharmacologic interventions for children's distress during painful medical procedures." *Journal of Consulting and Clinical Psychology* 55, 6:860–865, 1987.

Johnstone PA, Polston GR, Niemtzow RC, Martin PJ. "Integration of acupuncture into the oncology clinic." *Palliat Med.* 16(3):235–239, May 2002.

Joranson DE. "U.S. Senate hearing on pain management and improving end of life care. October 13, 1999. " See University of Wisconsin Pain & Policy Studies Group, http://www.medsch.wisc.edu/painpolicy.

Keefe FJ. "Cognitive behavioral therapy for managing pain." *The Clinical Psychologist 49*(3):4–5, 1996.

Koch ME, Kain ZN, Ayoub C, Rosenbaum SH. "The sedative and analgesic sparing effect of music." *Anesthesiology* 89:300–306, 1998.

Liossi C, Hatira P. "Clinical hypnosis in the alleviation of procedure-related pain in pediatric oncology patients." *Int J Clin Exp Hypn* 51(1):4–28, Jan. 2003.

"Longer-lasting pain relief—without pills." *Facts of Life: Issue Briefings for Health Reporters* 3, No. 6 (October 1998). Center for the Advancement of Health, 1998. Available at http://www.cfah.org/factsoflife/vol3no6.cfm.

Maclean CRK, Walton CG, et al. "Altered responses of cortisol, GH, TSH, and testosterone to acute stress after four months' practice of Transcendental Meditation (TM)." *Ann NY Acad Sci* 746:381–384, Nov. 1994.

Magill L. "The use of music therapy to address the suffering in advanced cancer pain." *Journal of Palliative Care* 17 (3):167–172, Autumn 2001.

Marchioro G, Azzarello G, Viviani F, Barbato F, Pavanetto M, Rosetti F, Pappagallo GL, Vinante O. "Hypnosis in the treatment of anticipatory nausea and vomiting in patients receiving cancer chemotherapy." *Oncology* 59, 2:100–104, August 2000.

Martinez M. "Acupuncture helps ease symptoms of many chronic illnesses." Associated Press Newswire. November 22, 2000.

McCarthy AM, Cool VA, Hanrahan K. "Cognitive behavioral interventions for children during painful procedures: research challenges and program development." *J Ped Nursing* 13, 1:55–63, 1998.

Molassiotis A. "A pilot study of the use of progressive muscle relaxation training in the management of post-chemotherapy nausea and vomiting." *European Journal of Cancer Care* 9 (4):230–234, Dec. 2000.

National Cancer Institute. "Depression PDQ." August 2002. Available at http://cancer.gov/cancerinfo/pdq/supportivecare/depression/healthprofessional.

National Institute of Nursing Research News Release. "Relaxation and music significantly reduce patients' postoperative pain." Bethesda, Md., May 7, 1999. Available at http://www.nih.gov/ninr/news-info/press/relaxation.html.

Pain management in children with cancer handbook. Texas Cancer Council, 1999. Available at http://www.childcancerpain.org/frameset_nogl.cfm?content=handbook.html.

Payne R. "At the end of life, color still divides." *Washington Post*, February 15, 2000.

Peterson C, Seligman ME, Vaillant GE. "Pessimistic explanatory style is a risk factor for physical illness: a thirty-five-year longitudinal study." *Journal of Personality and Social Psychology* 55:23–27, 1988.

Portenoy RK. "Morphine infusions at the end of life. The pitfalls in reasoning from anecdote." *J Pall Care* 12:44–46, 1996.

Quill TE, Dresser R, Brock DW. "The rule of double effect—a critique of its role in end-of-life decision making." *N Engl J Med* 337:1768–1771, 1997.

Redd WH, Montgomery GH, DuHamel KN. "Behavioral intervention for cancer treatment side effects." *Journal of the National Cancer Institute* 93, 11:810, June 6, 2001.

Roy DJ. "Need they sleep before they die?" *Journal of Palliative Care* 6:3–4, 1990.

Santiago-Palma J, Payne R. "Palliative care and rehabilitation." *Cancer* 92 (4 suppl.):1049–1052, August 15, 2001.

Schulz R, Bookwala J, Knapp J, et al. "Pessimism and mortality in young and old recurrent cancer patients." Paper presented at the American Psychosomatic Society annual meetings, Boston, April 15, 1994.

Seligman M. *Learned optimism.* New York: Pocket Books, 1990.

Seligman M. "Optimism, pessimism and mortality." *Mayo Clinic Proceedings* 75:133–143, 2000.

Sirkia K, Hovi L, Pouttu J, Saarinen-Pihkala UM. "Pain medication during terminal care of children with cancer." *J Pain Symptom Manage* 15, 4:220–226, 1998.

Smith C. "Herbal anti-inflammatories." University of Iowa College of Nursing. http://coninfo.nursing.uiowa.edu/sites/pedspain/NonPharm/HERBALpt.htm.

Solomon M, O'Donnell L, Jenning B, et al. "Decisions near the end of lfie: professional views of life-sustaining treatments." *American J Public Health.* 83:14–21, 1993.

Spiegel D, Bloom J. "Group therapy and hypnosis reduce metastatic breast carcinoma pain." *Psychosomatic Medicine* 45, 4:333–339, 1983.

Spiegel D, Moore R. "Imagery and hypnosis in the treatment of cancer patients." *Oncology (Hunting)* 11:1179–1195, 1997.

Syed IB. "Music therapy." Islamic Research Foundation International, Inc. Available at http://www.irfi.org/Islamic%20Articles%20Folder/music_therapy.htm.

Twycross RG. *Introducing palliative care.* 2nd ed. New York: Radcliffe Medical Press, 1995.

Walsh D. "Symptom control in advanced cancer: important drugs and routes of administration." *Semin Oncol* 27, 1:69–83, 2000.

Index